W9-BFQ-160

6th edition

comprehensive pharmacy review practice exams

EDITORS

Alan H. Mutnick, PharmD, RPh, FASHP
Assistant Director/ Clinical Pharmacy Services
Department of Pharmacy
University of Virginia Health System
Charlottesville, Virginia
Associate Clinical Professor
Department of Pharmacy Practice
Medical College of Virginia College of Pharmacy
Richmond, Virginia

Paul F. Souney, MS, RPh
National Director, Field Medical Affairs
Berlex Laboratories Affiliate of Schering AG
Wayne, New Jersey

Larry N. Swanson, PharmD, RPh, FASHP
Professor and Chairman
Department of Pharmacy Practice
Campbell University School of Pharmacy
Buies Creek, North Carolina

Leon Shargel, PhD, RPh
Applied Biopharmaceutics
Raleigh, North Carolina
Adjunct Associate Professor
Department of Pharmaceutical Sciences
University of Maryland School of Pharmacy
Baltimore, Maryland

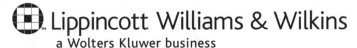 Lippincott Williams & Wilkins
a Wolters Kluwer business
Philadelphia • Baltimore • New York • London
Buenos Aires • Hong Kong • Sydney • Tokyo

Acquisitions Editor: David B. Troy
Managing Editor: Meredith L. Brittain
Marketing Manager: Marisa A. O'Brien
Production Editor: Jennifer P. Ajello
Designer: Stephen Druding
Compositor: Maryland Composition, Inc.
Printer: Data Reproductions Corporation

Copyright © 2008 Lippincott Williams & Wilkins
351 West Camden Street
Baltimore, MD 21201

530 Walnut Street
Philadelphia, PA 19106
All rights reserved. This book is protected by copyright. No part of this book may be
reproduced in any form or by any means, including photocopying, or utilized by any
information storage and retrieval system without written permission from the
copyright owner.
The publisher is not responsible (as a matter of product liability, negligence, or
otherwise) for any injury resulting from any material contained herein. This
publication contains information relating to general principles of medical care that
should not be construed as specific instructions for individual patients. Manufacturers'
product information and package inserts should be reviewed for current information,
including contraindications, dosages, and precautions.

Printed in the United States of America

Library of Congress Cataloging-in-Publication Data

Comprehensive pharmacy review practice exams / editors, Alan H. Mutnick ... [et al.].—6th ed.
    p. cm.
  ISBN-13: 978-0-7817-6997-6
  1. Pharmacy—Examinations, questions, etc. I. Mutnick, Alan H.
  [DNLM: 1. Pharmacy—Examination Questions.]
  RS97.P49 2007
  615'.1076—dc22

                        2006037709

The publishers have made every effort to trace the copyright holders for borrowed
material. If they have inadvertently overlooked any, they will be pleased to make the
necessary arrangements at the first opportunity.

To purchase additional copies of this book, call our customer service department at
(800) 638-3030 or fax orders to **(301) 223-2320.** International customers should call
(301) 223-2300.

Visit Lippincott Williams & Wilkins on the Internet: http://www.LWW.com.
Lippincott Williams & Wilkins customer service representatives are available from 8:
30 am to 6:00 pm, EST.

07 08 09 10 11
1 2 3 4 5 6 7 8 9 10

Contents

Preface

This practice exam booklet is a companion to *Comprehensive Pharmacy Review*. Whereas *Comprehensive Pharmacy Review* presents most of the subjects in the pharmacy curriculum in outline form with review questions interspersed, this booklet offers two examinations that are similar in format and coverage to those in the licensing examination required of all pharmacists.

Both patient profile–based and free-standing test items are included in the examinations. The questions are of two general types. In the first type (Example 1), the correct response most accurately completes a statement or answers a question. In the second type (Example 2), three statements are given. The correct answer may include one, two, or all three of these statements; these questions are to be answered according to the direction block that accompanies them.

Example 1 (Multiple-Choice)

Drugs that demonstrate nonlinear pharmacokinetics show which of the following properties?

A. A constant ratio of drug metabolites is formed as the administered dose increases.
B. The elimination half-life increases as the administered dose is increased.
C. The area under the curve (AUC) increases in direct proportion to an increase in the administered dose.
D. Both low and high doses follow first-order elimination kinetics.
E. The steady-state drug concentration increases in direct proportion to the dosing rate.

Example 2 (Multiple True–False)

Antimuscarinic agents are used in the treatment of Parkinson disease and in the control of some neuroleptic-induced extrapyramidal disorders. These agents include which of the following?

I. ipratropium
II. benztropine
III. trihexyphenidyl

A. I only
B. III only
C. I and II
D. II and III
E. I, II, and III

Allow a maximum of four hours for each examination. Answers, with explanations, are given at the end of each test. Also, several appendices are included at the back of the booklet for reference.

Taking a Test

One of the least attractive aspects of pursuing an education is the necessity of being examined on the material that has been presented. Instructors do not like to prepare tests, and students do not like to take them.

However, students are required to take many examinations during their learning careers, and little if any time is spent acquainting them with the positive aspects of tests and with systematic and successful methods for approaching them. Students perceive tests as punitive and sometimes feel as if they were merely opportunities for the instructor to discover what the student has forgotten or has never learned. Students need to view tests as opportunities to display their knowledge and to use them as tools for developing prescriptions for further study and learning.

While preparing for any exam, class and board exams as well as practice exams, it is important that students learn as much as they can about the subject they will be tested and are prepared to discover just how much they may not know. Students should study to acquire knowledge not just to prepare for tests. For the well-prepared student, the chances of passing far exceed the chances of failing.

Introduction to the NAPLEX

After graduation from an accredited pharmacy program, the prospective pharmacist must demonstrate the competency to practice pharmacy. The standards of competence for the practice of pharmacy are set by each state board of pharmacy. NAPLEX—The North American Pharmacist Licensure Examination—is the principal instrument used by the state board of pharmacy to assess the knowledge and proficiency necessary for a candidate to practice pharmacy. The National Association of Boards of Pharmacy (NABP) is an independent, international, and impartial association that assists member boards and jurisdictions in developing, implementing and enforcing uniform standards for the purpose of protecting the public health. NABP develops examinations that enable boards of pharmacy to assess the competence of candidates seeking licensure to practice pharmacy. Each state board of pharmacy may impose additional examinations. The two major examinations developed by NABP are

- The North American Pharmacist Licensure Examination (NAPLEX)
- Multistate Pharmacy Jurisprudence Examination (MPJE)

Registration information and a description of these computerized examinations may be found on the NABP Web site: www.nabp.net. Before submitting registration materials, the pharmacy candidate should contact the board of pharmacy for additional information regarding procedures, deadline dates, and required documentation.

The NAPLEX is a computer-adaptive test that measures a candidate's knowledge and ability by assessing the answers before presenting the next test question. If the answer is correct, the computer will select a more difficult question from the test item pool in an appropriate content area; if the answer is incorrect, an easier question will be selected by the computer. The NAPLEX score is based on the difficulty level of the questions answered correctly.

NAPLEX consists of 185 multiple-choice test questions. Of these, 150 questions are used to calculate the test score. The remaining 35 items serve as pretest questions and do not affect the NAPLEX score. Pretest questions are administered to evaluate the item's difficulty level for possible inclusion as a scored question in future exams. These pretest questions are dispersed throughout the exam and cannot be identified by the candidate.

A majority of the questions on the NAPLEX are asked in a scenario-based format (i.e., patient profiles with accompanying test questions). To properly analyze and answer the questions presented, the candidate must refer to the information provided in the patient profile. Some questions appear in a stand-alone format and should be answered solely from the information provided in the question.

All NAPLEX questions are based on competency statements that are reviewed and revised periodically. The NAPLEX Competency Statements describe the knowledge, judgment, and skills that the candidate is expected to demonstrate as an entry-level pharmacist. A complete description of the NAPLEX Competency Statements is published on the NABP Web site and is reproduced, with permission of NABP, in this edition (p. xiii). The NAPLEX examines three general areas of competence:

- Ensure safe and effective pharmacotherapy and optimize therapeutic outcomes
- Ensure safe and accurate preparation and dispensing of medications
- Provide healthcare information and promote public health

The NAPLEX *Candidates' Review Guide* is no longer available. NABP offers candidates who are preparing for the NAPLEX the Pre-NAPLEX, which is similar to the actual NAPLEX and allows candidates to gain experience in answering questions before examination day. The Pre-NAPLEX can be accessed via the Internet at the following URL: www.nabp.net/prenaplex/.

NAPLEX Blueprint

The NAPLEX Competency Statements

The NAPLEX Competency Statements provide a blueprint of the topics covered on the examination. They offer important information about the knowledge, judgment, and skills you are expected to demonstrate as an entry-level pharmacist. A strong understanding of the Competency Statements will aid in your preparation to take the examination.

Area 1: Assure safe and effective pharmacotherapy and optimize therapeutic outcomes (approximately 54% of test)

1.1.0 Obtain, interpret, and evaluate patient information to determine the presence of a disease or medical condition, assess the need for treatment and/or referral, and identify patient-specific factors that affect health, pharmacotherapy, and/or disease management.

1.1.1 Identify and assess patient information including medication, laboratory, and disease state histories.

1.1.2 Identify and/or use instruments and techniques related to patient assessment and diagnosis.

1.1.3 Identify and define the terminology, signs, and symptoms associated with diseases and medical conditions.

1.1.4 Identify and evaluate patient factors, genetic factors, biosocial factors, and concurrent drug therapy that are relevant to the maintenance of wellness and the prevention or treatment of a disease or medical condition.

1.2.0 Identify, evaluate, and communicate to the patient or health-care provider, the appropriateness of the patient's specific pharmacotherapeutic agents, dosing regimens, dosage forms, routes of administration, and delivery systems.

1.2.1 Identify specific uses and indications for drug products.

1.2.2 Identify the known or postulated sites and mechanisms of action of pharmacotherapeutic agents.

1.2.3 Evaluate drug therapy for the presence of pharmacotherapeutic duplications and interactions with other drugs, food, diagnostic tests, and monitoring procedures.

1.2.4 Identify contraindications, warnings and precautions associated with a drug product's active and inactive ingredients.

1.2.5 Identify physicochemical properties of drug substances that affect their solubility, pharmacodynamic and pharmacokinetic properties, pharmacologic actions, and stability.

1.2.6 Interpret and apply pharmacodynamic and pharmacokinetic principles to calculate and determine appropriate drug dosing regimens.

1.2.7 Interpret and apply biopharmaceutic principles and the pharmaceutical characteristics of drug dosage forms and delivery systems, to assure bioavailability and enhance patient compliance.

1.3.0 Manage the drug regimen by monitoring and assessing the patient and/or patient information, collaborating with other health care professionals, and providing patient education.

1.3.1 Identify pharmacotherapeutic outcomes and endpoints.

1.3.2 Evaluate patient signs and symptoms, and the results of monitoring tests and procedures to determine the safety and effectiveness of pharmacotherapy.

1.3.3 Identify, describe the mechanism of, and remedy adverse reactions, allergies, side effects and iatrogenic or drug-induced illness.

1.3.4 Prevent, recognize, and remedy medication non-adherence, misuse or abuse.

1.3.5 Recommend pharmacotherapeutic alternatives.

Area 2: Assure safe and accurate preparation and dispensing of medications (approximately 35% of test)

2.1.0 Perform calculations required to compound, dispense, and administer medication.

2.1.1 Calculate the quantity of medication to be compounded or dispensed; reduce and enlarge formulation quantities and calculate the quantity of ingredients needed to compound the proper amount of the preparation.

2.1.2 Calculate nutritional needs and the caloric content of nutrient sources.

2.1.3 Calculate the rate of drug administration.

2.1.4 Calculate or convert drug concentrations, ratio strengths, and/or extent of ionization.

2.2.0 Select and dispense medications in a manner that promotes safe and effective use.

2.2.1 Identify drug products by their generic, brand, and/or common names.

2.2.2 Determine whether a particular drug dosage strength or dosage form is commercially available, and whether it is available on a nonprescription basis.

2.2.3 Identify commercially available drug products by their characteristic physical attributes.

2.2.4 Interpret and apply pharmacokinetic parameters and quality assurance data to determine equivalence among manufactured drug products, and identify products for which documented evidence of inequivalence exists.

2.2.5 Identify and communicate appropriate information regarding packaging, storage, handling, administration, and disposal of medications.

2.2.6 Identify and describe the use of equipment and apparatus required to administer medications.

2.3.0 Prepare and compound extemporaneous preparations and sterile products.

2.3.1 Identify and describe techniques and procedures related to drug preparation, compounding, and quality assurance.

2.3.2 Identify and use equipment necessary to prepare and extemporaneously compound medications.

2.3.3 Identify the important physicochemical properties of a preparation's active and inactive ingredients; describe the mechanism of, and the characteristic evidence of incompatibility or degradation; and identify methods for achieving stabilization of the preparation.

Area 3: Provide health care information and promote public health (approximately 11% of test)

3.1.0 Access, evaluate, and apply information to promote optimal health care.

3.1.1 Identify the typical content and organization of specific sources of drug and health information for both health-care providers and consumers.

3.1.2 Evaluate the suitability, accuracy, and reliability of information from reference sources by explaining and evaluating the adequacy of experimental design and by applying and evaluating statistical tests and parameters.

3.2.0 Educate the public and health-care professionals regarding medical conditions, wellness, dietary supplements, and medical devices.

3.2.1 Provide health care information regarding the prevention and treatment of diseases and medical conditions, including emergency patient care.

3.2.2 Provide health care information regarding nutrition, lifestyle, and other non-drug measures that are effective in promoting health or preventing or minimizing the progression of a disease or medical condition.

3.2.3 Provide information regarding the documented uses, adverse effects, and toxicities of dietary supplements.

3.2.4 Provide information regarding the selection, use, and care of medical/surgical appliances and devices, self-care products, and durable medical equipment, as well as products and techniques for self-monitoring of health status and medical conditions.

Reprinted with permission from the National Association of Boards of Pharmacy, Mount Prospect, IL.

Test I

Use the patient profile below to answer questions 1–12.

MEDICATION PROFILE (COMMUNITY)

Patient Name: Rachel Honors

Address: 5 Duke Dog Ln.

Age: 55   Height: 5'4"

Sex: F   Race: white   Weight: 140 lb

Allergies: Aspirin-related products: anaphylaxis

DIAGNOSIS

Primary	(1)	Status post-STEMI, 9/15
Secondary	(1)	Hypertension
	(2)	Hypercholesterolemia
	(3)	Duodenal ulcer

MEDICATION RECORD (Prescription and OTC)

	Date	Rx No.	Physician	Drug and Strength	Quan	Sig	Refills
(1)	7/20	12233	Johnsie	Niacin 500 mg	30	i tab hs	6
(2)	7/20	12234	Johnsie	Simvastatin 40 mg	30	i tab hs	6
(3)	7/20	12235	Johnsie	Hydrochlorothiazide 25 mg	30	i tab AM	6
(4)	7/20	12236	Johnsie	Ecotrin 325 mg	100	i tab AM	12
(5)	8/21	14001	Johnsie	Doxazosin 2 mg	30	i tab AM	6
(6)	8/21	14002	Johnsie	Ramipril 5 mg	30	i tab AM	6
(7)	8/29	15005	Colon	Rabeprazole 20 mg	30	i tab AM	0
(8)	9/22	16500	Johnsie	Clopidogrel 75 mg	30	i tab AM	6
(9)	9/22	16501	Johnsie	Atenolol 50 mg	30	i tab AM	6
(10)	9/22	16502	Johnsie	Nitroglycerin 0.3 mg	100	as directed	6

PHARMACIST NOTES AND Other Patient Information

	Date	Comments
(1)	7/20	New patient received from another pharmacy.
(2)	7/20	Contacted physician regarding two potential problems with the current prescriptions.
(3)	7/20	Physician agreed with both suggestions and acknowledged the oversight.
(4)	7/20	Both medications were discontinued.
(5)	7/20	Contacted physician regarding new prescriptions received, based on findings from the ALLHAT and HOPE studies; however, Dr. Johnsie disagreed with suggestion to delete either of the prescriptions.
(6)	8/21	Patient instructed on proper technique to take blood pressure daily at the same time, before taking morning medications, and to make sure prescriptions are refilled promptly each month.
(7)	9/22	Updated patient medication profile to reflect current medications, including simvastatin, hydrochlorothiazide, doxazosin, ramipril, rabeprazole, clopidogrel, atenolol, and nitroglycerin SL.
(8)	9/22	Contacted Dr. Johnsie to reiterate findings from ALLHAT study, and this time he agreed to discontinue the medication.
(9)		
(10)		
(11)		
(12)		
(13)		
(14)		
(15)		

1. Which medications prompted the pharmacist to call Dr. Johnsie on 7/20 owing to potential problems?

    I. niacin
    II. simvastatin
    III. aspirin

    A. I only
    B. III only
    C. I and II
    D. II and III
    E. I, II, and III

2. Which of the prescriptions written by Dr. Johnsie on 8/21 was the pharmacist hoping to have discontinued, and which study demonstrated its potential negative effects in a hypertensive patient like Ms. Honors?

    A. doxazosin and Antihypertensive and Lipid-Lowering Treatment to Prevent Heart Attack Trial (ALLHAT) study
    B. ramipril and ALLHAT study
    C. doxazosin and Heart Outcomes Prevention Evaluation (HOPE) study
    D. ramipril and HOPE study
    E. both doxazosin and ramipril in the HOPE study

3. The seventh report of the Joint National Committee (JNC-7) guidelines for the treatment of hypertension include "compelling" indications that recommend the use of select drug therapies over standard therapy with a thiazide diuretic. Which of the following represent examples of compelling indications and their suggested therapy?

    I. heart failure (diuretics, β-blockers, angiotensin-converting enzyme [ACE] inhibitors)
    II. chronic kidney disease (ACE inhibitors, angiotensin II receptor blockers [ARBs])
    III. recurrent stroke prevention (diuretics, ACE inhibitors)

    A. I only
    B. III only
    C. I and II
    D. II and III
    E. I, II, and III

4. Which of the following statements would justify the prescription written on 9/22 for atenolol for Ms. Honors?

    I. treatment of hypertension in a patient who is post–myocardial infarction (MI) as a compelling indication
    II. prevention of sudden death in a post-MI patient
    III. secondary prevention of stroke

    A. I only
    B. III only
    C. I and II
    D. II and III
    E. I, II, and III

5. Which of the following agents, assuming no contraindications for use, was likely to have been given to Ms. Honors upon arrival to the hospital for the treatment of ST-segment elevated myocardial infarction (STEMI), assuming she arrived for treatment within 12 hr of her symptoms?

    I. alteplase (recombinant tissue-type plasminogen activator [rt-PA])
    II. reteplase (recombinant plasminogen activator [r-PA])
    III. tenecteplase (TNKase)

    A. I only
    B. III only
    C. I and II
    D. II and III
    E. I, II, and III

6. After her heart attack, Ms. Honors presents with a prescription for clopidogrel. What is the indication for clopidogrel in this patient?

    I. used as an alternative to aspirin because of aspirin allergy
    II. used in the prevention of acute coronary syndromes
    III. used in hypertensive patients who have a compelling indication

    A. I only
    B. III only
    C. I and II
    D. II and III
    E. I, II, and III

7. Ms. Honors is receiving rabeprazole for which of the following indications?

   A. post–myocardial infarction (MI) for prevention of sudden death
   B. duodenal ulcer
   C. hypercholesterolemia
   D. hypertension
   E. none of the above

8. Which of the following patient information items should be addressed when Ms. Honors receives the nitroglycerin prescription?

   I. The tablet should be dissolved under the tongue if it is difficult to swallow.
   II. The tablets should be placed in an easy-to-open plastic container for future use.
   III. The tablets should be taken for an acute angina attack or before an activity that might induce an attack (i.e., strenuous exercise, anxiety).

   A. I only
   B. III only
   C. I and II
   D. II and III
   E. I, II, and III

9. Based on the seventh report of the Joint National Committee (JNC-7) guidelines and the antihypertensive therapy being prescribed, which of the following best describes Ms. Honors's blood pressure classification?

   A. prehypertension
   B. stage I hypertension
   C. stage II hypertension
   D. stage III hypertension
   E. Malignant hypertension

10. Based on Ms. Honors's patient profile, which of the following medications would be contraindicated?

   A. Ecotrin
   B. ibuprofen
   C. celecoxib
   D. Relafen
   E. All of the above

11. Untreated hypertension can result in which of the following types of target organ damage?

   I. renal
   II. cerebral
   III. retinal

   A. I only
   B. III only
   C. I and II
   D. II and III
   E. I, II, and III

12. Which of the following agents would *not* be considered a first-line antihypertensive agent in an otherwise healthy patient with stage I hypertension?

   A. amiloride
   B. chlorthalidone
   C. chlorothiazide
   D. indapamide
   E. methyclothiazide

End of this patient profile; continue with the examination

---

13. Parenteral products, such as half-normal saline solution, with an osmotic pressure less than that of blood are referred to as

   A. isotonic solutions.
   B. hypotonic solutions.
   C. hypertonic solutions.
   D. iso-osmotic solutions.
   E. neutral solutions.

14. Epoetin α (Epogen) is used in chronic kidney disease to treat

   A. peripheral neuropathy.
   B. anemia.
   C. hyperphosphatemia.
   D. metabolic alkalosis.
   E. hyperuricemia.

15. Which of the following statements about insulin resistance are true?

    I. Insulin resistance is the need for > 200 U/day of insulin.
    II. Insulin resistance can be caused by a high concentration of circulating immunoglobulin G (IgG) anti-insulin antibodies.
    III. Insulin resistance can resolve spontaneously.

    A. I only
    B. III only
    C. I and II
    D. II and III
    E. I, II, and III

16. Lanolin is best described as

    I. a water-in-oil (w/o) emulsion containing approximately 25% water.
    II. an emulsion base that acts as an emollient, preventing water loss.
    III. a water-soluble base containing propylene glycol or polyethylene glycol, which increases evaporation.

    A. I only
    B. III only
    C. I and II
    D. II and III
    E. I, II, and III

17. Which products have been shown to be effective in the treatment of diarrhea?

    I. Donnagel-PG
    II. Kaopectate
    III. Pepto-Bismol

    A. I only
    B. III only
    C. I and II
    D. II and III
    E. I, II, and III

18. Levodopa is preferred to dopamine in the treatment of Parkinson disease because

    I. levodopa crosses the blood–brain barrier; dopamine does not.
    II. levodopa is a more potent agonist than dopamine at the receptor site in the substantia nigra.
    III. levodopa is decarboxylated in the gastrointestinal tract, whereas dopamine is not.

    A. I only
    B. III only
    C. I and II
    D. II and III
    E. I, II, and III

19. Conditions that might predispose a patient to toxicity from a highly protein-bound drug include which of the following?

    I. hypoalbuminemia
    II. hepatic disease
    III. malnutrition

    A. I only
    B. III only
    C. I and II
    D. II and III
    E. I, II, and III

20. The mechanism of action of salmeterol is that of a

    A. sympathomimetic agonist with high β_2 selectivity.
    B. sympathomimetic agonist with high β_1 selectivity.
    C. sympathomimetic antagonist with high β_2 selectivity.
    D. sympathomimetic antagonist with high β_1 selectivity.
    E. leukotriene receptor antagonist.

Use the patient profile below to answer questions 21–32.

MEDICATION PROFILE (COMMUNITY)

Patient Name: ___Alan Mutrick___

Address: ___5 Cinnamon Terrace___

Age: ___54___   Height: ___5'9"___

Sex: ___M___   Race: ___white___   Weight: ___175 lb___

Allergies: ___No known allergies___

DIAGNOSIS

Primary	(1)	Hypertension (9/10)
	(2)	Heart failure (8/10)
Secondary	(1)	Anemia (8/10)
	(2)	Chronic kidney disease (8/10)

MEDICATION RECORD (Prescription and OTC)

	Date	Rx No.	Physician	Drug and Strength	Quan	Sig	Refills
(1)	6/15	110555	Davis	Prednisone 10 mg	60	i bid	2
(2)	8/10	111002	Davis	Ferrous sulfate 325 mg	100	i tid	6
(3)	8/10	111003	Wonders	Lanoxin 0.25 mg	30	i q AM	6
(4)	8/10	111004	Wonders	Lasix 40 mg	30	i q AM	3
(5)	8/10	111005	Wonders	Slow-K 600 mg	90	i tid	3
(6)	9/10	113001	Wonders	Vasotec 5 mg	30	i qd	3
(7)	9/10	113002	Wonders	Hydrochlorothiazide 50 mg	30	i bid	3
(8)	9/10	113002	Wonders	Isordil 40 mg	120	i qid	3
(9)	9/10	113003	Wonders	Hydralazine 50 mg	60	i bid	3
(10)	12/1	200001	Wonders	Coreg 3.125 mg	30	i bid	0
(11)	12/1	200002	Wonders	Altace 2.5 mg	30	i q AM	0
(12)	12/15	200604	Wonders	Coreg 6.25 mg	30	i bid	0
(13)	1/2	201003	Wonders	Altace 5.0 mg	30	i q AM	3
(14)	1/2	201004	Wonders	Coreg 12.5 mg	60	i bid	0
(15)	1/16	203010	Wonders	Altace 10 mg	30	i q AM	6

PHARMACIST NOTES AND Other Patient Information

	Date	Comments
(1)	8/10	Pharmacist on duty contacted Dr. Wonders regarding the prescriptions just received with a question regarding one of the prescriptions; Slow-K is D.C.'d.
(2)	9/10	Patient presents with new prescriptions and tells pharmacist that Dr. Wonders wanted him to stop taking the Lanoxin.
(3)	9/10	Pharmacist contacted Dr. Wonders with questions about several of the prescriptions in patient profile as well as new prescriptions presented to pharmacy.
(4)	9/10	D.C. Lasix.
(5)	9/10	D.C. Lanoxin.
(6)	12/1	D.C. Isordil 40 mg, hydralazine 50 mg, and Vasotec 5 mg.
(7)	12/15	Pharmacist contacted Dr. Wonders regarding Coreg prescription initially filled on 12/1 and received requested verbal prescription.
(8)	1/2	Contacted Dr. Wonders regarding indication for increase in Altace prescription.
(9)		

21. Based on the medication profile presented on 8/10, which of the following describe potential causes for Mr. Mutrick's heart failure?

   I. low-output failure caused by anemia
   II. low-output failure caused by prednisone
   III. high-output failure caused by myocardial infarction

   A. I only
   B. III only
   C. I and II
   D. II and III
   E. I, II, and III

22. Which of the following statements describe the interaction that should have taken place when Mr. Mutrick was having his prescriptions filled on 8/10?

   I. No significant interaction is needed with the new prescriptions.
   II. The pharmacist should advise Dr. Wonders of the potential problem of giving a potassium supplement in a patient with chronic kidney disease.
   III. The pharmacist should call Dr. Wonders regarding the potential use of a β-blocker in this newly diagnosed heart failure patient.

   A. I only
   B. III only
   C. I and II
   D. II and III
   E. I, II, and III

23. Why did the pharmacist contact Dr. Wonders on 12/15 regarding the Coreg prescription?

   I. Coreg is an angiotensin II receptor blocker, which is currently not indicated in the treatment of heart failure.
   II. Coreg is a β-adrenergic blocker; in the treatment of heart failure, the dose must be closely titrated up to the optimal dose.
   III. β-Adrenergic blockers should not be abruptly discontinued in cardiac patients.

   A. I only
   B. III only
   C. I and II
   D. II and III
   E. I, II, and III

24. Which group of symptoms is most often associated with a patient who has signs of left-sided heart failure?

   A. shortness of breath, rales, paroxysmal nocturnal dyspnea
   B. jugular venous distention, hepatojugular reflux, pedal edema, shortness of breath
   C. hepatojugular reflux, jugular venous distention, pedal edema, abdominal distention
   D. paroxysmal nocturnal dyspnea, pedal edema, jugular venous distention, hepatojugular reflux
   E. fatigue, abdominal distention, hepatomegaly, rales

25. What is the therapeutic indication for ramipril (Altace) that might have prompted the pharmacist's call to Dr. Wonders on 1/2?

   I. hypertension
   II. renal dysfunction
   III. heart failure

   A. I only
   B. III only
   C. I and II
   D. II and III
   E. I, II, and III

26. How many milligrams of elemental iron does Mr. Mutrick receive with his daily dose of ferrous sulfate?

   A. 117 mg
   B. 195 mg
   C. 150 mg
   D. 322 mg
   E. 975 mg

27. Which action best describes how the drug Lasix would affect Mr. Mutrick?

   I. reduction of excess sodium and water in the patient
   II. direct pulmonary dilation
   III. increased preload through cytokine release

   A. I only
   B. III only
   C. I and II
   D. II and III
   E. I, II, and III

28. Which pharmacologic mechanisms relate primarily to the use of Vasotec in this patient?

    I. Angiotensin-converting enzyme (ACE) inhibitors indirectly reduce preload by decreasing aldosterone secretion.
    II. ACE inhibitors reduce afterload by decreasing angiotensin II production.
    III. ACE inhibitors decrease levels of bradykinin.

    A. I only
    B. III only
    C. I and II
    D. II and III
    E. I, II, and III

29. What is the major difference between Lanoxin tablets and Lanoxicaps capsules?

    I. The digoxin contained in Lanoxicaps capsules is more potent than the digoxin contained in Lanoxin tablets.
    II. The digoxin contained in Lanoxicaps capsules is more completely absorbed than is the digoxin in Lanoxin tablets.
    III. Digoxin absorption from Lanoxicaps capsules is less variable than is the digoxin absorption from Lanoxin tablets.

    A. I only
    B. III only
    C. I and II only
    D. II and III only
    E. I, II, and III

30. Which drug used in the treatment of heart failure has been associated with systemic lupus erythematosus?

    A. Apresoline
    B. Lanoxin
    C. Vasotec
    D. Lasix
    E. Isordil

31. Which of the following drugs were recently given a Class III recommendation—"conditions for which there is evidence and/or general agreement that a procedure/therapy is not useful/effective and in some cases may be harmful"—in the treatment of heart failure?

    I. Inocor
    II. Dobutrex
    III. dopamine

    A. I only
    B. III only
    C. I and II
    D. II and III
    E. I, II, and III

32. Which statements best represent the actions that a pharmacist should take if presented with a prescription for a nonsteroidal anti-inflammatory drug (NSAID) for Mr. Mutrick?

    I. Contact the physician regarding the history of anemia in the patient and the current disease profile.
    II. Contact with the physician is not necessary.
    III. Fill the prescription and counsel the patient on the correct method for taking the NSAID with meals.

    A. I only
    B. III only
    C. I and II
    D. II and III
    E. I, II, and III

End of this patient profile; continue with examination

33. Which of the following statements does *not* accurately describe the current role that β-adrenergic blockers play in the treatment of heart failure?

    A. β-Adrenergic blockers have been shown to decrease the risk of death and hospitalization as well as to improve the clinical status of heart failure patients.
    B. Current guidelines recommend the use of β-adrenergic blockers in all patients with stable heart failure as a result of left ventricular dysfunction, unless they have a contraindication to their use or are unable to tolerate their effects owing to hypotension, bradycardia, bronchospasm, and the like.
    C. β-Adrenergic blockers are generally used in conjunction with diuretics and angiotensin-converting enzyme (ACE) inhibitors.
    D. Side effects to β-adrenergic blockers may occur during the early days of therapy but do not generally prevent their long-term use, and progression of the disease may be reduced.
    E. β-Adrenergic blockers are contraindicated in the treatment of heart failure because of their strong negative inotropic effects, which further reduce cardiac output.

34. The use of atropine sulfate in the treatment of sinus bradycardia centers around its anticholinergic activity. What hemodynamic response should be monitored for when the drug is administered?

    A. Initial doses may cause constipation.
    B. High doses will cause pupillary constriction.
    C. Initial doses may exacerbate the bradycardia.
    D. High doses will cause diarrhea.
    E. Initial doses will cause extreme sweating.

35. Which cardiac drugs are available in extended-release dosage forms?

    I. Quinaglute
    II. Coreg
    III. Plendil

    A. I only
    B. III only
    C. I and II
    D. II and III

36. Which agents would be an alternative therapy in an intensive care unit (ICU) patient nonresponsive to dopamine or dobutamine?

    A. Blocadren
    B. Calan
    C. Norpace
    D. Inocor
    E. Tenormin

37. Which agent works by irreversibly blocking the proton pump of parietal cells, thereby inhibiting basal gastric acid secretion?

    A. Tagamet
    B. Carafate
    C. Sandostatin
    D. Prevacid
    E. Pepcid

38. The serum creatinine level, along with the age, weight, and gender of the patient, may be used to estimate creatinine clearance. Creatinine clearance is a measurement of

    A. glomerular filtration rate (GFR).
    B. active tubular secretion.
    C. muscle metabolism.
    D. hepatic function.
    E. effective renal plasma flow.

39. Which of the following agents may induce an acute attack of gout?

    I. low-dose aspirin
    II. nicotinic acid
    III. cytotoxic drugs

    A. I only
    B. III only
    C. I and II
    D. II and III
    E. I, II, and III

40. When used as a topical decongestant, oxymetazoline

    I. is recommended for administration every 12 hr.
    II. has limited use, generally ≤ 3 days.
    III. acts as a direct-acting parasympathomimetic agent.

    A. I only
    B. III only
    C. I and II
    D. II and III
    E. I, II, and III

41. The elimination half-life for a newly released antimicrobial agents is approximately 2 hr. The drug has been shown to demonstrate first-order elimination characteristics. What percent of this drug would be eliminated from the body 6 hr after it is administered as an intravenous (IV) bolus dose?

    A. 12.5%
    B. 25%
    C. 50%
    D. 75%
    E. 87.5%

42. The culture and sensitivity report from a sputum specimen indicates the following minimum inhibitory concentrations (MICs) against a gram-negative bacterial isolate:

    ceftazidime 8 μg/mL
    gentamicin 4 μg/mL
    cefepime 1 μg/mL
    meropenem 2 μg/mL
    ciprofloxacin 32 μg/mL
    Based on the results of the report, which of the listed antimicrobials is the most potent single agent against this specific bacterial isolate?

    A. ceftazidime
    B. gentamicin
    C. cefepime
    D. meropenem
    E. ciprofloxacin

Use the patient profile below to answer questions 43–58.

MEDICATION PROFILE (COMMUNITY)

Patient Name: Chuck Johnson

Address: 245 Conway St.

Age: 66   Height: 5'9"

Sex: M   Race: white   Weight: 172 lb

Allergies: No known allergies

DIAGNOSIS

Primary	(1)	Diabetes mellitus	
	(2)	Osteoarthritis	
	(3)	Insomnia	
Secondary	(1)	Hx of peptic ulcer disease	

MEDICATION RECORD (Prescription and OTC)

	Date	Rx No.	Physician	Drug and Strength	Quan	Sig	Refills
(1)	1/12			Tylenol 500 mg	100	1–2 prn	OTC
(2)	1/30			Nytol QuickGels 50 mg	24	1 hs prn	OTC
(3)	2/10	20101	Jones	Sonata 5 mg	20	1 hs prn	1
(4)	3/6	21134	Jones	Glyburide 5 mg	30	1 q am	3
(5)	6/19	22453	Jones	Metformin 500 mg	60	1 bid	3
(6)	6/19		Jones	Tylenol 500 mg	100	2 q6h max	OTC
(7)	7/12			Alka Seltzer Plus Nighttime Cold and Cough Liquid-Gels	12	as directed	OTC
(8)	8/30	23100	Jones	Tramadol 50 mg	40	1\2 tab to start	2
(9)	9/7	25398	Jones	Acarbose 25 mg	90	1 tid	3

PHARMACIST NOTES AND Other Patient Information

	Date	Comments
(1)	1/12	Patient complains of some pain in his right knee; he indicates that there is no redness or swelling; recommended Tylenol to treat.
(2)	1/30	Patient complains of insomnia; recommended Nytol 50 mg.
(3)	3/6	Patient has oral glucose tolerance test.
(4)	7/12	Patient reports symptoms of a common cold.
(5)	9/7	Patient reports SMBG high after meals.
(6)		
(7)		
(8)		
(9)		
(10)		
(11)		
(12)		
(13)		
(14)		
(15)		
(16)		
(17)		
(18)		

43. There are four clinical classes of diabetes mellitus. Which of the following *best* identifies three of these four clinical classes?

    A. type 1, type 2, hyperglycemia
    B. prediabetes, hyperglycemic hyperosmolar nonketotic syndrome (HHNK), type 3
    C. gestational diabetes mellitus, type 1, type 2
    D. Cushing syndrome, diabetic ketoacidosis, thiazide diuretic diabetes
    E. prediabetes, gestational diabetes mellitus, ketonemia

44. Diagnostic criteria used to make the diagnosis of diabetes mellitus in this patient would include

    I. a fasting plasma glucose level of ≥ 126 mg/dL.
    II. a random plasma glucose level ≥ 200 mg/dL, with the classic symptoms of diabetes of polydipsia, polyuria, and polyphagia, and weight loss.
    III. a 2-hr plasma glucose level of 140 mg/dL during an oral glucose tolerance test using 75 g anhydrous glucose dissolved in water.

    A. I only
    B. III only
    C. I and II
    D. II and III
    E. I, II, and III

45. Mr. Johnson indicates to you that his physician said something about a "hemoglobin-type test to check how my blood sugar was doing." Which of the following applies to hemoglobin A_{1C} in diabetes?

    I. A value of < 7% (based on 6% as the upper limit of normal) would be a desired therapeutic endpoint.
    II. Another name for this is the glycosylated hemoglobin test.
    III. This reflects the average blood glucose level over the preceding 2–3 months.

    A. I only
    B. III only
    C. I and II
    D. II and III
    E. I, II, and III

46. Glyburide is an example of

    I. an oral insulin secretagogue.
    II. an oral hypoglycemic agent.
    III. a sulfonylurea.

    A. I only
    B. III only
    C. I and II
    D. II and III
    E. I, II, and III

47. Glyburide is also known as

    I. DiaBeta.
    II. Micronase.
    III. Glucotrol.

    A. I only
    B. III only
    C. I and II
    D. II and III
    E. I, II, and III

48. Which of the following information applies to the prescription for metformin given to Mr. Johnson?

    I. It can be used in combination with glyburide.
    II. It is classified as an insulin sensitizer.
    III. It is contraindicated in situations that have the potential for increased risk of lactic acidosis.

    A. I only
    B. III only
    C. I and II
    D. II and III
    E. I, II, and III

49. Why would acarbose be added to the other agents used to treat this patient?

    I. Mr. Johnson probably has significant postprandial hyperglycemia.
    II. This agent helps lower the baseline blood glucose level.
    III. This agent has a similar mechanism of action as metformin.

    A. I only
    B. III only
    C. I and II
    D. II and III
    E. I, II, and III

50. Mr. Johnson is interested in a blood glucose monitor that allows him to test at other sites besides the finger. Using an alternate site would *not* be appropriate

    I. when he wakes in the morning.
    II. when he has an episode of hypoglycemia.
    III. immediately after a meal.

    A. I only
    B. III only
    C. I and II
    D. II and III
    E. I, II, and III

51. Mr. Johnson apparently has osteoarthritis in his right knee. Which of the following are characteristic of osteoarthritis?

    I. It was formerly known as degenerative joint disease.
    II. It is the most common form of arthritis.
    III. It has a significant inflammatory component.

    A. I only
    B. III only
    C. I and II
    D. II and III
    E. I, II, and III

52. Mr. Johnson requested something to help him with his sleep problem. Which of the following applies to Mr. Johnson and his use of Nytol QuickGels?

    I. This product contains diphenhydramine as the active ingredient.
    II. This product should be used cautiously in the elderly because of potential adverse central anticholinergic effects.
    III. As an elderly man, Mr. Johnson may have prostate enlargement, and this agent may produce polyuria, which could confuse the interpretation of his diabetes symptoms.

    A. I only
    B. III only
    C. I and II
    D. II and III
    E. I, II, and III

53. Mr. Johnson was prescribed Sonata for his insomnia. Which of the following applies to this agent?

    I. It has a long half-life and is therefore useful for patients who have difficulty staying asleep.
    II. It would be particularly useful for patients having difficulty falling asleep.
    III. He has received the lower strength of this agent, which is probably good because he is an elderly gentleman.

    A. I only
    B. III only
    C. I and II
    D. II and III
    E. I, II, and III

54. Which of the following agents is considered the first-line therapy for osteoarthritis?

    A. ibuprofen
    B. acetaminophen
    C. naproxen
    D. codeine
    E. celecoxib

55. Is the dose selected for this patient on 6/19, an appropriate one to treat the osteoarthritis?

    A. yes
    B. no

56. Which of the following applies to tramadol?

    I. Mr. Johnson was likely begun on this agent instead of a non-steroidal anti-inflammatory drug (NSAID) because of his history of peptic ulcer disease.
    II. Tramadol is considered a good choice when the patient cannot take an NSAID.
    III. Although not considered an opioid, its side effects are similar.

    A. I only
    B. III only
    C. I and II
    D. II and III
    E. I, II, and III

57. Giving Alka Seltzer Plus Cold and Cough Liguid-gels to Mr. Johnson to treat his common cold symptoms would not be recommended because

    I. the oral decongestant in this product may cause an elevation in his blood sugar.
    II. it is shotgun therapy; one should usually treat specific symptoms with single-agent products.
    III. it contains acetaminophen, which may push Mr. Johnson into a toxic dose.

    A. I only
    B. III only
    C. I and II
    D. II and III
    E. I, II, and III

58. Which of Mr. Johnson's diabetes medications are prone to primary and secondary failure?

    I. glyburide
    II. metformin
    III. acarbose

    A. I only
    B. III only
    C. I and II
    D. II and III
    E. I, II, and III

End of this patient profile; continue with examination

---

59. Jean, a regular customer in your pharmacy, shows you her newborn baby's head and asks you to recommend treatment. Upon examining the baby, you notice that he has an accumulation of skin scales on the scalp. You tell her that the baby has cradle cap and recommend that she treat the baby by

    A. washing the baby's head with coal tar solution daily for 2 weeks.
    B. washing his head with an antifungal shampoo (Nizoral AD).
    C. applying topical antibiotics such as Neosporin daily until resolved.
    D. massaging the scalp with baby oil followed by washing his head with a mild shampoo, such as Johnson & Johnson's baby shampoo.
    E. applying a moisturizer to the scalp daily until resolved.

60. Sunscreens should generally not be used in children < 6 months of age because

    A. the products commonly cause a severe rash in this age group.
    B. infants produce too much sweat, which can dilute the sunscreen.
    C. the metabolic and excretory systems of infants are not fully developed.
    D. overexposure to the sun can interfere with vitamin D production.
    E. infants have a lot of dermal melanin, which causes them to burn more easily.

61. Common warts are treated with which acid?

    A. glycolic acid
    B. salicylic acid
    C. lactic acid
    D. muriatic acid
    E. galactic acid

62. Which virus is responsible for common warts?

    A. herpes simplex virus (HSV)
    B. Epstein-Barr virus
    C. coronavirus
    D. HIV
    E. human papillomavirus

PATIENT RECORD (INSTITUTION/NURSING HOME)

Patient Name: Salvatore Torres

Address: 369 Cherry St.

Age: 59

Sex: M   Race: white

Height: 5'10"

Weight: 170 lb

Allergies: Sulfa drug–induced Stevens-Johnson syndrome

DIAGNOSIS

Primary	(1)	Hypertension
Secondary	(1)	Drug-induced erythema multiforme
	(2)	Status post acute coronary syndrome
	(3)	Asthma

LAB/DIAGNOSTIC TESTS

	Date	Test
(1)	11/3	WBC 5500/mm^3
(2)	11/3	BUN 15 mg/dL
(3)	11/3	Cr 1.0 mg/dL
(4)	11/3	Blood pressure 170/100 mm Hg
(5)	11/3	Electrolytes within normal limits
(6)	11/5	Total cholesterol 250 mg/dL; elevated LDL

MEDICATION ORDERS (Including Parenteral Solutions)

	Date	Drug and Strength	Route	Sig
(1)	11/3	Atenolol 50 mg	po	i bid
(2)	11/3	Hydrochlorothiazide (HCTZ) 50 mg	po	i q AM
(3)	11/3	Nitroglycerin 1/150	sl	prn
(4)	11/3	Spironolactone 50 mg	po	i bid
(5)	11/3	Theo-Dur 200 mg	po	i tid
(6)	11/5	Irbesartan 150 mg	po	i qd
(7)	11/5	Simvastatin 40 mg	po	i hs
(8)	11/5	Nitroprusside infusion	IV	i µg/kg/min titrated
(9)	11/5	Morphine sulfate	IM	prn chest pain

ADDITIONAL ORDERS

	Date	Comments
(1)		
(2)		

DIETARY CONSIDERATIONS (Enteral and Parenteral)

	Date	Comments
(1)	11/3	Low-fat American Heart Association diet.
(2)	11/3	Limit sodium intake to no additional salt with meals.

PHARMACIST NOTES AND Other Patient Information

	Date	Comments
(1)	11/3	D.C. HCTZ and replace with spironolactone.
(2)	11/5	Blood pressure not responding to initial therapy; begin nitroprusside infusion.
(3)	11/5	Begin lipid-lowering therapy.
(4)	11/5	Schedule for coronary catheterization in the morning.

63. Which of the following represents the medication of choice for the initial therapy of stage I hypertension in an otherwise healthy individual with no compelling indications?

    A. hydrochlorothiazide
    B. spironolactone
    C. doxazosin
    D. hydralazine
    E. clonidine

64. The decision to discontinue hydrochlorothiazide therapy and begin spironolactone therapy was based on which of the following?

    I. inappropriate therapeutic effect by thiazide diuretics in hypertensive patients
    II. lack of proven benefit in reducing mortality rates with diuretics in treating hypertension
    III. patient's documented allergy to sulfa drug–induced Stevens-Johnson syndrome

    A. I only
    B. III only
    C. I and II
    D. II and III
    E. I, II, and III

65. Which of the following is *not* a major determinant of myocardial oxygen demand?

    A. heart rate
    B. myocardial contractility
    C. coronary blood flow
    D. left ventricular volume
    E. myocardial wall tension

66. Which of the following represents an example of an acute coronary syndrome?

    I. unstable angina
    II. ST-segment elevated myocardial infarction (STEMI)
    III. non-ST-segment elevated myocardial infarction (NSTEMI)

    A. I only
    B. III only
    C. I and II
    D. II and III
    E. I, II, and III

67. Theophylline serum levels are increased by all of the following *except*

    A. pneumonia.
    B. ciprofloxacin.
    C. heart failure.
    D. smoking.
    E. cor pulmonale.

68. Because Mr. Torres has a secondary diagnosis of asthma, which of the following medications might need to be avoided owing to a potential contraindication in asthmatic patients?

    I. spironolactone
    II. irbesartan
    III. atenolol

    A. I only
    B. III only
    C. I and II
    D. II and III
    E. I, II, and III

69. Which of the following agents slows electrical conduction through the atrioventricular node of the heart and has been used for treating hypertension and tachyarrhythmias as well as angina pectoris?

    A. amlodipine
    B. nifedipine
    C. felodipine
    D. verapamil
    E. isradipine

70. Which of the following currently available agents have been shown to be effective in reducing low-density lipoprotein (LDL) cholesterol levels with a resultant reduction in the mortality rate from coronary artery disease in patients with hypercholesterolemia?

    I. rosuvastatin
    II. pravastatin
    III. simvastatin

    A. I only
    B. III only
    C. I and II
    D. II and III
    E. I, II, and III

71. Olmesartan represents which of the following drug classes currently available for the treatment of hypertension?

    I. centrally acting α-adrenergic agonist
    II. cardiospecific β-adrenergic receptor blocking agent
    III. angiotensin II type 1 receptor antagonist

    A. I only
    B. III only
    C. I and II
    D. II and III
    E. I, II, and III

End of this patient profile; continue with examination

Use the patient profile below to answer questions 72–82.

PATIENT RECORD (INSTITUTION/NURSING HOME)

Patient Name: Eunice Lee

Address: 3549 Lakeside Dr.

Age: 73

Sex: F   Race: white

Height: 5'2"

Weight: 125 lb

Allergies: No known allergies

DIAGNOSIS

Primary	(1)	2-year history Parkinson disease
Secondary	(1)	Narrow-angle glaucoma
	(2)	30-year history of hypertension
	(3)	Gastroesophageal reflux disease

LAB/DIAGNOSTIC TESTS

	Date	Test
(1)	6/20	Na 135 mEq/L; K 3.6 mEq/L; Cl 95 mEq/L; CO_2 24 mEq/L; BUN 18 mg/dL; Cr 1.3 mg/dL
(2)	6/20	Occult blood in stool negative
(3)	6/20	Blood pressure 150/85 mm Hg

MEDICATION ORDERS (Including Parenteral Solutions)

	Date	Drug and Strength	Route	Sig
(1)	6/20	Acetazolamide SR 500 mg	po	i qd
(2)	6/20	Levodopa/Carbidopa 25/250	po	i tid
(3)	6/20	Pilocarpine 4%	ophthalmic	gtt i ou q6h
(4)	6/20	Reserpine 0.25 mg	po	i qd
(5)	6/20	Diltiazem 30 mg	po	i tid
(6)	6/20	Vitamin B complex w/ vitamin C	po	i qd
(7)	7/20	Entacapone tablets	po	200 mg daily
(8)	12/20	Tolcapone	po	100 mg tid

ADDITIONAL ORDERS

	Date	Comments
(1)	12/20	Baseline LFTs.

DIETARY CONSIDERATIONS (Enteral and Parenteral)

	Date	Comments
(1)		
(2)		

PHARMACIST NOTES AND Other Patient Information

	Date	Comments
(1)	12/20	D.C. entacapone tablets.
(2)		
(3)		
(4)		
(5)		
(6)		

72. Ms. Lee has Parkinson disease, which is a slowly progressive, degenerative, neurologic disease characterized by tremor, rigidity, bradykinesia, and postural instability. Although this disease is primarily idiopathic in origin, secondary parkinsonism may be caused by

    I. dopamine antagonists (e.g., phenothiazines, butyrophenones).
    II. poisoning by chemicals (e.g., carbon monoxide poisoning, manganese, mercury).
    III. infectious diseases (e.g., viral encephalitis, syphilis).

    A. I only
    B. III only
    C. I and II
    D. II and III
    E. I, II, and III

73. Ms. Lee's physician wants to initiate antihistamine therapy to treat the mild tremor that was the initial parkinsonian symptom experienced. Which antihistamines would be suitable?

    I. amantadine
    II. trihexyphenidyl
    III. diphenhydramine

    A. I only
    B. III only
    C. I and II
    D. II and III
    E. I, II, and III

74. The physician selects biperiden rather than the antihistamine to treat Ms. Lee's initial symptoms. The usual daily dosage range for biperiden is

    A. 1.0–6.0 mg.
    B. 1.5–4.5 mg.
    C. 2.0–8.0 mg.
    D. 300–600 mg.
    E. 200–1600 mg.

75. Upon the monthly medical record review by the local pharmacist, a notation is made to follow up with the medical staff on the recent order written for entacapone on 7/20. What place does entacapone have in the treatment of Parkinson disease?

    I. Entacapone is indicated as an adjunct to levodopa/carbidopa to treat patients with end-of-dose "wearing-off" symptoms.
    II. Entacapone is an enhancer of the bioavailability of levodopa.
    III. Entacapone is a precursor to dopamine indicated in the treatment of refractory Parkinson disease.

    A. I only
    B. III only
    C. I and II
    D. II and III
    E. I, II, and III

76. The physician has some concerns regarding the use of anticholinergics in Ms. Lee. Of what precautions in their use should the pharmacist inform the physician?

    A. complications of narrow-angle glaucoma
    B. consequences of fluid loss from diarrhea
    C. urinary incontinence
    D. excessive salivation
    E. excessive central nervous system excitation

77. Typical side effects associated with the use of levodopa include

    I. gastrointestinal effects, such as anorexia, nausea and vomiting, and abdominal distress.
    II. cardiovascular effects, such as postural hypotension and tachycardia.
    III. musculoskeletal effects, such as dystonia or choreiform muscle movements.

    A. I only
    B. III only
    C. I and II
    D. II and III
    E. I, II, and III

78. When using anticholinergic therapy for the treatment of this patient's parkinsonian tremor, which therapeutic considerations are applicable?

    I. Anticholinergic agents are best used in combination to maximize benefits.
    II. Trihexyphenidyl is generally the most effective anticholinergic agent for the treatment of parkinsonian tremor.
    III. Changing to another anticholinergic agent may not prove helpful if the therapeutic effect of the first agent is unsatisfactory, but changing to a different drug class may be beneficial.

    A. I only
    B. III only
    C. I and II
    D. II and III
    E. I, II, and III

79. Based on the patient's medical history before admission, the physician concludes that anticholinergic or antihistamine therapy is insufficient. Dopaminergic therapy could be instituted in the form of

    A. chlorpheniramine.
    B. biperiden.
    C. mesoridazine.
    D. pergolide.
    E. perphenazine.

80. Levodopa is metabolized to dopamine by dopa-decarboxylase both centrally and peripherally. This metabolism could be a potential complication for this patient because of

    A. concomitant vitamin B complex therapy.
    B. elevated serum creatinine level.
    C. concomitant diltiazem therapy.
    D. concomitant vitamin C therapy.
    E. elevated blood pressure.

81. In choosing dopaminergic therapy for Ms. Lee, the physician considers giving the combination of carbidopa and levodopa therapy. This combination

    I. inhibits peripheral decarboxylation of levodopa to dopamine.
    II. increases the required dose of levodopa by approximately 25%.
    III. decreases the amount of levodopa available for transport to the brain.

    A. I only
    B. III only
    C. I and II
    D. II and III
    E. I, II, and III

82. An adjunctive therapeutic regimen for Ms. Lee, relative to her previous "on–off" history, would be

    A. monthly interruption of levodopa therapy (drug holiday) on either an inpatient or an outpatient basis.
    B. addition of bromocriptine in a dosage range of 2.5–40 mg/day.
    C. addition of amantadine in a dose tailored to the level of renal function.
    D. addition of a monoamine oxidase inhibitor.
    E. addition of haloperidol in a dosage range of 2.5–15 mg/day.

End of this patient profile; continue with examination

83. The effects of food and antacid on the bioavailability of a new antihypertensive agent were studied in 24 men, using a three-way crossover design. The results of this study are summarized in the table below.

Treatment	C_{max} (µg/mL)[a]	AUC (0–24 hr; µg × hr/mL)[a]	T_{max} (hr)[a]
Fasting	95 ± 10	450 ± 115	1.5 ± 1.1
With antacid	106 ± 18	498 ± 123	1.0 ± 1.2
With high-fat breakfast	75 ± 11[b]	423 ± 110	2.4 ± 1.3

[a]Results are expressed as the mean ± SD.
[b]Compared with fasting, $p \leq .05$.

Compared with fasting, what results did the study show?

I. The high-fat breakfast had no significant effect on the bioavailability of the drug.
II. The antacid significantly increased the extent of systemic drug absorption.
III. The high-fat breakfast treatment decreased the rate of systemic drug absorption.

A. I only
B. III only
C. I and II
D. II and III
E. I, II, and III

84. An example of a nitrogen mustard is

A. chlorambucil.
B. busulfan.
C. melphalan.
D. mechlorethamine.
E. doxorubicin.

85. A controlled-release dosage form by which the mechanism for drug release is the result of an osmotically active drug core is known as

A. Dospan.
B. OROS.
C. TDDS.
D. Pennkinetic.
E. HBS.

86. All of the following are quinolone antimicrobials *except*

A. moxifloxacin.
B. levofloxacin.
C. clarithromycin.
D. ciprofloxacin.
E. gatifloxacin.

87. Which immunosuppressive agents are used after kidney transplantation?

I. azathioprine
II. basiliximab
III. cyclosporine

A. I only
B. III only
C. I and II
D. II and III
E. I, II, and III

PATIENT RECORD (INSTITUTION/NURSING HOME)

Patient Name: Joel Melvin
Address: 345 Bimini Ct.
Age: 54
Sex: M   Race: white
Height: 5'8"
Weight: 190 lb
Allergies: Quinidine: tinnitus, blurred vision, headache, nausea; Diuril: rash

DIAGNOSIS

Primary	(1)	Acute myocardial infarction
Secondary	(1)	Hypertension
	(2)	Chronic kidney disease

LAB/DIAGNOSTIC TESTS

	Date	Test
(1)	3/20	EKG stat and then at completion of TNKase therapy; baseline ST segment increase in II, III, and aVF
(2)	3/20	CBC: WBC count 12,000/mm^3
(3)	3/20	Platelet count 240,000 µL
(4)	3/20	Chem 20
(5)	3/20	Cardiac enzymes stat and then at 6 and 12 hr; baseline 1500 IU, peak 2566 IU
(6)	3/20	CK-MB fraction stat and then at 6 and 12 hr; baseline 32 IU, peak 166 IU
(7)	3/20	INR, aPTT stat and then at 6 and 12 hr after completion of t-PA; aPTT at baseline 30 sec, 6 hr > 120; INR at baseline 1
(8)	3/20	Urinalysis stat and then at 6 hr; baseline within normal limits
(9)	3/23	+ S$_3$, short of breath, bradycardia (55), fatigued

MEDICATION ORDERS (Including Parenteral Solutions)

	Date	Drug and Strength	Route	Sig
(1)	3/20	Chewable ASA 80 mg	po	ASAP
(2)	3/20	Heparin 5000 U	IV	as one-time only bolus
(3)	3/20	Heparin 1000 U	IV	qh as continuous infusion
(4)	3/20	TNKase 50 mg	IVP	over 5–10 sec
(5)	3/20	Atenolol 5 mg	IV	over 5 min, repeated in 10 min
(6)	3/20	Atenolol 50 mg	po	10 min after last IV dose
(7)	3/20	Ramipril 5 mg	po	i qd
(8)	3/20	Docusate 50-mg capsules	po	ii hs
(9)	3/20	Reduce heparin infusion to 800 U	IV	qh
(10)	3/20	Continue amiodarone as at home 200 mg	po	ii qd
(11)	3/23	Ramipril 10 mg	po	i qd
(12)	3/23	Atenolol 25 mg	po	i bid
(13)	3/23	Spironolactone 25 mg	po	i tid

DIETARY CONSIDERATIONS (Enteral and Parenteral)

	Date	Comments
(1)	3/20	Low-salt, low-fat diet.
(2)	3/22	Extra fiber.

PHARMACIST NOTES AND Other Patient Information

	Date	Comments
(1)	3/20	BP 150/100, pulse 120, respirations 20/min.
(2)	3/20	ST segment elevation in II, III, and aVF.
(3)	3/20	aPTT at 6 hr > 120 sec.
(4)	3/20	aPTT at 12 hr 65 sec.
(5)	3/21	Urine output OK.
(6)	3/22	Pulmonary rales, S$_3$.
(7)	3/23	BP increased, patient appears irritable, anxious, heart rate 120.
(8)	3/24	Appears well, good color, no chest pain, shortness of breath.

88. From the medication orders written for Mr. Melvin, it appears that ramipril was prescribed shortly after the acute period of the heart attack. Based on the patient's profile, what is the most logical reason for including ramipril in this setting?

    I. adjunctive therapy to prevent left ventricular dysfunction after acute myocardial infarction (MI)
    II. additive therapy to help bring the patient's blood pressure down
    III. treatment of suspected renal dysfunction

    A. I only
    B. III only
    C. I and II
    D. II and III
    E. I, II, and III

89. Creatinine clearance may be calculated from serum creatinine by using the

    A. Cockcroft and Gault equation.
    B. Fick's law.
    C. law of mass action.
    D. Henderson-Hasselbalch equation.
    E. Noyes-Whitney equation.

90. On 3/23, Mr. Melvin appears to be demonstrating signs and symptoms consistent with cardiac decompensation. On examination, his heart rate is found to be 55, he is short of breath, and fatigued,. Which of the following might be contributing to these symptoms?

    I. atenolol
    II. heart failure post–myocardial infarction (MI)
    III. ramipril

    A. I only
    B. III only
    C. I and II
    D. II and III
    E. I, II, and III

91. The half-life of amiodarone is

    A. 1 hr.
    B. 6 hr.
    C. 24 hr.
    D. 50 hr.
    E. Up to 50 days

92. Propranolol is administered to patients with hyperthyroidism because it

    I. helps reduce tachycardia, sweating, and tremor associated with the condition.
    II. inhibits the peripheral conversion of thyroxine (T_4) to triiodothyronine (T_3).
    III. suppresses the production of T_4.

    A. I only
    B. III only
    C. I and II
    D. II and III
    E. I, II, and III

93. Which of the following best summarize the use of tenecteplase (TNKase) in the acute management of Mr. Melvin's myocardial infarction?

    I. TNKase is the least expensive medication given compared to tissue plasminogen activator (t-PA) and reteplase in the acute management of myocardial infarction.
    II. TNKase is the easiest of the routinely available agents to administer in the acute management of myocardial infarction.
    III. The "open artery hypothesis" has been proven correct; and the earlier an infarcted artery is reopened after occlusion, the lower the mortality rate after an acute coronary occlusion and the better the long-term patency of the artery.

    A. I only
    B. III only
    C. I and II
    D. II and III
    E. I, II, and III

94. Atenolol is prescribed for the acute management of Mr. Melvin's myocardial infarction for which of the following reasons?

    I. It is used as an adjunctive treatment that prevents angina pectoris and potentially significant atrial tachyarrhythmias.
    II. Atenolol is used in this patient to decrease the patient's blood pressure.
    III. β-Adrenergic blockers have been shown to be effective in post–myocardial infarction patients in the prevention of mortality owing to sudden cardiac death.

    A. I only
    B. III only
    C. I and II
    D. II and III
    E. I, II, and III

95. From the allergy history presented on admission by Mr. Melvin, it appears that he has had some problems in the past taking quinidine as an antiarrhythmic. Are there ways to prevent these reactions?

    I. No, there has yet to be documented any method to desensitize the patient so that quinidine can be administered at a later date or time.
    II. Yes, administer aluminum hydroxide gel to prevent the reactions.
    III. Yes, the signs and symptoms reported reflect cinchonism, which can be prevented by reducing the dose of quinidine administered.

    A. I only
    B. III only
    C. I and II
    D. II and III
    E. I, II, and III

End of this patient profile; continue with examination

MEDICATION PROFILE (COMMUNITY)

Patient Name: Jon Rones

Address: 11 Cherry Ln.

Age: 65

Sex: M   Race: white

Height: 5'10"

Weight: 230 lb

Allergies: Sulfonamides, penicillin; both cause rash

DIAGNOSIS

Primary   (1)   Acute renal failure

              (2)   Hyperkalemia

Secondary   (1)   Hypertension

              (2)   Heart failure

              (3)   Sinus congestion

MEDICATION RECORD (Prescription and OTC)

	Date	Rx No.	Physician	Drug and Strength	Quan	Sig	Refills
(1)	6/8	245320	Sadler	Hydrochlorothiazide 50 mg	30	i qd	6
(2)	6/8	245321	Sadler	Moexipril 7.5 mg	30	i qd	6
(3)	6/8	245322	Sadler	Slow-K 8 mEq	100	i tid	6
(4)	6/15	246100	Frisch	Sudafed	100	i q6h	12
(5)	6/15	246101	Frisch	Tenuate Dospan	30	1 qd	5
(6)	11/7	278900	Sadler	Isoptin SR 120 mg	60	i bid	0
(7)	11/7	278901	Sadler	Tenormin 50 mg	60	i bid	0
(8)	11/7	278902	Sadler	Isordil 40 mg	120	i qid	5
(9)	11/7	278903	Sadler	Lanoxin 0.25 mg	30	i qd	0
(10)	12/5	279100	Frisch	Tenuate Dospan	30	i qd	5
(11)	2/5	280001	Sadler	Capoten 25 mg	100	i tid	1
(12)	2/5	280002	Sadler	Aldactone 25 mg	100	i tid	1
(13)	3/15	290016	Sadler	Vasotec 5 mg	60	i bid	6
(14)	3/15	290017	Sadler	Lanoxin 0.125 mg	30	i qd	6

PHARMACIST NOTES AND Other Patient Information

	Date	Comments
(1)	11/7	D.C. HydroDIURIL 50 mg.
(2)	11/7	D.C. Moexipril 7.5 mg.
(3)	11/7	D.C. Slow-K 8 mEq.
(4)	2/5	D.C. Lanoxin 0.25 mg.
(5)	2/5	D.C. Isoptin SR 120 mg.
(6)	2/5	D.C. Tenormin 50 mg.
(7)	3/5	D.C. Capoten 25 mg.
(8)	3/5	D.C. Aldactone 25 mg.
(9)	3/5	D.C. Sudafed.
(10)	3/5	D.C. Tenuate Dospan.
(11)		
(12)		
(13)		
(14)		

96. Based on the patient's medication profile, which condition(s) are potential underlying causes of the acute renal failure (ARF) in Mr. Rones?

    I. heart failure
    II. hypertension
    III. hyperkalemia

    A. I only
    B. III only
    C. I and II
    D. II and III
    E. I, II, and III

97. Based on Mr. Rones's allergies, which medication can he receive safely?

    A. hydrochlorothiazide
    B. V-Cillin-K
    C. Bactrim
    D. Septra
    E. None of the above

98. Based on the patient information, which medications would warrant a call to the physician before the pharmacist dispensed them to Mr. Rones?

    I. Slow-K
    II. Sudafed
    III. moexipril

    A. I only
    B. III only
    C. I and II
    D. II and III
    E. I, II, and III

99. According to the guidelines from the seventh report of the Joint National Committee (JNC-7), which agents are suitable alternatives to a thiazide diuretic for the initial treatment of stage I hypertension in this patient?

    I. atenolol
    II. ramipril
    III. candesartan

    A. I only
    B. III only
    C. I and II
    D. II and III
    E. I, II, and III

100. All of the following measures can be used in the prevention and treatment of digoxin-induced toxicity *except*

    A. maintaining normal concentrations of potassium in the serum.
    B. routinely monitoring renal function to determine digoxin elimination.
    C. administering Kayexalate solutions.
    D. administering lidocaine.
    E. None of the above.

101. Which of the following accurately describes the agents listed and the drug class they belong to?

    I. Felodipine: β-adrenergic receptor blocker; ramipril: angiotensin-converting enzyme (ACE) inhibitor; losartan: calcium channel blocker; propranolol: β-adrenergic receptor blocker
    II. felodipine: calcium channel blocker; losartan: angiotensin II receptor antagonist; ramipril: ACE inhibitor; enalapril: ACE inhibitor
    III. atenolol: β-adrenergic receptor blocker; carvedilol: β-adrenergic receptor blocker; isradipine: calcium channel blocker; enalapril: ACE inhibitor

    A. I only
    B. III only
    C. I and II
    D. II and III
    E. I, II, and III

102. Which of the following would not be considered appropriate treatment for this patient's hyperkalemia?

    A. dialysis
    B. calcium chloride or calcium gluconate
    C. regular insulin with dextrose
    D. sodium polystyrene sulfonate
    E. spironolactone

103. When dispensing the prescription for Isoptin and Tenormin, the pharmacist should advise Mr. Rones to

    I. check his heart rate regularly for brady-cardia.
    II. report swelling, shortness of breath, and fatigue.
    III. report orthopnea, dyspnea on exertion, and paroxysmal nocturnal dyspnea.

    A. I only
    B. III only
    C. I and II
    D. II and III
    E. I, II, and III

104. Which reference text could a pharmacist use to determine the indications and dosage for a relatively newly released medication for the treatment of hypertension?

    A. *Merck Index*
    B. American Hospital Formulary Service (AHFS)
    C. *Trissel's*
    D. *Hansten's*
    E. *Physicians' Desk Reference (PDR)*

105. The use of Lanoxin 0.125 mg for Mr. Rones centers around its ability to

    A. decrease the chronotropic actions of the heart, thereby reducing blood pressure.
    B. increase the chronotropic actions of the heart, thereby reducing blood pressure.
    C. increase renal blood flow, thereby improving urinary output.
    D. increase the inotropic actions of the heart, thereby increasing cardiac output.
    E. decrease the inotropic actions of the heart, thereby decreasing cardiac output.

106. Digoxin has an elimination half-life of 36 hr and 4.5 days in patients who have normal renal function and in those who are anephric, respectively. If no loading doses were used in Mr. Rones and he is anephric, the time to reach steady-state serum digoxin (Lanoxin) concentrations would be

    A. 2–3 days.
    B. 3–5 days.
    C. 6–8 days.
    D. 10–15 days.
    E. 15–20 days.

107. Which medication might provide benefit as an alternative to Inderal in a hypertensive patient who also suffers from bronchospastic lung disease and noncompliance?

    A. Inderal LA
    B. Blocadren
    C. Brevibloc
    D. Corgard
    E. Sectral

108. Which statements about the treatment of heart failure in Mr. Rones are correct?

    I. Isordil is probably being used as a pre-load reducing agent.
    II. Dopamine would be an appropriate alternative to Lanoxin in this patient.
    III. Dobutrex would be an appropriate alternative to Lanoxin in this patient.

    A. I only
    B. III only
    C. I and II
    D. II and III
    E. I, II, and III

End of this patient profile; continue with examination

---

109. A patient has just returned from England, where she received a drug to treat her asthma. She asks for the U.S. equivalent for this drug. What is the best resource for identifying this drug?

    A. *Facts and Comparisons*
    B. *Martindale's Extra Pharmacopoeia*
    C. *Identidex*
    D. *Physicians' Desk Reference (PDR)*
    E. *Drug Information 1990*

110. Peritoneal dialysis is useful for removing drugs from an intoxicated person if the drug

    A. is polar.
    B. is lipid soluble.
    C. is highly bound to plasma proteins.
    D. is nonpolar.
    E. has a large apparent volume of distribution.

111. Which of the following groups of herbal medicines are considered unsafe by the FDA because of their ability to cause damage to various organ systems?

    I. tonka bean, heliotrope, and periwinkle, causing hepatotoxicity
    II. mistletoe, spindle tree, and wahoo, causing seizures
    III. jimson weed and sweet flag, causing hallucinations

    A. I only
    B. III only
    C. I and II
    D. II and III
    E. I, II, and III

112. The percentage of elemental iron in ferrous gluconate is

    A. 10%.
    B. 12%.
    C. 20%.
    D. 30%.
    E. 33%.

113. In the extemporaneous compounding of an ointment, the process of using a suitable nonsolvent to reduce the particle size of a drug before its incorporation into the ointment is known as

    A. geometric dilution.
    B. levigation.
    C. pulverization by intervention.
    D. spatulation.
    E. trituration.

114. An antibiotic for IV infusion is supplied in 50-mL vials at a concentration of 5 mg/mL. How many vials are required for a 80-kg patient who needs an adult dose at a suggested infusion rate of 2.5 mg/kg/hr for 6 hr?

    A. 1
    B. 2
    C. 3
    D. 4
    E. 5

115. The bioavailability of a drug from an immediate-release tablet dosage form is most often related to the

    A. disintegration of the tablet.
    B. dissolution of the drug.
    C. elimination half-life of the drug.
    D. plasma protein binding of the drug.
    E. size of the tablet.

116. Which of the following is a list of protease inhibitors used in the treatment of HIV?

    I. amprenavir, indinavir, and nelfinavir
    II. zalcitabine, stavudine, lamivudine
    III. delavirdine, efavirenz, nevirapine

    A. I only
    B. III only
    C. I and II
    D. II and III
    E. I, II, and III

117. The rate of dissolution of a weak acid drug may be increased by

    I. increasing the pH of the medium.
    II. increasing the particle size of the solid drug.
    III. increasing the viscosity of the medium.

    A. I only
    B. III only
    C. I and II
    D. II and III
    E. I, II, and III

Use the patient profile below to answer questions 118–128.

PATIENT RECORD (INSTITUTION/NURSING HOME)

Patient Name: Bernard Hayley
Address: 2983 North Circle Dr.
Age: 29   Height: 5'11"
Sex: M   Race: white   Weight: 200 lb
Allergies: Reaction to contrast media; hives

DIAGNOSIS
Primary   (1)   Bipolar disorder
Secondary   (1)   Prehypertension
               (2)   History of epilepsy

LAB/DIAGNOSTIC TESTS
	Date	Test
(1)	8/10	Lithium 0.9 mEq/L
(2)	8/10	WBC 14,000/mm^3

MEDICATION ORDERS (Including Parenteral Solutions)
	Date	Drug and Strength	Route	Sig
(1)	8/10	Lithium carbonate (Lithobid) 300 mg	po	i q12h
(2)	8/10	Tegretol 200 mg	po	i tid
(3)	8/10	Hydrochlorothiazide (HCTZ) 25 mg	po	i q AM
(4)	8/10	Ambien 10 mg	po	1 q hs prn
(5)	8/10	Acetaminophen 500 mg	po	i–ii q4h prn

ADDITIONAL ORDERS
	Date	Comments
(1)		
(2)		

DIETARY CONSIDERATIONS (Enteral and Parenteral)
	Date	Comments
(1)	8/10	Salt-restricted diet.

PHARMACIST NOTES AND Other Patient Information
	Date	Comments
(1)		
(2)		
(3)		
(4)		
(5)		
(6)		
(7)		
(8)		
(9)		
(10)		
(11)		

118. Which of the following statements is/are correct concerning Mr. Hayley's primary diagnosis?

    I. This condition is also known as manic depression.
    II. Bipolar disorder may be classified as bipolar I disorder, bipolar II disorder, cyclothymia, and rapid cycling.
    III. Mood stabilizers have historically been the mainstays of therapy for this condition.

    A. I only
    B. III only
    C. I and II
    D. II and III
    E. I, II, and III

119. Which statement concerning lithium is true?

    A. It is the drug of choice for the acute and maintenance treatment of mania and hypomania.
    B. It is classified as an anxiolytic.
    C. It is a serum electrolyte similar to sodium and is relatively free of serious adverse effects and drug interactions.
    D. It is commonly used as an antidepressant.
    E. It is similar to haloperidol in neuroleptic activity.

120. The molecular weight of lithium carbonate, Li_2CO_3, is 73.89. How many milliequivalents of lithium are there in a 300-mg tablet of lithium carbonate?

    A. 1.24
    B. 2.46
    C. 4.06
    D. 8.12
    E. 12.18

121. The admitting physician had suspected that the patient was noncompliant with lithium therapy before admission. When interpreting the admission lithium level, the physician should consider

    I. the sample draw time with respect to the time of the last scheduled lithium dose.
    II. concomitant drug therapy.
    III. the acute manic condition of the patient.

    A. I only
    B. III only
    C. I and II
    D. II and III
    E. I, II, and III

122. For monitoring this patient's serum lithium concentrations, the most appropriate serum drug concentration that can be conveniently sampled is the

    I. minimum (trough) serum drug concentration.
    II. average serum drug concentration.
    III. peak serum drug concentration.

    A. I only
    B. III only
    C. I and II
    D. II and III
    E. I, II, and III

123. During the first 3 days of hospitalization, the patient began to experience symptoms of gastrointestinal (GI) upset, a fine hand tremor, polyuria, polydipsia, and dry mouth. Which statement represents the most rational approach for addressing this situation?

    A. The patient's dose should be doubled as these symptoms occur with subtherapeutic levels.
    B. A repeat lithium level should be obtained as the patient may be experiencing dose-related adverse effects.
    C. The patient should be placed on a special diet because he may be exhibiting signs and symptoms of diabetes mellitus.
    D. The patient is likely experiencing an interaction with tyramine-containing foods and should avoid wine and cheese.
    E. The patient's lithium therapy should be immediately stopped as he is experiencing severe lithium toxicity.

124. The hydrochlorothiazide order for Mr. Hayley might affect his serum lithium concentration by

    A. altering the glomerular filtration of lithium.
    B. increasing the absorption of lithium in the loop of Henle.
    C. increasing the absorption of lithium and sodium in the gastrointestinal tract.
    D. interfering with sodium reabsorption in the kidney.
    E. decreasing lithium reabsorption in the distal tubule.

125. Assuming Mr. Hayley was already taking each of the agents noted on his profile at admission, what drug would likely explain the white blood cell (WBC) count reported on admission?

    A. acetaminophen
    B. hydrochlorothiazide
    C. Ambien
    D. lithium

126. Based on the patient profile, if the physician were to initiate therapy with a tricyclic antidepressant, caution should be exercised with Mr. Hayley because of which potentially life-threatening adverse effect?

    A. mydriasis
    B. tachycardia
    C. dry mouth
    D. lowered seizure threshold
    E. systemic lupus erythematosus

127. Recent literature has supported the use of atypical antipsychotics as monotherapy or adjunctive treatment in bipolar mania. Which of the following is *not* an atypical antipsychotic?

    A. Zyprexa (olanzapine)
    B. Seroquel (quetiapine)
    C. Abilify (aripiprazole)
    D. Thorazine (chlorpromazine)
    E. Risperdal (risperidone)

128. Symbyax is the trade name of a combination product of an atypical antipsychotic and another agent and is approved for depressive episodes in bipolar disorder. What are the two agents that make up this product?

    A. olanzapine/fluoxetine
    B. aripiprazole/amitriptyline
    C. chlorpromazine/fluoxetine
    D. quetiapine/paroxetine

End of this patient profile; continue with examination

---

129. Methotrexate is used alone or in combination for the treatment of various neoplastic diseases. A recommended IV loading dose of methotrexate for the treatment of acute lymphoblastic leukemia is 200 mg/m^2 for the pediatric patient. What would be the loading dose for an 8-year-old patient whose body surface area is 0.89 m^2?

    A. 224 mg
    B. 150 mg
    C. 178 mg
    D. 200 mg
    E. 295 mg

130. The diuretic action of furosemide is the result of

    A. osmotic activity within the renal tubules.
    B. inhibition of sodium and chloride reabsorption at the distal segment of the nephron.
    C. inhibition of carbonic anhydrase at the nephron.
    D. inhibition of sodium reabsorption at the ascending limb of the loop of Henle.
    E. inhibition of aldosterone at the distal segment of the nephron.

131. Nonprescription decongestants used for topical application to the nasal passages include

    I. phenylephrine.
    II. oxymetazoline.
    III. pseudoephedrine.

    A. I only
    B. III only
    C. I and II
    D. II and III
    E. I, II, and III

132. According to the seventh report of the Joint National Committee (JNC-7), first-line drugs in the treatment of Stage I hypertension, in the absence of other disease states, include

    I. Diuril.
    II. Tenormin.
    III. Catapres.

    A. I only
    B. III only
    C. I and II
    D. II and III
    E. I, II, and III

133. To minimize the risk of tardive dyskinesia in a patient receiving antipsychotic drug therapy, the patient should be

    I. given the lowest possible dose of antipsychotic agent for the shortest duration possible.
    II. monitored closely for signs or symptoms of tardive dyskinesia.
    III. given second-generation agents (atypical antipsychotics) as first-line therapy.

    A. I only
    B. III only
    C. I and II
    D. II and III
    E. I, II, and III

134. Which of these agents would produce a significant drug–drug interaction in a patient who is taking Parnate?

    I. Demerol
    II. morphine
    III. ketorolac

    A. I only
    B. III only
    C. I and II
    D. II and III
    E. I, II, and III

135. Which agent is a selective antagonist of serotonin and has been shown to prevent the nausea and vomiting caused by highly emetogenic cancer chemotherapy?

    A. Zyban
    B. Zoloft
    C. Zyvox
    D. Zofran
    E. Zocor

136. Which of the following drugs is an antipsychotic agent?

    A. aripiprazole
    B. rabeprazole
    C. butoconazole
    D. clotrimazole

137. Which vitamin or other agent is often given along with a calcium supplement to aid in its absorption?

    A. Citracal
    B. vitamin D
    C. ascorbic acid
    D. vitamin E
    E. pantothenic acid

Use the patient profile below to answer questions 138–148.

MEDICATION PROFILE (COMMUNITY)

Patient Name: Barbara Szymuniak

Address: 200 Hawkins Dr.

Age: 60

Sex: F   Race: white

Height: 5'10"

Weight: 150 lb

Allergies: Penicillin, codeine

DIAGNOSIS

Primary	(1)	Rheumatoid arthritis (RA), diagnosed 1/5
Secondary	(1)	Community-acquired pneumonia, 1/15
	(2)	Urinary tract infection, 4/5

MEDICATION RECORD (Prescription and OTC)

	Date	Rx No.	Physician	Drug and Strength	Quan	Sig	Refills
(1)	1/5	209356	Cook	Motrin 800 mg	90	i tid	2
(2)	1/15	209490	Cook	Clarithromycin 500 mg	20	i po bid	0
(3)	2/15	211323	Cook	Plaquenil 200 mg	60	i bid	3
(4)	2/15	211324	Cook	Prednisone 5 mg	30	i qd	1
(5)	3/21	215855	Cook	Vitamin B_{12} 250 μg	30	i q AM	0
(6)	3/21	215856	Cook	Folic acid 1 mg	30	i q AM	0
(7)	3/21	215857	Cook	Ferrous sulfate 325 mg	30	i q tid	0
(8)	4/1	216092	Cook	Arthrotec 50 mg	120	i qid	0
(9)	4/5	216143	Cook	Ceftin 125 mg	20	i bid for 10 days	0
(10)	4/15	216614	Cook	Celebrex 100 mg	60	i bid	1
(11)	5/1	217851	Cook	Enbrel 50 mg SQ	1 box	once/week	2

PHARMACIST NOTES AND Other Patient Information

	Date	Comments
(1)	1/15	Pneumonia.
(2)	3/21	Called MD to discuss rationale for anemia medications; he agreed that these should not be filled.
(3)	4/1	D.C. Motrin; begin Arthrotec.
(4)	4/5	UTI.
(5)	4/15	D.C. Arthrotec; begin Celebrex.
(6)		
(7)		
(8)		
(9)		
(10)		
(11)		
(12)		
(13)		
(14)		
(15)		
(16)		
(17)		
(18)		

138. Which of the agents listed in the patient profile is a macrolide antibiotic?

     I. Ceftin
     II. Celebrex
     III. clarithromycin

     A. I only
     B. III only
     C. I and II
     D. II and III
     E. I, II, and III

139. Pharmacists will encounter patients with various types of arthritis. To make the diagnosis of rheumatoid arthritis, at least four of seven criteria need to be met. Which of the following would Ms. Szymuniak have likely experienced?

     I. morning stiffness in and around the joint lasting at least 1 hr before improvement
     II. arthritis of hand joints
     III. asymmetric involvement of the body joints

     A. I only
     B. III only
     C. I and II
     D. II and III
     E. I, II, and III

140. Which of the following arthritis medications in Ms. Szymuniak's profile require(s) close monitoring by an ophthalmologist to prevent adverse effects on the eyes?

     I. Motrin
     II. Celebrex
     III. Plaquenil

     A. I only
     B. III only
     C. I and II
     D. II and III
     E. I, II, and III

141. All of the following agents could be used to replace Plaquenil *except*

     A. Plavix.
     B. Ridaura.
     C. Rheumatrex.
     D. Depen.
     E. Aurolate.

142. Which agent(s) would be (an) appropriate alternative(s) for Motrin when it was originally prescribed (1/5) for Ms. Szymuniak?

     I. Celebrex
     II. Naprosyn
     III. nabumetone

     A. I only
     B. III only
     C. I and II
     D. II and III
     E. I, II, and III

143. Which of the following nonsteroidal anti-inflammatory drugs are correctly matched by brand and generic names?

     I. Lodine/sulindac
     II. Voltaren/celecoxib
     III. Naprosyn/naproxen

     A. I only
     B. III only
     C. I and II
     D. II and III
     E. I, II, and III

144. Which of the following apply to Ms. Szymuniak's prescriptions written on 2/15?

     I. The prednisone is likely used as a bridge therapy as Ms. Szymuniak is begun on a disease-modifying antirheumatic drug (DMARD).
     II. The prednisone appears to be dosed appropriately (lowest effective dose to minimize adverse effects).
     III. Plaquenil was begun within the recommended time frame after diagnosis of rheumatoid arthritis (RA).

     A. I only
     B. III only
     C. I and II
     D. II and III
     E. I, II, and III

145. On 3/21, Ms. Szymuniak was given prescriptions for three medications used to treat anemia. Patients with rheumatoid arthritis may have an anemia associated with their disease, which is unrelated to drug therapy. Would any of these medications be appropriate for this anemia?

     A. Yes
     B. No

146. The prescription that Dr. Cook wrote for Ms. Szymuniak on 4/1 was most likely given

    I. for treatment of her constipation.
    II. as an additional disease-modifying anti-rheumatic drug (DMARD).
    III. because of concern about potential gastrointestinal damage caused by Motrin.

    A. I only
    B. III only
    C. I and II
    D. II and III
    E. I, II, and III

147. On 4/15, Ms. Szymuniak was placed on Celebrex and the Arthrotec was discontinued. These two products represent approaches to the prevention of peptic ulcer disease induced by non-steroidal anti-inflammatory drugs (NSAIDs). Which of the following could also be considered?

    I. H_2-receptor antagonist co-therapy with a nonselective NSAID
    II. proton pump inhibitor cotherapy with a nonselective NSAID
    III. two nonselective NSAIDs given together

    A. I only
    B. III only
    C. I and II
    D. II and III
    E. I, II, and III

148. Finally, Ms. Szymuniak was placed on Enbrel. All of the following are correct statements concerning the use of this agent **except** which one?

    A. It is a biological response modifier for slowing the progression of rheumatoid arthritis.
    B. It is an agent that inhibits only the cyclooxygenase 2 receptor.
    C. The agent is given by subcutaneous injection.
    D. It is a great deal more expensive than traditional disease-modifying antirheumatic drugs (DMARDs).
    E. Agents such as this can be used when other traditional DMARDs fail.

End of this patient profile; continue with examination

---

149. Pyrantel pamoate is indicated for the treatment of pinworms. Besides treatment with this agent, other precautions must be used when a child has pinworms. Related to the treatment of this condition, all the following are correct **except** which one?

    A. Pyrantel pamoate paralyzes the worms through depolarization of muscle.
    B. All household members should be treated.
    C. All bedrooms should be thoroughly swept with a broom.
    D. Clothes and linens should be washed in hot water.
    E. Children should take showers rather than baths.

150. Sally, a regular customer in your pharmacy, wants some advice on an over-the-counter (OTC) treatment for itchy, odorous feet. Upon questioning, you discover that in between her toes, the skin is whiter than usual, thick, and scaly. She tells you that she swims competitively and often uses public showers at the pool. What condition is Sally most likely suffering from?

    A. tinea cruris
    B. tinea capitis
    C. tinea pedis
    D. tinea corporis
    E. tinea unguium

151. All of the following over-the-counter (OTC) agents are considered safe and effective for treating Sally's condition (see question 150) **except**

    A. terbinafine.
    B. clotrimazole.
    C. tolnaftate.
    D. hexylresorcinol.
    E. miconazole.

152. What are the two over-the-counter (OTC) antihistamines approved by the FDA for insomnia?

    A. diphenhydramine and doxylamine
    B. chlorpheniramine and loratadine
    C. doxylamine and brompheniramine
    D. thonzylamine and pheniramine
    E. dexbrompheniramine and chlorpheniramine

153. Mr. Conway, a 45-year-old who drives cross-country for a trucking company, complains of a runny nose, sneezing, and watery eyes that typically occur about this time of year. He knows it is allergies but cannot remember what medication he took for his allergies last year. Which of the following would be the best initial over-the-counter (OTC) recommendation for Mr. Conway to take for this condition this year?

    A. pseudoephedrine 60 mg twice a day
    B. loratadine 10 mg every day
    C. diphenhydramine 25 mg every 6 hr
    D. no OTC recommendation; refer the patient to a physician for a prescription for a nonsedating antihistamine

154. On a slow Sunday afternoon, you spot a teenager in the analgesic aisle and ask if there's anything you can help her find. She blushes a bit and blurts, "I just started my period and I think I'm going to die if I don't take something pretty quick here!" You hide your surprise (after all, this is the 12-year-old daughter of one of your friends at church) and offer to help. Which of the following medications is **not** an option for this girl?

    A. ketoprofen
    B. acetaminophen
    C. ibuprofen
    D. naproxen
    E. aspirin

155. Your pharmacy student pulls you aside and says, "I'm trying to counsel Mrs. Pound on the nonprescription medication treatment options to take care of her daughter's head lice." Which of the following products could be recommended over the counter (OTC)?

    I. a synergized pyrethrins product
    II. a product containing permethrin
    III. a product containing lindane

    A. I only
    B. III only
    C. I and II
    D. II and III
    E. I, II, and III

156. There are a large number of insulin products. What is the composition of Novolin 70/30?

    A. 70% regular insulin, 30% NPH insulin
    B. 70% Humalog insulin, 30% NPH insulin
    C. 70% NPH insulin, 30% regular insulin
    D. 70% NPH insulin, 30% Humalog insulin

Use the patient profile below to answer questions 157–168.

MEDICATION PROFILE (COMMUNITY)

Patient Name: Fanny Urmeister

Address: 24555 Colonial Estates

Age: 79   Height: 5'2"

Sex: F   Race: black   Weight: 178 lb

Allergies: Aspirin

DIAGNOSIS

Primary   (1)   Arrhythmias

Secondary   (1)   Status post-NSTEMI

               (2)   Smoking

               (3)   Obesity

MEDICATION RECORD (Prescription and OTC)

	Date	Rx No.	Physician	Drug and Strength	Quan	Sig	Refills
(1)	10/5	111345	Lamb	Tambocor 50 mg	60	i bid	6
(2)	10/5	111346	Lamb	Docusate 100 mg	60	ii hs	6
(3)	10/5	111347	Lamb	Ecotrin 325 mg	30	i q AM	6
(4)	10/5	111348	Lamb	Coumadin 2.5 mg	30	i q AM	6
(5)	10/5	111349	Troys	NicoDerm Patches	1	as directed	0
(6)	10/26	111941	Troys	Procan SR 500 mg	60	i qid	6
(7)	10/26	111942	Lamb	Isordil 20 mg	120	i q6h	3
(8)	11/2	112300	Cold	Isuprel Inhalation	1	as directed	4
(9)	11/2	112301	Cold	Dimetane 4 mg	30	i q8h	0
(10)	11/5	112589	Lamb	Quinidex 300 mg	60	i q8h	6
(11)	11/5	112590	Lamb	Robitussin-DM	120	i tsp q4h	0
(12)	11/5	112591	Lamb	Imodium 2 mg	30	as directed	0

PHARMACIST NOTES AND Other Patient Information

	Date	Comments
(1)	10/26	D.C. Tambocor.
(2)	11/5	D.C. Procan SR.
(3)	11/5	D.C. Imodium.
(4)		
(5)		
(6)		
(7)		
(8)		
(9)		
(10)		
(11)		
(12)		
(13)		
(14)		
(15)		
(16)		
(17)		

157. Based on Ms. Urmeister's allergies, which medications may be filled by the pharmacist?

    I. Tambocor
    II. Coumadin
    III. Ecotrin

    A. I only
    B. III only
    C. I and II
    D. II and III
    E. I, II, and III

158. Which medications best represent class I antiarrhythmics?

    I. quinidine, procainamide, and disopyramide
    II. lidocaine, tocainide, and mexiletine
    III. flecainide, propafenone, and moricizine

    A. I only
    B. III only
    C. I and II
    D. II and III
    E. I, II, and III

159. What are the advantages of Procan SR tablets over Pronestyl capsules?

    I. Procan SR tablets provide more procainamide per dose.
    II. Procan SR tablets are taken less frequently.
    III. After Procan SR treatment, the plasma procainamide hydrochloride levels have smaller fluctuations between peak and trough levels.

    A. I only
    B. III only
    C. I and II
    D. II and III
    E. I, II, and III

160. Which medications would be appropriate for Ms. Urmeister during the first several hours after her myocardial infarction?

    I. reteplase
    II. metoprolol
    III. heparin

    A. I only
    B. III only
    C. I and II
    D. II and III
    E. I, II, and III

161. Which treatments for Ms. Urmeister are likely to include Isordil?

    I. treatment of heart failure after a myocardial infarction
    II. treatment of the increased oxygen demand causing angina pectoris
    III. acute treatment of hypertension

    A. I only
    B. III only
    C. I and II
    D. II and III
    E. I, II, and III

162. Which of the following may result in increased oxygen demand by the myocardium and, therefore, may cause a problem in Ms. Urmeister?

    I. isoproterenol
    II. smoking
    III. acebutolol

    A. I only
    B. III only
    C. I and II
    D. II and III
    E. I, II, and III

163. The physician would like the pharmacist to dispense a generic drug product that is bioequivalent to Quinidex. This generic drug product should have

    I. the same drug bioavailability.
    II. an equal or better rate and extent of systemic drug absorption.
    III. an equal or better C_{max}, area under the curve (AUC), and T_{max}.

    A. I only
    B. III only
    C. I and II
    D. II and III
    E. I, II, and III

164. Which agent would be a suitable first-line oral drug to use in this patient, who needs maintenance therapy for ventricular tachycardia?

    A. Tambocor
    B. Enkaid
    C. lidocaine
    D. Tikosyn
    E. Mexitil

165. Which agents are most likely to be responsible for Ms. Urmeister's use of Imodium on 11/5?

    I. Tambocor
    II. Procan SR
    III. Quinidex

    A. I only
    B. III only
    C. I and II
    D. II and III
    E. I, II, and III

166. Which agent is effective in reducing pain, anxiety, and cardiac workload in the myocardial infarction patient?

    A. aspirin
    B. morphine
    C. furosemide
    D. digoxin
    E. lidocaine

167. Which agents are effective in preventing sudden death in post-myocardial infarction patients?

    I. Procan SR
    II. Blocadren
    III. Tenormin

    A. I only
    B. III only
    C. I and II
    D. II and III
    E. I, II, and III

168. All of the following are correctly matched by brand and generic names *except* which one?.

    A. quinidine sulfate/Quinidex
    B. warfarin/Coumadin
    C. nitroglycerin patches/NicoDerm Patches
    D. disopyramide/Norpace
    E. diltiazem/Cardizem

End of this patient profile; continue with examination

---

169. A 30-year-old male comes into your pharmacy complaining of difficulty falling asleep at night. He hands you a list of all the drugs he is currently taking. Which one of these medications is the most likely culprit responsible for this sleep problem?

    A. Metamucil
    B. Sudafed
    C. Flonase
    D. Benadryl
    E. aspirin

170. Which of the following conditions can be treated with nonprescription products?

    A. water-clogged ears
    B. otitis media
    C. swimmer's ear
    D. impacted cerumen
    E. Both A and D

171. Which of the following topical nasal decongestant agents has a 12-hr duration of action and, therefore, is administered twice daily for adult patients?

    A. oxymetazoline
    B. naphazoline
    C. phenylephrine
    D. ephedrine
    E. propylhexedrine

172. Jim, a technician working in your pharmacy, asks you to recommend a sunscreen for him to take to the beach for spring break. He has fair skin and states that he usually burns after only 10 min in the sun. If you recommend a sun protection factor (SPF) of 15 and assume Jim applies this product correctly, for how long will Jim be protected?

     A. 30 min
     B. 21\2 hr
     C. 6 hr
     D. 45 min
     E. 11\2 hr

173. A 21-year-old male walks up to you at the counter with a bottle of 5% minoxidil in hand. He proceeds to ask you about how to effectively apply this product. All of the following are appropriate points to cover in counseling this patient *except* which one?

     A. Double the dose if you miss an application.
     B. Apply or spray about 1 mL of the product onto the affected area of the scalp twice daily.
     C. This strength is indicated for only men, not women.
     D. This product must be used continuously to maintain any hair regrowth.
     E. Allow 4 hr for the drug to penetrate the scalp before showering or going swimming.

174. Which of the following nonprescription ingredients does *not* have proven safety/efficacy for the treatment of acne?

     A. benzoyl peroxide
     B. sulfur
     C. triclosan
     D. salicylic acid
     E. sulfur and resorcinol

175. A teenage girl and her mother are at your counseling window in the pharmacy. The mother explains that her daughter has had acne for a few months now and has used a couple of over-the-counter (OTC) agents (benzoyl peroxide cream and face wash), and asks you to recommend a product to help treat the acne. You examine the girl's face and count over a dozen papules and pustules along with some mild scarring. The girl says she has a few more on her trunk. What do you recommend for this patient?

     A. Use Oxy Balance Deep Action Night Formula (benzoyl peroxide 2.5%) each evening.
     B. Use Clearasil Clearstick Maximum Strength (salicylic acid 2%) each morning.
     C. Wash face at least four to five times daily with SAStid Soap (precipitated sulfur 10%).
     D. No further OTC product recommendations can be made at this time; advise the girl to see a physician or dermatologist.
     E. Wash face no more than twice daily with a product such as Oxy 10 Balance Maximum Medicated Face Wash (benzoyl peroxide 10%).

176. Which one of the following best describes the mechanism of action of benzoyl peroxide for acne?

     A. porolytic—allows the pores to "open up"
     B. keratolytic only
     C. antibacterial only
     D. releases oxygen to destroy the anaerobic *P. acnes;* causes peeling of outer layer of skin
     E. dries out lesions by decreasing sebum production by sebaceous glands

177. Rhinitis medicamentosa is an adverse effect associated with overuse of which agents?

     A. oral decongestants
     B. antihistamines
     C. topical decongestants
     D. expectorants
     E. cough suppressants

178. The pharmacist should advise a patient not to crush tenuate Dospan because crushing this tablet

    I. destroys the active drug in this dosage form.
    II. allows immediate absorption of the active drug.
    III. destroys the integrity of the delivery system.

    A. I only
    B. III only
    C. I and II
    D. II and III
    E. I, II, and III

179. A first-order reaction is characterized by

    I. $da / dt = -k$.
    II. $A = A_0 e^{-kt}$.
    III. $t_{1\backslash 2} = 0.693 / k$.

    A. I only
    B. III only
    C. I and II
    D. II and III
    E. I, II, and III

180. FluMist is approved for use in

    I. children ages 6 months to $<$ 5 years.
    II. children ages 5–17.
    III. adults ages 18–49.

    A. I only
    B. III only
    C. I and II
    D. II and III
    E. I, II, and III

181. Calcium is available for oral administration in all of the following salt forms *except*

    A. chloride.
    B. lactate.
    C. gluconate.
    D. phosphate.
    E. carbonate.

182. All of the following are side effects of prednisone *except*

    A. osteonecrosis.
    B. hyperglycemia.
    C. leukopenia.
    D. fluid retention.
    E. cataracts.

183. Which of the following is *not* a protease inhibitor for treatment of HIV infection?

    A. saquinavir
    B. ritonavir
    C. cidofovir
    D. indinavir
    E. Crixivan

184. Pyrogen testing of parenteral solutions is a quality control procedure used to check that the product

    I. does not contain fever-producing substances.
    II. is sterile.
    III. does not contain particulate matter.

    A. I only
    B. III only
    C. I and II
    D. II and III
    E. I, II, and III

185. Common laboratory tests to assess kidney disease include

    I. blood urea nitrogen (BUN) and serum creatinine.
    II. lactic dehydrogenase (LDG), aspartate aminotransferase (AST; formerly SGOT), and alanine aminotransferase (ALT; formerly SGPT).
    III. red blood count (RBC) and white blood count (WBC).

    A. I only
    B. III only
    C. I and II
    D. II and III
    E. I, II, and III

186. Treatment of chemotherapy-induced nausea and vomiting includes all of the following drugs *except*

    A. Zofran.
    B. Reglan.
    C. Inapsine.
    D. Tagamet.
    E. Marinol.

187. Laboratory findings in acute renal failure include all of the following conditions *except*

    A. hypophosphatemia.
    B. hyperuricemia.
    C. hyperkalemia.
    D. metabolic acidosis.
    E. hypocalcemia.

188. Which trace element, if deficient, is responsible for cretinism in children?

    A. zinc
    B. copper
    C. chromium
    D. selenium
    E. iodine

189. All of the following are true of omalizumab *except* which one?

    A. It is an immunoglobulin (Ig) monoclonal antibody that blocks the IgE receptor and thereby decreases allergic reactions.
    B. It is administered orally twice a day.
    C. It is approved for adults and adolescents with steroid-resistant asthma.
    D. It requires refrigeration during storage.
    E. Benefits may take several weeks to be noticeable.

190. All of the following would be good recommendations to prevent poison ivy contact dermatitis *except* which one?

    A. Wash hands with soap and water within 10 min of exposure to poison ivy.
    B. Apply bentoquatam 5% solution at least 15 min before possible plant contact.
    C. Apply bentoquatam 5% solution immediately after contact with the poison ivy plant to exposed area of skin.
    D. Avoid the poison ivy plant.
    E. Identify the poison ivy plant in books, on TV, and so forth so the patient will know what it looks like and how to avoid it.

TEST 1 ANSWERS AND EXPLANATIONS

1. The answer is E (I, II, III).
The two potential problems were (1) the drug interaction between niacin and simvastatin and (2) the use of aspirin in a patient with a history of an aspirin allergy. The combination of niacin and simvastatin may increase the risk of myopathy and rhabdomyolysis (additive effects) and should be brought to the prescriber's attention. Aspirin is contraindicated in patients who are hypersensitive to it, as stated in Ms. Honors' profile.

2. The answer is A.
Doxazosin in doses of 2–8 mg/day was one of the treatment arms in ALLHAT, and the treatment was discontinued prematurely owing to an apparent 25% increase in the incidence of combined cardiovascular disease outcomes compared to patients in the control group receiving the diuretic chlorthalidone. The added risks for heart failure, stroke, and coronary heart disease were the major outcomes of the doxazosin arm. The HOPE project was one of the first clinical trials demonstrating the benefits of angiotensin-converting enzyme inhibitors (ramipril) in reducing cardiovascular death, myocardial infarction, and stroke in patients who were at high risk for or had vascular disease in the absence of heart failure. Ramipril in doses of 10 mg/day, demonstrated substantial clinical benefits that could not be explained through its blood pressure-lowering effects alone.

3. The answer is E (I, II, III).
The JNC-7 provided a table of "compelling" indications that suggested specific drug therapy in select patients rather the use of standard suggested guidelines. Included as compelling indications, and their respective therapy, are heart failure (diuretics, β-blockers, ACE inhibitors, ARBs, aldosterone antagonists), post–myocardial infarction (β-blockers, ACE inhibitors, aldosterone antagonists), high coronary disease risk (diuretics, β-blockers, ACE inhibitors, calcium channel blockers), diabetes (diuretics, β-blockers, ACE inhibitors, ARBs, calcium channel blockers), chronic kidney disease (ACE inhibitors, ARBs), and recurrent stroke prevention (diuretics, ACE inhibitors).

4. The answer is C (I, II).
β-Adrenergic blockers such as atenolol are indicated in post-MI patients, where they have been shown to significantly reduce sudden death and overall mortality. In addition, they have been suggested by the JNC-7 guidelines as therapeutic options in hypertensive patients with the following compelling indications for their use instead of standard suggested therapy: heart failure, post-MI, high-risk coronary disease patients, and diabetes. Ms. Honors, as a post-MI patient with hypertension, would be a candidate for atenolol.

5. The answer is E (I, II, III).
Thrombolytic agents (rt-PA, r-PA, TNKase) have been used in patients with STEMI who have had chest pain for < 6–12 hr. Successful early reperfusion has been shown to reduce infarct size, improve ventricular function, and improve mortality. Benefits may be seen in patients using thrombolytic therapy as late as 12 hr after pain starts. The use of thrombolytics may restore blood flow in an occluded artery if administered within 12 hr of an acute MI, although < 6 hr is optimal. The goal of treatment of STEMI patients is to initiate thrombolytic therapy within 30–60 min of arrival in an emergency room. Most studies have shown that each agent, when used early, can reopen (reperfuse) occluded coronary arteries and reduce mortality from STEMI. However, considerations such as ease of use, onset of action, incidence of bleed, and cost are important in determining which agent is used in a given hospital and given patient.

6. The answer is C (I, II).
Clopidogrel is a thienopyridine derivative related to ticlopidine, but it possesses antithrombotic effects that are greater than those of ticlopidine. Clopidogrel is a therapeutic option in patients who cannot take aspirin owing to contraindications. A dosage of 75 mg/day is recommended to prevent the development of acute coronary syndromes.

7. The answer is B.
Rabeprazole is a proton pump inhibitor (PPI), which among other indications (gastroesophageal reflux disease, erosive gastritis, hypersecretory conditions, and treatment of *Helicobacter pylori* infections) is also indicated for the treatment of duodenal ulcer. Current recommendations suggest a dosage of 20 mg by mouth daily for 4 weeks, which may be repeated for an additional 4 weeks if needed.

8. The answer is B (III).
Sublingual nitroglycerin is indicated for the acute treatment of angina pectoris as well as for the prophylaxis of angina pectoris. The tablets are to be placed under the tongue, where they dissolve and demonstrate a quick onset of action of 2–5 min. Sublingual nitroglycerin tablets are not to be swallowed or placed in easy-to-open plastic containers and should remain in the manufacturer's bottle to reduce loss of potency. Patients should also be warned that they may become light-headed or dizzy after taking a tablet and should either sit down or support themselves against a solid object to prevent falls. Patients should also be informed that nitroglycerin tablets can cause a headache and routinely cause a slight burning sensation when placed under the tongue.

9. The answer is C.
JNC-7 guidelines include four blood pressure classes (normal, prehypertension, stage I hypertension, and stage II hypertension); the classes are based on patient blood pressure readings and are linked to current treatment recommendations. Normal (systolic < 120 and diastolic < 80 mm Hg) requires no treatment. Prehypertension (systolic 120–139 or diastolic of 80–89 mm Hg) again requires no antihypertensive treatment unless the patient has a compelling indication. In stage I hypertension (systolic 140–159 or diastolic 90–99 mm Hg), thiazide-type diuretics are indicated for most patients, though patients with compelling indications would be candidates for other agents. In stage II hypertension (systolic ≥ 160 or diastolic ≥ 100 mm Hg), two-drug combinations are indicated for most patients (thiazide-type diuretic and ACE inhibitor, ARB, or β-blocker, or calcium channel blocker). Ms. Honors, who is currently receiving a diuretic, a β-blocker, and an ACE inhibitor and depends on most recent blood pressure readings, could be considered to have stage II hypertension.

10. The answer is E.
The patient profile states that the patient has an allergy to aspirin, which has resulted in an anaphylactic reaction. Consequently, all salicylates such as Ecotrin would be contraindicated. In addition, all nonsteroidal anti-inflammatory drugs (NSAIDs)—ibuprofen-like as well as the cyclooxygenase 2 (COX-2) selective agents such as celecoxib, and meloxicam—are contraindicated and should not be given to this patient.

11. The answer is E (I, II, III).
Untreated hypertension has been shown to cause target organ damage to four major organ systems. *Cardiac effects:* left ventricular hypertrophy compensates for the increased cardiac workload, resulting in signs and symptoms of heart failure, and increased oxygen requirements of the enlarged heart may produce angina pectoris. Hypertension can be caused by accelerated atherosclerosis. Atheromatous lesions in the coronary arteries lead to decreased blood flow, resulting in angina pectoris and myocardial infarction; sudden death may ensue. *Renal effects:* decreased blood flow leads to an increase in renin-aldosterone secretion, which heightens the reabsorption of sodium and water and increases blood volume. Accelerated atherosclerosis decreases the oxygen supply, leading to renal parenchymal damage, with decreased filtration capability and azotemia. The atherosclerosis also decreases blood flow to the renal arterioles, leading to nephrosclerosis and, ultimately, renal failure (acute as well as chronic). *Cerebral effects:* decreased blood flow, decreased oxygen supply, and weakened blood vessel walls lead to transient ischemic attacks, cerebral thromboses, and the development of aneurysms with hemorrhage. There are alterations in mobility along with weakness, paralysis, and memory deficits. *Retinal effects:* decreased blood flow with retinal vascular sclerosis and increased arteriolar pressure with the appearance of exudates and hemorrhage result in visual defects (e.g., blurred vision, spots, blindness).

12. The answer is A.
In an otherwise healthy patient with stage I hypertension, thiazide diuretics are considered the first-line treatment of choice for most patients. In patients who might have a compelling indication, such as renal disease, stroke, high-risk cardiovascular disease, or diabetes mellitus, other agents have been recommended. Amiloride is referred to as a potassium-sparing diuretic that inhibits distal convoluted tubule aldosterone-induced sodium resorption and is not generally indicated over thiazide diuretics as first-line therapy. Chlorthalidone, chlorothiazide, indapamide, and methyclothiazide are all thiazide diuretics; and though they may have different pharmacokinetic profiles and different costs, they should all be considered first-line antihypertensives.

13. The answer is B.
Isotonic and iso-osmotic solutions have osmotic pressures that are equal to blood. Normal saline solution, 0.9% sodium chloride, usually is given as an example of an isotonic solution. Hypertonic solutions have osmotic pressures greater than blood (e.g., high concentrations of dextrose used in total parenteral therapy). Half-normal saline solution (0.45% sodium chloride) has an osmotic pressure less than that of blood and is referred to as a hypotonic solution.

14. The answer is B.
Anemia is a common complication of chronic kidney disease, caused by a decrease in erythropoietin an endocrine product produced in the kidney. Erythropoietin, stimulates red blood cell production in the bone marrow. This is reflected by an increase in hematocrit and hemoglobin and a decrease in the need for blood transfusions.

15. The answer is E (I, II, III).
Insulin resistance is defined as the need for > 200 U of insulin per day in the absence of ketoacidosis. Causes include obesity, infection, glucocorticoid therapy, and circulating IgG anti-insulin antibodies. Insulin resistance may resolve without treatment, by insulin switching, or with prednisone therapy.

16. The answer is C (I, II).
Lanolin (hydrous wool fat) has been used as an emulsion base. whereas occlusive films can prevent water loss from the skin through evaporation.

17. The answer is D (II, III).
Kaopectate and Pepto-Bismol are considered effective in the treatment of diarrhea. Donnagel-PG is an opiate-containing antidiarrheal that exerts a direct musculotropic effect, which inhibits propulsive intestinal movements. Its value as an antidiarrheal is unproven. Both Kaopectate (attapulgite) and Pepto-Bismol (bismuth salts) are considered adsorbents, which are nonabsorbable inert powders that absorb bacteria, toxins, and gases.

18. The answer is A (I).
Dopamine does not cross the blood–brain barrier, but its precursor levodopa does. Levodopa is metabolized centrally and peripherally to dopamine by dopa-decarboxylase. Carbidopa does not cross the blood–brain barrier and inhibits peripheral decarboxylation of levodopa. Therefore, more levodopa is available for transport to the brain, and the peripheral side effects are reduced. Sinemet combines the antiparkinsonian effects of levodopa with the dopamine metabolism-inhibiting effects of carbidopa.

19. The answer is E (I, II, III).
Drugs that are highly bound to albumin will have higher concentrations of free drug circulating in the blood if albumin levels are reduced. Hypoalbuminemia, liver (hepatic) disease, malnutrition, and cancer are several of the more common conditions that result in decreased albumin levels, which necessitate alterations in dosage in highly albumin-bound drugs.

20. The answer is A.
The action of salmeterol is that of a sympathomimetic agonist with high β_2 selectivity. The lung contains β_2-receptors, which are responsible for the relaxation of tracheal and bronchial muscles. In contrast, β_1-receptors are in the heart and are responsible for chronotropic (rate) and inotropic (contraction force) effects. Salmeterol gives the asthmatic patient maximal bronchodilation with minimal stimulation of cardiac receptors.

21. The answer is A (I).
Different age groups have common underlying causes for the development of heart failure. The patient in this case is 54 years of age and has no history of myocardial infarction as a possible cause, which is a leading cause of heart failure in people aged 40–50 years. Drugs such as corticosteroids have been implicated as causative agents in the development of heart failure owing to their ability to cause sodium and water retention. In both of these cases, metabolic demands placed on the heart normally do not increase; however, the heart is still unable to meet them (low output). Mr. Mutrick has a secondary diagnosis of anemia (possibly caused by steroid use), which increases the metabolic demands placed on a heart that is already unable to meet such demands (high output).

22. The answer is D (II, III).
On receiving the prescriptions on 8/10, the pharmacist should have called the physician's office for assurance that the potassium supplement was truly warranted owing to the documentation of chronic kidney disease. Potassium elimination depends on the kidney, and declining function means the ability to excrete potassium is reduced. In addition, based on updated treatment guidelines, the pharmacist would be justified in discussing the potential role for a β-adrenergic blocker in this type of patient. Its merits may very well extend beyond those appreciated in heart failure, including hypertension as "compelling" condition.

23. The answer is D (II, III).
Carvedilol (Coreg) is a β-adrenergic receptor blocker that is indicated in the treatment of hypertension and heart failure. When used in the treatment of heart failure, as in Mr. Mutrick, doses must be slowly and closely titrated up to the maximal dosage every 2 weeks as tolerated. The pharmacist was able to identify that there were no prescriptions on file for Mr. Mutrick for Coreg and there were no refills provided with the initial prescription of Coreg 3.125 mg. This has the potential for leaving the patient without his medication at the end of the 2-week period. Cardiac patients receiving β-adrenergic receptor blockers should not have their β-blocker discontinued abruptly, as this may induce an acute coronary event caused by the lack of β-blockade.

24. The answer is A.
A patient with left-sided heart failure presents with symptoms and signs of fluid backing up behind a failed left ventricle. Mr. Mutrick would initially present with complaints involving the pulmonary system (e.g., rales, shortness of breath, paroxysmal nocturnal dyspnea). Peripheral signs and symptoms (e.g., jugular venous distention, hepatojugular reflux, pedal edema, abdominal distention, and hepatomegaly) are more the consequence of the backup of fluid behind the failing right ventricle, characteristically seen in right-sided heart failure. It is important to recognize that, because the circulatory system is closed, patients rarely present with strictly left-sided signs or right-sided signs; rather, they present with a combination of signs and symptoms that reflect global circulatory problems.

25. The answer is E (I, II, III).
Ramipril (Altace) is an angiotensin-converting enzyme (ACE) inhibitor. Recent clinical guidelines recommend the use of ACE inhibitors in all patients with heart failure owing to left ventricular systolic dysfunction, unless they have a contraindication to their use or have demonstrated intolerance to their use. Currently, these drugs are considered the first-line agents in the treatment of heart failure and have been shown to have a beneficial effect on cardiac remodeling. The Heart Outcomes Prevention Evaluation (HOPE) trial demonstrated that the ACE inhibitor ramipril (10 mg/day) reduced cardiovascular death, myocardial infarction, and stroke in patients > 55 years of age who were at high risk for or had vascular disease in the absence of heart failure. ACE inhibitors have also been shown to be beneficial in patients who have chronic kidney disease, in whom they can reduce the onset of deteriorating renal function. Each of the three conditions—hypertension, heart failure, and chronic kidney disease—have now been shown to benefit from the use of ACE inhibitors such as ramipril. However, caution is still required; patients should be monitored for elevations in potassium levels and a potential reduction in renal function indicators (serum creatinine).

26. The answer is B.
Ferrous sulfate is available in the hydrous form as a 325-mg tablet. The preparation contains 20% elemental iron. Consequently, 325 mg given three times a day would equal 0.20 × 3 × 325 mg, or 195 mg per day. Other available salts that contain varying degrees of elemental iron are ferrous gluconate, 12%; ferrous fumarate, 33%; and ferrous sulfate (desiccated), 30%.

27. The answer is C (I, II).
All diuretics are capable of reducing total body and sodium reabsorption through their diuretic effects on the kidney. These effects reduce venous return to the heart and decrease preload. Lasix (furosemide) has an additional benefit, in the acute situation, of causing a direct dilating effect on the lung, and it is a useful agent for the rapid reversal of pulmonary congestion. Current national guidelines recommend the use of a diuretic for patients with heart failure accompanied by fluid retention (edema) and those who have had fluid retention in the past with heart failure. Lasix has yet to show any significant effect on cytokines and their subsequent release.

28. The answer is C (I, II).
Enalapril (Vasotec), captopril (Capoten), lisinopril (Zestril and Prinivil), benazepril (Lotensin), fosinopril (Monopril), quinapril (Accupril), ramipril (Altace), moexipril (Univasc), and trandolapril (Mavik) are the ACE inhibitors currently on the market. The agents as a group have the same general pharmacologic effects by blocking the actions of the converting enzyme, which converts angiotensin I to angiotensin II (a potent vasoconstrictor), thereby reducing afterload and stimulating aldosterone release from the adrenal gland. Currently, ACE inhibitors are considered the first-line agents in the treatment of heart failure and have been shown to have a beneficial effect on cardiac remodeling.

29. The answer is D (II, III).
Digoxin molecules in tablet or capsule form have the same potency. Lanoxicaps is a liquid-filled capsule containing digoxin dissolved in a solvent composed of polyethylene glycol 400 USP, ethyl alcohol (8%), propylene glycol USP, and purified water. The systemic absorption of digoxin from the capsule is practically complete (F 90–100%) and less variable than the systemic absorption of digoxin from the tablet (F 60–80%). Digitalis, specifically digoxin, is now recommended in conjunction with diuretics, an angiotensin-converting enzyme (ACE)inhibitor, and a β-adrenergic blocker to improve the symptoms and clinical status of patients with heart failure as a result of left ventricular systolic dysfunction.

30. The answer is A.
Hydralazine (Apresoline) is an arteriolar dilator that has been used in hypertension. However, by decreasing peripheral vascular resistance, it also has been shown to reduce afterload in patients with heart failure. A Veterans Administration study has shown that the combination of hydralazine and isosorbide dinitrate significantly reduced mortality in heart failure patients unresponsive to digitalis and diuretics. Long-term therapy with hydralazine has been associated with the development of systemic lupus erythematosus, which presents as fatigue, malaise, low-grade fever, and joint aches and pains. Baseline and serial blood counts for antinuclear antibody titers should be performed; if systemic lupus erythematosus develops, discontinuation of the drug results in reversal of the symptoms over time.

31. The answer is E (I, II, III).
Inocor (inamrinone), Dobutrex (dobutamine), and dopamine are inotropic agents. Inotropic agents have been used in the emergency treatment of patients with heart failure and in patients refractory to, or unable to take, digitalis. However, current guidelines provide a Class III recommendation for these drugs. In addition, current guidelines provide a Class IIb recommendation—"conditions for which there is conflicting evidence and/or a divergence of opinion about the usefulness/efficacy of performing the procedure/therapy and that the usefulness/efficacy is less well established by evidence/opinion"—for the use of continuous intravenous infusion of a positive inotropic agent for palliation of heart failure symptoms.

32. The answer is A (I).
NSAIDs have been reported to cause gastrointestinal erosions and ulcers. This patient could have a major problem because of a report of anemia. In addition, the physician should be given an update from the pharmacist regarding the current disease conditions to reinforce caution for such agents owing to the patient's history of hypertension and chronic kidney disease.

33. The answer is E.
Similar to ACE inhibitors, β-adrenergic blockers work through actions of the endogenous neurohormonal system. Unlike ACE inhibitors, which work strictly by blocking the effects of the renin–angiotensin system, β-adrenergic blockers work by interfering with the sympathetic nervous system. This has prompted the use of three different types of β-adrenergic blockers: those that are relatively selective toward β_1-receptors (e.g., metoprolol); those that are selective to both β_1- and β_2-receptors (e.g., propranolol and bucindolol); and those that are selective to β_1-, β_2-,and α_1-receptors (e.g., carvedilol). β-adrenergic blockers, similar to ACE inhibitors, have been shown to decrease the risk of death and hospitalization as well as improve the clinical status of heart failure patients. Current guidelines recommend the use of a β-adrenergic blocker in all patients with stable heart failure owing to left ventricular dysfunction, unless they have a contraindication to their use or are unable to tolerate their effects because hypotension, bradycardia, bronchospasm, and the like.

34. The answer is C.
Atropine in therapeutic doses inhibits cholinergic impulses and increases the heart rate. When treatment is initiated in a patient with sinus bradycardia, initial small doses may actually stimulate cholinergic receptors and therefore increase the degree of bradycardia. Constipation, dry mouth, decreased secretions, and pupillary dilation are all side effects associated with anticholinergic drugs. Rarely do single doses of atropine cause constipation.

35. The answer is A (I).
Quinidine is a class I$_A$ antiarrhythmic agent, which has gastrointestinal intolerance as one of its side effects. Sustained-release products such as Quinaglute have been shown to reduce this effect by lowering the peak blood levels of quinidine. This reduction causes a more consistent, prolonged effect. Carvedilol (Coreg) is a β-adrenergic blocker and is indicated in the treatment of heart failure but is not available as a sustained-release product, nor is it indicated as an antiarrhythmic. Felodipine (Plendil) is not available as an extended-release product but it does have an extended half-life, which allows less frequent dosing in the treatment of hypertension. It is one of the second-generation calcium channel blocking agents and is not indicated as an antiarrhythmic agent.

36. The answer is D.
Inamrinone (Inocor) is a bipyridine agent that has both positive inotropic effects and vasodilating effects. It does offer an alternative to dopamine and dobutamine and is given as an IV infusion of 5–10 μg/kg/min. Timolol (Blocadren) and atenolol (Tenormin) are β-adrenergic blockers, verapamil (Calan) is a calcium channel blocker, and disopyramide (Norpace) is a class I$_A$ antiarrhythmic agent; all have negative inotropic activities. Their use could create a problem in a patient who requires inotropic support. β-adrenergic blockers are currently recommended as first-line agents in patients with stable heart failure, unless they have a contraindication to their use or cannot tolerate their effects because hypotension, bradycardia, bronchospasm, and the like.

37. The answer is D.
Lansoprazole (Prevacid) is a proton pump inhibitor used for the short-term treatment of refractory duodenal ulcer, severe erosive esophagitis, and poorly responsive gastroesophageal reflux disease. Cimetidine (Tagamet) and famotidine (Pepcid) are H$_2$-receptor antagonists that work by inhibiting the actions of histamine at the parietal cell receptor sites. Sucralfate (Carafate) is a nonabsorbable mucosal protectant that adheres to the base of ulcer craters. Octreotide (Sandostatin) is a long-acting synthetic octapeptide that works like somatostatin by inhibiting serotonin, gastrin, vasoactive intestinal polypeptide, insulin, glucagon, growth hormone, and other agents.

38. The answer is A.
Creatinine is formed during muscle metabolism, and creatinine clearance is the most common method for the measurement of GFR. When only the serum creatinine level and the patient's age, weight, and gender are known, creatinine clearance may be determined by the Cockroft and Gault equation.

39. The answer is E (I, II, III).
Low doses of aspirin and other salicylates inhibit the tubular secretion of uric acid, which may result in uric acid accumulation and gout. Nicotinic acid competes with uric acid for excretion in the kidney tubule, resulting in greater retention of uric acid and the possibility of a gout attack. Cytotoxic drugs, by nature of their ability to increase nucleic acid turnover (uric acid is a byproduct of nucleic acid), cause an increase in uric acid and the potential for a gout attack.

40. The answer is C (I, II).
Oxymetazoline is a sympathomimetic vasoconstrictor; its effect lasts up to 12 hr. This agent is administered twice daily for up to 3 days.

41. The answer is E.
For any first-order process, 50% of the initial amount of drug is eliminated at the end of the first half-life, and 50% of the remaining amount of drug (i.e., 75% of the original amount) is eliminated at the end of the second half-life. Since the half-life of the drug is 2 hr, in 2 hr 50% is eliminated, at 4 hr (an additional half-life) 75%, and at 6 hr (a third half-life) 87.5% of the drug is eliminated.

42. The answer is C.
The MIC for an antimicrobial indicates the lowest concentration of antibiotic that prevents microbial growth after 18–24 hr of incubation. The report states that the antimicrobial agent cefepime, at a concentration of 1 μg/mL is able to prevent such growth. This is in contrast to ciprofloxacin, which requires a concentration of 32 μg/mL, ceftazidime (8 μg/mL), gentamicin (4 μg/mL), and meropenem (2 μg/mL). Typically, for antimicrobials that demonstrate concentration-dependent antimicrobial activity, the peak antibiotic concentration at the site of infection must be four to five times the MIC to be considered therapeutic and effective.

43. The answer is C.
The four clinical classes of diabetes mellitus are type 1, type 2, gestational diabetes mellitus, and secondary diabetes. Hyperglycemia is elevated blood sugar but is not identified as a clinical class of diabetes mellitus. Hyperglycemic nonketotic syndrome can occur in type 2 diabetes, when blood glucose levels increase but without the breakdown of fats because some insulin is present. Diabetic ketoacidosis may occur in patients with type 1 diabetes. This results in hyperglycemia and the breakdown of fats because of insulin insufficiency. Ketonemia (accumulation of ketone bodies in the blood) results from the breakdown of adipose tissue when there is insulin deficiency in type 1 diabetes. Thiazide diuretics and Cushing syndrome may result in hyperglycemia (secondary diabetes). There is no such thing as type 3 diabetes.

44. The answer is C (I, II).
Choices I and II describe the diagnostic criteria for nonpregnant adults. To meet the diagnostic criteria for an oral glucose tolerance test, the plasma glucose level at the 2-hr mark must be at least 200 mg/dL. The pharmacist did not record any symptoms for Mr. Johnson. Because he received an oral glucose tolerance test, apparently his level was > 200 mg/dL.

45. The answer is E (I, II, III).
Hemoglobin A_{1C} is a useful long-term monitoring tool to measure glycemic control. It is usually tested at least once or twice per year in patients under good control and at least quarterly for therapy changes and for those who are in poor control.

46. The answer is E (I, II, III).
Glyburide is chemically classified as a sulfonylurea. These agents stimulate the pancreatic secretion of insulin (insulin secretagogue) and, therefore, result in lowered blood glucose (hypoglycemic agent).

47. The answer is C (I, II).
DiaBeta, Micronase, and Glynase (not listed as a choice) are trade names for glyburide. Glucotrol is glipizide, another sulfonylurea agent.

48. The answer is E (I, II, III).
Glucovance is a trade name for the combination product of glyburide and metformin. These two individual drugs can be used successfully in combination to treat type 2 diabetes. Metformin has several mechanisms of action, but it is generally recognized as an insulin sensitizer. Situations such as renal dysfunction and chronic or binge alcohol ingestion can increase the risk for developing lactic acidosis.

49. The answer is A (I).
Acarbose is an α-glucosidase inhibitor in the intestine and acts by reducing the absorption of carbohydrates (complex carbohydrate absorption requires the action of α-glucosidase). Postprandial blood glucose levels are, therefore, lower. This agents has little effect on preprandial or fasting blood glucose levels, and it has an entirely different mechanism of action from metformin.

50. The answer is D (II, III).
Other test sites such as the forearm, upper arm, thigh, calf, and other areas of the hand should not be used when a patient feels an episode of hypoglycemia coming on or immediately after a meal. Alternate site testing is approved only for the fasting state, 2 hr after a meal, or 2 hr after exercise. Blood flow to the fingers is 3–5 times faster than any other site; alternate sites are not able to detect rapid changes in blood glucose.

51. The answer is C (I, II).
Osteoarthritis, formerly known as degenerative joint disease, is the most common form of arthritis. There is little, if any, inflammation in the osteoarthritic joint.

52. The answer is C (I, II).
The product contains the antihistamine diphenhydramine. Diphenhydramine and doxylamine are the two FDA-approved over-the-counter (OTC) agents indicated for insomnia. Diphenhydramine may produce adverse central anticholinergic effects in the elderly, including confusion, disorientation, impaired short-term memory, and sometimes visual and tactile hallucinations. Because of its anticholinergic properties, diphenhydramine may cause restriction in the urinary outflow in a male patient with an enlarged prostate and should be avoided in this situation. It would not cause polyuria.

53. The answer is D (II, III).
Sonata (zaleplon) has a short terminal half-life (about 1 hr) and decreases sleep latency; at this dose, it would be more useful for individuals having difficulty falling asleep. The 5-mg dose is appropriate for an elderly man. Sonata should not be taken unless the patient is able to get ≥ 4 hr of sleep before he or she is to be active again.

54. The answer is B.
Because there is little, if any, inflammation in the osteoarthritic joint, acetaminophen has been shown to be as efficacious as ibuprofen and naproxen in patients with mild to moderate osteoarthritic pain. It is considered by the American College of Rheumatology as first-line therapy for osteoarthritis of the hip or knee. It generally has fewer side effects than the nonsteroidal anti-inflammatory drugs (NSAIDs), and usually it is given initially to patients with this disease. Mr. Johnson was initially prescribed acetaminophen for this condition, which was the correct choice.

55. The answer is A.
The dose should be adequate to control the patient's pain. Hepatotoxicity, the main concern, can occur in patients taking > 4 g acetaminophen per day. Symptoms can include nausea, vomiting, abdominal pain, malaise, and diaphoresis.

56. The answer is E (I, II, III).
Elderly patients and those with a history of peptic ulcer disease are at increased risk for gastrointestinal toxicity when taking NSAIDs. Tramadol is considered a good choice, after acetaminophen, in patients who cannot tolerate NSAID use. Tramadol is not a narcotic analgesic, but side effects such as nausea, constipation, and somnolence occur with both tramadol and opioids.

57. The answer is E (I, II, III).
Alka Seltzer Plus Cold and Cough Liquid-Gels contains acetaminophen, phenylephrine, chlorpheniramine, and dextromethorphan. Before recommending an over-the-counter (OTC) product for the treatment of the common cold, it is important to know what symptoms the patient is experiencing and then target the therapy to those symptoms—most likely with a single-ingredient product. Because he is experiencing what he describes as a common cold and it is summertime, is it truly a common cold or is he experiencing symptoms of seasonal allergic rhinitis? Phenylephrine administration may result in increasing Mr. Johnson's blood sugar, so this agent should be used cautiously (if at all) in patients with diabetes. This product does contain 325 mg acetaminophen, which may push Mr. Johnson over the 4 g maximum daily allotment of acetaminophen.

58. The answer is A (I).
The insulin secretagogues (e.g., the sulfonylurea, glyburide) may not work to control blood sugar during the first 4 weeks of therapy (primary). This is likely the result of the insufficient number of functioning β cells in the pancreas. Secondary failure occurs when the drug controls hyperglycemia initially but fails to maintain the control. In most cases, this represents a progression of the diabetes rather than a drug failure.

59. The answer is D.
Massaging with oil and shampooing treat this form of seborrhea of the scalp in the newborn. This procedure will gently remove the accumulated scaly skin.

60. The answer is C.
It is generally believed that the absorptive characteristics of the skin in children < 6 months of age are different from those of adults. The metabolic and excretory systems of these young children may not be able to handle the sunscreen agent that does get absorbed.

61. The answer is B.
Salicylic acid is a keratolytic agent and is considered safe and effective for the treatment of warts by the FDA. It is also used for the treatment of corns and calluses.

62. The answer is E.
Human papillomavirus is the cause of common warts. HSV 1 is responsible for cold sores; HSV-2, for genital herpes. The Epstein-Barr virus is the usual cause of infectious mononucleosis. Coronavirus is one of the viruses responsible for the common cold. HIV is the human immunodeficiency virus.

63. The answer is A.
According to the recommendations of the JNC-7 (a multidisciplinary, national collaborative group), drug therapy is usually initiated with a thiazide diuretic in patients with stage I hypertension not associated with any of the "compelling" indications. However, additional recommendations include alternative therapy with angiotensin-converting enzyme (ACE) inhibitors, angiotensin II receptor blockers, β-adrenergic receptor blockers, or calcium channel blockers for patients who are unable to tolerate a thiazide diuretic or who do not respond appropriately to them. Spironolactone is a potassium-sparing diuretic that antagonizes aldosterone receptors within the distal convoluted tubule and has minor diuretic effects. Doxazosin is a peripherally acting α-adrenergic blocker that demonstrated potentially negative clinical effects in the Antihypertensive and Lipid-Lowering Treatment to Prevent Heart Attack Trial (ALLHAT) study. Hydralazine is a vasodilator that directly dilates peripheral arteries to reduce blood pressure. Clonidine is a centrally acting antihypertensive that stimulates α_2-adrenergic receptors to decrease sympathetic outflow to lower blood pressure. None of these agents is considered an alternative to thiazide diuretics as initial therapy for stage I hypertension.

64. The answer is B (III).
The individual reviewing the orders identified that hydrochlorothiazide (HCTZ) is a sulfa derivative and, because of the nature of the previously documented allergy—specifically Stevens-Johnson syndrome (a type of erythema multiforme reaction)—was able to inform the prescriber, so that spironolactone, which is not a sulfa derivative (although it is considerably less potent than HCTZ), was prescribed. Previous studies have demonstrated the benefit of thiazide diuretics on mortality rates in hypertensive patients. However, additional considerations in the current patient should include the potential use of angiotensin-converting enzyme (ACE) inhibitors, angiotensin II receptor blockers, β-adrenergic receptor blockers, and/or calcium channel blockers because this patient cannot take a thiazide diuretic.

65. The answer is C.
The development of ischemic heart disease involves the relationship between oxygen supplied to the heart and oxygen demanded by the heart. Similar to a balance, when these two parameters are equal, the heart is able to provide oxygen to the metabolizing tissues, which they need to maintain normal bodily functions. However, the inability for the supply of oxygen to increase as demands placed on the heart are increased can result in an acute coronary syndrome. Heart rate, cardiac contractility, fluid volume within the cardiac ventricles, and the wall tension within the cardiac ventricles directly reflect the oxygen demands placed on the heart. Coronary blood flow is a direct reflection of the degree of oxygen supplied to the heart. As oxygen supply is reduced, coronary blood flow is reduced (atherosclerosis, vasospasm); as oxygen demand is increased (increased heart rate, increased ventricular size, increased cardiac contractility), the balance between supply and demand is altered and can result in ischemic heart disease in predisposed patients.

66. The answer is E (I, II, III).
Acute ischemic (coronary) syndromes is a term that has evolved as a way to describe a group of clinical symptoms representing acute myocardial ischemia. The clinical symptoms include acute myocardial infarction, which might be STEMI or NSTEMI, a Q wave or non-Q wave infarction, or unstable angina. Current terminology has not included angina pectoris as one of the acute coronary syndromes.

67. The answer is D.
Theophylline serum levels are increased by conditions that decrease theophylline elimination. Smoking increases the rate of theophylline elimination by increasing the rate of metabolism, resulting in a reduced serum theophylline level. Pneumonia, ciprofloxacin, cor pulmonale, and heart failure decrease the rate of theophylline elimination, resulting in an increased serum theophylline level.

68. The answer is B (III).
Atenolol is a β-adrenergic blocking agent, which is referred to as a relatively cardioselective agent. However, no β-adrenergic blocking agent is entirely safe in an asthmatic patient such as Mr. Torres, because it might induce a bronchospastic attack. Spironolactone, a potassium-sparing diuretic, and irbesartan, an angiotensin II receptor blocker, can be prescribed for patients with asthma because they do not affect the respiratory system.

69. The answer is D.
All of the agents listed are calcium channel blockers and have been used successfully in the treatment of hypertension. However, within the calcium channel blockers, there are three different chemical groups; amlodipine, nifedipine, felodipine, and isradipine are referred to as dihydropyridine derivatives, which do not slow impulses within the atrioventricular (AV) node. Verapamil has been shown to effectively slow impulses within the AV node and has been used in the treatment of tachyarrhythmias, angina pectoris, and hypertension.

70. The answer is D (II, III).
All three of the agents are referred to collectively as β-hydroxy-β-methylglutaryl-coenzyme A (HMG-CoA) reductase inhibitors. Additional agents include lovastatin, fluvastatin, and atorvastatin. To date, several studies have shown that pravastatin and simvastatin can reduce the mortality rate from coronary artery disease when administered to patients with hypercholesterolemia.

71. The answer is B (III).
Olmesartan is a member of a large class of agents referred to as angiotensin II type 1 receptor antagonists, which decrease the conversion of angiotensin I to angiotensin II. This results in a reduction in the release of aldosterone as well as a reduction in the powerful vasoconstrictor effects of angiotensin II. Centrally acting α-adrenergic agonists, such as clonidine, have been available for several years, but the identification of a purely cardiospecific β-adrenergic blocker has yet to occur. Several β-blockers have been shown to be relatively cardioselective, which results in greater $β_1$ inhibition within the myocardium than $β_2$ inhibition within the peripheral vascular system and pulmonary system. However, cardioselective properties are dose dependent, and to date no β-adrenergic blocker has been shown to possess strictly $β_1$-inhibiting properties.

72. The answer is E (I, II, III).
In most patients, the cause of Parkinson disease is unknown (idiopathic); however, a small percentage of cases are secondary, and many of these cases are curable. Secondary parkinsonism may be caused by drugs such as dopamine antagonists (phenothiazine, butyrophenones such as haloperidol, reserpine), poisoning by chemicals such as carbon monoxide and heavy metals (such as manganese and mercury), infectious diseases such as viral encephalitis and syphilis, and other causes (arteriosclerosis, degenerative diseases of the central nervous system, and various metabolic disorders).

73. The answer is B (III).
Diphenhydramine is an antihistaminic agent that has some mild anticholinergic effects and is used for symptomatic relief of mild tremor. Amantadine is a dopaminergic agent. Trihexyphenidyl is an anticholinergic agent. Treatment of Parkinson disease usually involves the use of antihistaminic drugs, anticholinergic agents, and dopaminergic agents. Owing to its adverse reaction within the central nervous system, diphenhydramine should be used with caution in the elderly.

74. The answer is C.
Biperiden is an anticholinergic agent used in the treatment of Parkinson disease; the daily dosage range is 2–8 mg. Benztropine, another anticholinergic agent, has a daily dosage range of 1–6 mg. Pramipexole, referred to as a nonergot dopamine agent, has a daily dosage range of 1.5–4.5 mg. Tolcapone (300–600 mg/day) and entacapone (200–1600 mg/day) are referred to as catechol-*O*-methyltransferase (COMT) inhibitors.

75. The answer is C (I, II).
Entacapone, a catechol-*O*-methyltransferase (COMT) inhibitor, works by delaying the metabolism of levodopa and, therefore, prolonging its availability. It is thus indicated as an adjunctive treatment to levodopa in patients who suffer from a wearing-off effect.

76. The answer is A.
Caution is needed when introducing anticholinergics in this patient who has narrow-angle glaucoma. Anticholinergic agents may aggravate certain other underlying conditions and, therefore, should also be used with caution in patients with obstructions of the gastrointestinal or genitourinary tracts or severe cardiac disease. Side effects usually include dry mouth, blurred vision, constipation, urinary retention, and tachycardia. Central nervous system side effects may include hallucinations, ataxia, mental slowing, confusion, and memory impairment.

77. The answer is E (I, II, III).
Levodopa is capable of causing adverse drug reactions within the gastrointestinal, cardiovascular, and musculoskeletal systems. Additional organ systems with associated adverse reactions include the central nervous system (confusion, memory changes, depression, hallucinations, and psychosis) and the hematologic system (hemolytic anemia, leukopenia, and agranulocytosis).

78. The answer is B (III).
Anticholinergic agents should be given one drug at a time. Several agents are available for therapy, and they all appear to be equally effective. One of the principles of drug therapy is that if a patient does not respond to an agent in one class, try another class. The exception includes the use of dopamine agonists bromocriptine, and pergolide; patients who do not respond to one of the agents may not respond to the other.

79. The answer is D.
Of the drugs listed, only pergolide is a dopaminergic agent. Available dopaminergic agents and their mechanisms include levodopa, which exogenously replenishes striatal dopamine; bromocriptine, which directly stimulates dopamine receptors; amantadine, which stimulates presynaptic dopamine release; pergolide, which directly stimulates dopamine receptors in the nigrostriatal system; selegiline, which selectively inhibits monoamine oxidase type B and selectively prevents the breakdown of dopamine in the brain; pramipexole and ropinirole, which are considered non-ergot dopamine agents; and tolcapone and entacapone, referred to as catechol-*O*-methyltransferase (COMT) inhibitors, which delay the breakdown of dopamine in the brain.

80. The answer is A.
Levodopa must be converted to dopamine, and this conversion must occur centrally, for therapeutic effect. Because dopamine does not readily cross the blood–brain barrier, it is important that only minimal amounts of levodopa be converted to dopamine peripherally. The enzyme for this metabolic reaction is dopa-decarboxylase, for which pyridoxine (vitamin B_6) is a coenzyme. Exogenous pyridoxine can, therefore, increase the peripheral metabolism of levodopa, making less dopamine available centrally for the desired effect.

81. The answer is A (I).
Carbidopa inhibits the peripheral decarboxylation of levodopa to dopamine. Carbidopa does not cross the blood–brain barrier, therefore making more levodopa available for transport to the brain. This situation minimizes the risk of peripheral side effects and may lower the required dose of levodopa by approximately 75%.

82. The answer is B.
The on–off phenomenon refers to swings in drug response to levodopa or dopamine agonists. Loss of drug effectiveness is characteristic of off periods. Bromocriptine, a dopamine agonist, has been shown to be effective in patients who have responded poorly to levodopa or who have experienced a severe on–off phenomenon. It is often used as an adjunct to levodopa therapy. Pergolide is a similarly acting agent that has been shown to be 1000 times more potent than bromocriptine on a milligram basis.

83. The answer is B (III).
Significance is generally determined by using an analysis of variance. A probability of $p < .05$ indicates a statistically significant difference (i.e., one that is not the result of chance alone). Thus the high-fat breakfast treatment had a longer T_{max} and a lower C_{max}, indicating a delay in absorption. The slower rate of systemic drug absorption may have been caused by a delay in stomach emptying time owing to the ingestion of fat.

84. The answer is D.
Mechlorethamine (Mustargen) is nitrogen mustard, which serves as an alkylating agent. Chlorambucil (Leukeran), busulfan (Myleran), and melphalan (Alkeran) are all considered water-soluble compounds that alkylate (alkylating agents) DNA. Doxorubicin (Adriamycin) is an example of a tetracyclic amino sugar-linked antibiotic.

85. The answer is A.
Dospan is an erosion-core tablet that employs insoluble plastics, hydrophilic polymers, or fatty compounds to create a matrix device. The slowly dissolving tablet releases the majority of a dose after the primary dose is released from the tablet coating. OROS is an osmotic delivery system. The transdermal drug delivery system (TDDS) is designed to support the passage of drug substances from the skin surface. Pennkinetic is an ion-exchange resin. The hydrodynamically balanced system (HBS) represents a hydrocolloid system.

86. The answer is C.
Moxifloxacin, levofloxacin, ciprofloxacin, and gatifloxacin are all quinolone derivatives. Clarithromycin is a macrolide antibiotic claimed to be slightly more active than erythromycin against select gram-positive bacteria.

87. The answer is E (I, II, III).
Immunosuppressive agents are administered to prevent graft rejection after renal transplantation. Azathioprine interferes with DNA and RNA synthesis so that it may reduce cell-mediated and humoral immune responses. Basiliximab is a chimeric monoclonal antibody that binds to block the interleukin 2 receptor on the surface of activated T lymphocytes, thus preventing T lymphocyte activation and acute rejection. Cyclosporine inhibits T cell activation in the early stage of immune response to foreign antigen such as a graft.

88. The answer is A (I).
Ramipril represents the class of drugs referred to as angiotensin-converting enzyme (ACE) inhibitors, which have been shown to provide a beneficial effect when given in the post-MI stage to reduce morbidity and mortality from the MI and prevent left ventricular dysfunction. The Survival and Ventricular Enlargement (SAVE) trial was the first major study to show the direct benefits of ACE inhibitors in post-MI patients. In Mr. Melvin's case, the order for ramipril was written approximately 3 days after his heart attack and the dose was slowly titrated upward to prevent untoward hypotensive effects of the drug. Recent studies show that ACE inhibitors have a beneficial effect in certain patient populations (diabetes mellitus) in the prevention of renal nephropathy, but Mr. Melvin is not receiving ramipril for this reason. In addition, ACE inhibitors do have a blood pressure-lowering effect, and although Mr. Melvin may have received the drug for high blood pressure, he most likely received the drug for prevention of left ventricular dysfunction after the acute myocardial infarction.

89. The answer is A

The Cockcroft and Gault equation is a common method for estimating creatinine clearance. This equation is based on the serum creatinine concentration and patient characteristics, including age, weight, and gender. Fick's law describes drug diffusion by passive transport from a region of high drug concentration to a region of lower drug concentration. The law of mass action describes the rate of a chemical reaction in terms of the concentrations of the reactants. The Henderson-Hasselbalch equation describes the relationship among pK_a, pH, and the extent of ionization of a weak acid or a weak base. The Noyes-Whitney equation describes the rate of dissolution of a solid drug.

90. The answer is C (I, II).

The patient is experiencing symptoms suggesting heart failure, which may occur as a consequence of the acute coronary syndrome (myocardial infarction) or of the patient receiving too much of the β-blocker atenolol, or a combination of the two. Ramipril, an angiotensin converting enzyme (ACE) inhibitor, was initiated in this patient to reduce cardiac consequences, as demonstrated in the Heart Outcomes Prevention Evaluation (HOPE) trial. In this setting, the physician opted to cut back on the atenolol dose with the hope of reducing the β-blocking side effects while still providing the drug, which has shown to be beneficial post-MI. In addition, the dose of ramipril was increased to try to maximize its contributions to the patient's treatment.

91. The answer is E.

Amiodarone has an extremely long half-life—up to 50 days. The therapeutic effect of amiodarone may be delayed for weeks after oral therapy begins, and adverse reactions may persist up to 4 months after therapy ends.

92. The answer is C (I, II).

Propranolol is a β-adrenergic blocking agent that helps reduce some peripheral manifestations of hyperthyroidism (e.g., tachycardia, sweating, tremor). In addition to providing symptomatic relief, propranolol inhibits the peripheral conversion of thyroxine (T_4) to triiodothyronine (T_3).

93. The answer is E (I, II, III).

Numerous large, multisite studies have been conducted comparing the various thrombolytic agents used in the management of acute coronary syndromes (acute myocardial infarction). Cost issues continue to be significant in the selection of an ideal thrombolytic agent. Currently, there is not much difference in the costs associated with t-PA, reteplase, and TNKase. However, the ease of administration of TNKase has made it an acceptable agent in the acute management of coronary syndromes, when time is especially critical. A single IV bolus dose is administered over several seconds, and there is no need for the follow up infusions, titrations, and so on needed with t-PA.

94. The answer is B (III).

β-adrenergic blockers have been shown to be effective in the acute management of myocardial infarction patients in the prevention of sudden cardiac death owing to acute myocardial infarction. They are also indicated in the treatment of angina pectoris, hypertension, and tachyarrhythmias along with numerous other drug-specific indications. However, the acute administration of a β-blocker (primarily atenolol and metoprolol) has become an important part of the treatment of acute MI. Whichever agent is used, usually a series of IV administrations of the drug are given over a short period of time, and then the patient is converted to oral medication daily thereafter. The parameters that need to be evaluated in these patients include blood pressure (if too low, the patient cannot receive a β-blocker), heart rate (if too low, the patient cannot receive a β-blocker), and pulmonary/left ventricular function (though indicated in the treatment of heart failure, patients must be monitored carefully when receiving β-blocker therapy).

95. The answer is B (III).

The patient has a reported allergy history that is consistent with quinidine-induced cinchonism, a consequence of an elevated quinidine serum level. If left unaltered, it can progress to delirium and psychosis, but the therapy of choice is to reduce the dose of quinidine, with a resultant decrease in the quinidine serum level and a potential reduction in symptoms. Aluminum hydroxide gel has been shown effective in the prevention of diarrhea, which has been reported to occur in up to 30% of patients receiving quinidine. Desensitization of patients to quinidine by administering very small doses of quinidine over an accelerated period of time has not become a standard of practice for patients with reported allergies to quinidine. Most patients can be successfully maintained on an alternative antiarrhythmic agent.

96. The answer is C (I, II).

There are numerous causes for ARF, which is a sudden, potentially reversible interruption of kidney function, resulting in the retention of nitrogenous waste products in body fluids. ARF is classified according to its cause. In prerenal ARF, impaired renal perfusion occurs as a result of dehydration, hemorrhage, vomiting, urinary losses from excessive diuresis, decreased cardiac output owing to heart failure, or severe hypotension. Intrarenal ARF reflects structural kidney damage owing to nephrotoxins such as aminoglycosides, severe hypotension, malignant hypertension, and radiation. Postrenal ARF occurs because of obstruction of urine flow along the urinary tract as a result of uric acid crystals, thrombi, bladder obstruction, etc. Mr. Rones has a history of heart failure and hypertension, which are both capable of causing ARF. Hyperkalemia does not cause ARF, but rather ARF is associated with hyperkalemia, which might be considered a medical emergency.

97. The answer is E.

Mr. Rones has reported allergies to sulfonamides and penicillin, so he should not be given any of the medications. Penicillin V potassium (V-Cillin-K) is a penicillin. Although the pharmacist may not know the exact nature of the reported allergy, a conversation with the physician would answer the question of whether an allergy exists. Trimethoprim-sulfamethoxazole (Bactrim, Septra) and hydrochlorothiazide are both sulfonamide derivatives; again, the pharmacist may not know the exact nature of the reported allergy, but a follow-up conversation with the physician should take place before filling either of these prescriptions for the patient.

98. The answer is E (I, II, III).

Slow-K is a potassium supplement used to prevent hypokalemia. However, Mr. Rones is diagnosed as having hyperkalemia, probably secondary to acute renal failure, and he should not receive the prescription. In addition, moexipril, an angiotensin-converting enzyme (ACE) inhibitor, is contraindicated in hyperkalemia owing to its potassium-retaining properties. Sudafed (pseudoephedrine HCl) is an indirect-acting sympathomimetic that stimulates receptors, resulting in the release of adrenergic amines; it must be used with great caution in this hypertensive patient. The pharmacist should contact the physician before dispensing either of these prescriptions to determine whether the physician does indeed want to use them.

99. The answer is A (I).

Mr. Rones has heart failure as a "compelling" indication, which would suggest the use of diuretics, angiotensin-converting enzyme (ACE) inhibitors (ramipril), angiotensin II receptor blockers (candesartan), β-adrenergic blockers (atenolol), or an aldosterone antagonist such as spironolactone. However, because of to the presence of hyperkalemia in this patient, ramipril and candesartan should be avoided if possible.

100. The answer is C.

Situations that favor the development of hypokalemia—use of non-potassium-sparing diuretics, failure to administer potassium supplements, administration of agents that decrease serum potassium (Kayexalate, sodium polystyrene sulfonate)—have been reported to be able to cause digoxin toxicity because of the development of hypokalemia. Phenytoin and lidocaine have both been shown to be effective in the treatment of digoxin toxicity–induced arrhythmias. Digoxin is primarily eliminated in the active form via the kidney, but when renal function decreases, as in advancing age, the elimination of the drug is decreased. Monitoring for renal function can help prevent the development of digoxin toxicity.

101. The answer is D (II, III).

Felodipine and isradipine are referred to as second-generation dihydropyridine derivatives, similar in action to nifedipine, which make up the class of calcium channel blockers. Ramipril and enalapril are two examples of ACE inhibitors. Losartan is an example of the class of drugs referred to as angiotensin II receptor antagonists; and atenolol, carvedilol, and propranolol are examples of the β-adrenergic receptor antagonist class of drugs.

102. The answer is E.
Patients such as Mr. Rones who have renal failure lose their ability to eliminate potassium from the kidney, and consequently elevations in serum potassium should be expected. Situations that favor the reabsorption of potassium by the kidney (administration of potassium supplements, use of potassium-sparing diuretics [spironolactone, ACE inhibitors, angiotensin II receptor blockers]) should be avoided. However, hyperkalemia can be treated by the removal of potassium by the body (dialysis), potassium-removing resin (sodium polystyrene sulfonate), pharmacologic antagonists (calcium chloride or gluconate), and shifting potassium intracellularly (regular insulin with dextrose).

103. The answer is E (I, II, III).
Verapamil (Isoptin) and atenolol (Tenormin) are representatives of the calcium channel blocker and β-adrenergic blocker groups and, as such, possess negative inotropic and negative chronotropic effects. Patients should be advised to check their heart rates and report any symptoms that represent side effects from the negative inotropic effects of these agents. This helps prevent the development of signs of heart failure.

104. The answer is B.
The AHFS provides yearly updates on available products along with dosage forms, indications, adverse drug reactions, and other information on products available in the United States. In addition, throughout the year, AHFS publishes supplements that provide updates on newly released agents. Newly released agents are not immediately described in the AHFS, but they do appear in supplements shortly after their release. Of the resources listed, AHFS offers the greatest benefit. AHFS is now available in a personal digital assistant (PDA) format, and updates are provided regularly. *Merck Index, Trissel's, Hansten's,* and the *PDR* do not provide updates throughout the year, so they would not provide much help on a newly released product. *Trissel's* focuses on injectable drug products; *Hansten's,* on drug interactions.

105. The answer is D.
Digoxin (Lanoxin) had previously been widely considered the mainstay in the treatment of heart failure. However, its use, particularly in chronic heart failure, has become somewhat controversial, and recent guidelines have limited its use to the short-term management of acute symptoms. Current recommendations favor the use of angiotensin-converting enzyme (ACE) inhibitors as primary therapy, with the addition of a diuretic if accompanied by shortness of breath, and the use of β-adrenergic blockers. Digoxin does possess two pharmacologic effects that reflect its concentration within the body. With lower total body stores (8–12 mg/kg), digoxin exerts a positive inotropic effect on the myocardium: an increase in cardiac output and renal blood flow and a decrease in cardiac filling pressure, venous and capillary pressures, heart size, and fluid volume. With higher total body stores (15–18 mg/kg), digoxin produces negative chronotropic effects—a reduction in electrical impulse conduction from the sinoatrial node throughout the atria into the atrioventricular node.

106. The answer is E.
It takes 4–5 half-lives, with no loading doses given, for a patient to reach steady-state serum digoxin concentrations. For an anephric patient, who has a terminal half-life of 3.5–4.5 days, 15–20 days would be required to reach a steady state. If the patient is in acute heart failure, the treatment of choice is rapid loading of enough digoxin to obtain total body stores of 8–12 mg/kg over a 12-hr period, followed by daily maintenance doses. The patient who has normal renal function needs 6–8 days of daily maintenance doses to reach steady state, if loading doses are not given.

107. The answer is E.
Acebutolol (Sectral) is a long-acting, relatively cardioselective agent that may be beneficial in patients who have lung disease and need to receive fewer doses per day to increase compliance. All β-adrenergic blockers have the potential to cause bronchospasm in patients with suspected lung disease, but the cardioselective agents may provide benefit in lower doses. Timolol (Blocadren) lacks cardioselectivity but is longer-acting. Esmolol (Brevibloc) is available only in intravenous form and has a very short half-life of approximately 9 min. Nadolol (Corgard) is a long-acting agent without cardioselective properties. Propranolol (Inderal LA) would offer no more cardioselective properties than those of Inderal.

108. The answer is A (I).
Isosorbide dinitrate (Isordil) and other nitrates have been shown to reduce pulmonary congestion and increase cardiac output by reducing preload and perhaps afterload. Nitrates generally cause venous dilation, with a resultant increase in venous pooling and a reduction in venous return and preload. The combination of nitrates with hydralazine (arteriole dilator) has been shown to reduce morbidity and mortality in patients with heart failure. However, the combination should not be used as initial therapy over angiotensin-converting enzyme (ACE) inhibitors but should be considered in patients who are intolerant of ACE inhibitors. Dopamine and dobutamine are inotropic agents, and current guidelines provide a Class III recommendation ("conditions for which there is evidence and/or general agreement that a procedure/therapy is not useful/effective and in some cases may be harmful"). In addition, current guidelines provide a Class IIb recommendation for the use of continuous intravenous infusion of a positive inotropic agent for palliation of heart failure symptoms ("conditions for which there is conflicting evidence and/or a divergence of opinion about the usefulness/efficacy of performing the procedure/therapy and that the usefulness/efficacy is less well established by evidence/opinion").

109. The answer is B.
Martindale's Extra Pharmacopoeia is an international publication that may help identify products from markets outside the United States. *Facts and Comparisons, Identidex,* the *PDR,* and *Drug Information 1990* focus on products available in the United States.

110. The answer is A.
Peritoneal dialysis is not practical for drugs that are highly bound to plasma or tissue proteins, are nonpolar or lipid soluble, or have a large volume of distribution. Drugs that are polar and have a small apparent volume of distribution tend to have a larger concentration in plasma and highly perfused tissues. These polar drugs are more easily dialyzed in the case of drug intoxication.

111. The answer is E (I, II, III).
An important potential problem with the use of herbal medications is the inability to retrieve up-to-date information on many substances currently available through various vendors. Previously, the FDA's Center for Food Safety and Applied Nutrition created the "Special Nutritional Adverse Event Monitoring System" Web site for dietary supplements. Unfortunately, that site was not updated after 1999 and is currently no longer available. Before the site's removal, the center developed an extensive list of supplements considered unsafe by the FDA because of reported damage to various organ systems.

112. The answer is B.
Iron is available in different oral forms as ferrous gluconate, ferrous sulfate, and ferrous fumarate. Each form has a different iron content. Ferrous gluconate contains 12% elemental iron, ferrous sulfate 20%, and ferrous fumarate 33%.

113. The answer is C.
In extemporaneous compounding, various methods may be used to reduce the particle size of a drug, including levigation, pulverization by intervention, spatulation, and trituration. Geometric dilution is a method of mixing a small amount of a drug with a large amount of powder in a geometric progression so that the final powder mixture is homogeneous. Pulverization by intervention uses the addition of nonsolvent.

114. The answer is E.
The total dose is 2.5 mg/kg/hr = 1200 mg. At a strength of 5 mg/L, each 50-mL vial contains 250 mg. The number of vials needed for this patient can be calculated by dividing the total dose (1200 mg) by the amount of antibiotic per vial (250 mg) to get 4.8 vials (5 vials).

115. The answer is B.
For most drugs with poor aqueous solubility, the dissolution rate (the rate at which the drug is solubilized) is the rate-limiting step for systemic drug absorption. Disintegration is the fragmentation of a solid dosage form into smaller pieces.

116. The answer is A (I).

Amprenavir, indinavir, and nelfinavir are referred to as protease inhibitors and are used in the treatment of HIV infection in combination with other groups of antiretroviral agents. Ritonavir and saquinavir are additional agents in this group of drugs. Zalcitabine, lamivudine, and stavudine are referred to as nucleoside reverse transcriptase inhibitors and are used in combination with protease inhibitors in the treatment of HIV. Delavirdine, efavirenz, and nevirapine are referred to as nonnucleoside reverse transcriptase inhibitors and are used in the treatment of HIV as well.

117. The answer is A (I).

The rate of dissolution of a weak acid drug is directly influenced by the surface area of the solid particles, the water in oil partition coefficient, and the concentration gradient between the drug concentrations in the stagnant layer and the bulk phase of the solvent. An increase in the pH of the medium will make the medium more alkaline, and the weak acid will convert to the ionized species, becoming more water soluble. Increasing the particle size decreases the effective surface area of the solid drug. Increasing the viscosity of the medium slows the diffusion of drug molecules into the solvent.

118. The answer is E (I, II, III).

All three of these statements are correct. The further classifications of bipolar disorder relate to the type and frequency of hypomanic, manic, and depressive episodes. Mood stabilizers—lithium, valproic acid, and carbamazepine—have historically been the mainstays of therapy.

119. The answer is A.

While the mechanism of action for lithium remains virtually unknown, this agent remains the therapy of choice for the acute and maintenance treatment of mania and hypomania. Membrane stabilization, inhibition of norepinephrine release, accelerated norepinephrine metabolism, increased presynaptic reuptake of norepinephrine and serotonin, and decreased receptor sensitivity appear to be therapeutic properties of lithium.

120. The answer is D.

Equivalent weight (Li_2CO_3) = molecular weight/valence = 73.89/2 = 36.945. Milliequivalents = drug (mg)/equivalent weight (mg) = 300/36.945 = 8.12 mEq

121. The answer is E (I, II, and III).

Lithium therapy is monitored effectively by periodic determinations of serum lithium levels. Lithium has a narrow therapeutic index, with a therapeutic range of 0.5–1.2 mEq/L. A variety of factors can affect serum lithium levels; important among these are the time between the last dose and the taking of the blood sample and the concomitant drug therapy (e.g., thiazide diuretics may increase serum lithium levels; extra sodium in the diet may decrease lithium levels [note the salt-restricted diet in order]). If the patient were acutely manic on admission, it might indicate that he was not taking his lithium medication as prescribed. Patients presenting with acute mania generally require levels in the higher end of the therapeutic range.

122. The answer is A (I).

The minimum, or trough, serum drug concentration is the most appropriate of the three; it is always lowest just before the administration of the next dose. The best time to monitor serum lithium levels is 12 hr after the last dose—that is, just before the first dose of the day. The exact times for the peak drug concentration and the average drug concentration are uncertain for any individual patient. The drawing of a sample to obtain a "peak" serum level uses an approximate time for maximum absorption of the drug. The average serum drug concentration cannot be obtained directly but is approximated by dividing the area under the curve (AUC) dosing interval by the time (T) of the dosage interval.

123. The answer is B.

Before any other measures are taken, a repeat lithium level should be obtained to assess the patient's situation. Adverse effects of lithium are usually related to the serum lithium level. Early-onset adverse effects of lithium, such as GI distress, polyuria and polydipsia, fine hand tremor, and dry mouth, are usually associated with lithium serum concentrations < 1.5 mEq/L. A repeat level will determine if a dosing adjustment is needed. Other symptoms, such as persistent GI distress, coarse hand tremor, hyperirritability, slurred speech, confusion, and somnolence, may be warning signs of toxicity and are evident with serum levels between 1.5 and 2.5 mEq/L. Severe lithium toxicity usually occurs when levels exceed 3.0 mEq/L; levels this high may be life threatening.

124. The answer is D.
Lithium is eliminated renally by glomerular filtration and competes with sodium for reabsorption in the renal tubules. Thiazide diuretics interfere with sodium reabsorption and, therefore, may favor lithium reabsorption, leading to elevated lithium levels. If the hydrochlorothiazide is being used to "treat" the prehypertension, it should be discontinued now until the patient's manic episode is stabilized. Blood pressure monitoring would need to be continued to determine if drug therapy is even needed at all.

125. The answer is D.
Lithium can cause a leukocytosis (elevated WBC count) as an early-onset adverse effect. The other agents do not cause this effect.

126. The answer is D.
Tricyclic antidepressants appear to lower the seizure threshold; therefore, caution must be exercised when using these preparations in patients with a history of seizures. The incidence of seizures remains low and is usually associated with high doses of these agents. Lithium may enhance the neurotoxic effect of the tricyclic antidepressants. Mr. Hayley is apparently taking Tegretol for his seizure disorder although this agent has also been used for bipolar disorder.

127. The answer is D.
Chlorpromazine (Thorazine) is a traditional (first-generation) antipsychotic agent. The others listed are considered atypical (second-generation) antipsychotics.

128. The answer is A.

129. The answer is C.
Loading dose $= 200 \text{ mg/m}^2 \times 0.89 \text{ m}^2 = 178 \text{ mg}$.

130. The answer is D.
Furosemide (Lasix) is a loop diuretic that acts principally at the ascending limb of the loop of Henle, where it inhibits the cotransport of sodium and chloride from the luminal filtrate. Loop diuretics increase the excretion of water, sodium, and chloride.

131. The answer is C (I, II).
Topical over-the-counter (OTC) nasal decongestants are sympathomimetic amines and include, among others, phenylephrine (e.g., Neo-Synephrine) and oxymetazoline (e.g., Afrin). Pseudoephedrine is an oral decongestant and is not available as a topical nasal decongestant.

132. The answer is C (I, II).
The JNC-7 recommendations include thiazide-type diuretics (chlorothiazide [Diuril]), either alone or in combination with one other agent (e.g., ACE inhibitor, angiotensin receptor blocker, β-blocker, or calcium channel blocker), for first-line treatment of Stage I hypertension, if there are no indications for another type of drug. Tenormin (atenolol), a β-blocker, would therefore be considered as a first-line agent. Catapres (clonidine) is an α_2-adrenergic agonist and is not part of this first-line list.

133. The answer is E (I, II, III).
Tardive dyskinesia is characterized by a mixture of orofacial dyskinesia, tics, chorea, and athetosis. Signs and symptoms usually appear while patients are receiving first-generation antipsychotic agents. Recommendations for avoiding the onset of tardive dyskinesia include using antipsychotic agents only when clearly indicated, keeping the daily dose as low as possible and for as short a duration as possible, monitoring patients closely for signs and symptoms of tardive dyskinesia. and using atypical antipsychotics as first-line agents (which have little or no propensity to cause tardive dyskinesia). Also, chronic use of anticholinergic agents is not recommended because these agents may increase the risk of tardive dyskinesia.

134. The answer is A (I).
Parnate (tranylcypromine) is a monoamine oxidase (MAO) inhibitor. Serious adverse drug reactions have been reported in patients receiving MAO inhibitors with opioid drugs. These serious interactions (hypotension, hyperpyrexia, coma) have occurred in patients receiving MAO inhibitors with meperidine (Demerol) but have not been reported to occur with morphine. Meperidine should be considered contraindicated in patients receiving MAO inhibitors. Nonsteroidal anti-inflammatory drugs (NSAIDs), a group that includes ketorolac, do not produce adverse interactions with MAO inhibitors. If a narcotic is necessary, morphine may be used cautiously, although waiting 14 days between the onset of morphine therapy and the discontinuation of MAO inhibitor therapy would be judicious.

135. The answer is D.
Ondansetron (Zofran) is a selective 5-HT$_3$-receptor antagonist, blocking serotonin both peripherally on vagal nerve terminals and centrally at the chemoreceptor trigger zone for chemotherapy-induced and special postoperative cases of nausea and vomiting. Bupropion (Zyban) is available for use as an aid in smoking cessation. Sertraline (Zoloft) is a selective inhibitor of serotonin reuptake and an agent prescribed for the treatment of depression. Linezolid (Zyvox) is used in the treatment of resistant gram-positive bacterial infections such as vancomycin-resistant enterococcus. Simvastatin (Zocor) is a β-hydroxy-β-methylglutaryl-coenzyme A (HMG-CoA) reductase inhibitor used in the treatment of hyper-cholesterolemia.

136. The answer is A.
Aripiprazole (Abilify) is an atypical antipsychotic approved for the treatment of schizophrenia. Rabeprazole (AcipHex) is a proton pump inhibitor commonly used for gastroesophageal reflux disease and peptic ulcer disease. Butoconazole is an antifungal approved for use in the treatment of vulvovaginal candidiasis. Clotrimazole is an antifungal agent used in the treatment of susceptible fungal infections.

137. The answer is B.
Vitamin D increases the absorption of calcium. Citracal is a brand name for calcium citrate. Ascorbic acid (vitamin C), vitamin E, and pantothenic acid are other vitamins.

138. The answer is B (III).
Clarithromycin is classified as a macrolide antibiotic. Ceftin is a cephalosporin antibiotic. Celebrex is a cyclooxygenase 2 (COX-2) nonsteroidal anti-inflammatory drug (NSAID).

139. The answer is C (I, II).
According to the guidelines established by the American College of Rheumatology, patients are diagnosed as having rheumatoid arthritis if they have satisfied at least four of the following seven criteria, with the first four continuing for at least 6 weeks: (1) morning stiffness, (2) arthritis in three or more joint areas, (3) arthritis of hand joints, (4) symmetric arthritis, (5) subcutaneous nodules (rheumatoid nodules), (6) abnormal serum rheumatoid factor, and (7) radiologic changes with erosion or bone decalcification of involved joints.

140. The answer is B (III).
Hydroxychloroquine (Plaquenil) is a disease-modifying antirheumatic drug (DMARD); its therapeutic benefit may take up to 6 months to develop. Hydroxychloroquine is given in dosages of 400 mg/day and has been associated with severe and sometimes irreversible adverse effects on the eyes, skin, central nervous system, and bone marrow. Because the drug may have severe effects on the eyes, an ophthalmologist should check visual acuity every 3–6 months, and therapy should be discontinued at the first signs of retinal toxicity.

141. The answer is A.
Plavix (clopidogrel bisulfate) is an antiplatelet drug indicated for the reduction of atherosclerotic events (myocardial infarction, stroke, and vascular death) in patients with atherosclerosis documented by recent stroke, recent myocardial infarction, or established peripheral arterial disease. Several agents are collectively referred to as disease-modifying antirheumatic drugs (DMARDs), including the commonly used hydroxychloroquine; sulfasalazine (Azulfidine), and methotrexate (Rheumatrex); penicillamine (Depen, Cuprimine) and gold salts (Ridaura) are used less frequently. Like hydroxychloroquine (Plaquenil), they are added to first-line therapy to slow or delay progression of the disabling symptoms and effects of rheumatoid arthritis.

142. The answer is E (I, II, and III).
Celebrex (celecoxib) represents a class of nonsteroidal anti-inflammatory drugs (NSAIDs) referred to as cyclooxygenase 2 (COX-2) receptor inhibitors. Currently, they are indicated in the treatment of rheumatoid arthritis or osteoarthritis, similar to previous NSAIDs (COX-1 inhibitors), to manage the symptoms associated with these diseases. Current literature suggests that they might offer a benefit over traditional NSAIDs by reducing the gastrointestinal consequences associated with use of these agents. Naproxen (Naprosyn) is an NSAID that is also used in the treatment of rheumatoid arthritis. Relafen (nabumetone), another NSAID agent, is believed to have a greater specificity for the COX-2 receptor than the COX-1 receptor; it has also been used in the symptomatic control of rheumatoid arthritis. Each agent could be a suitable alternative for ibuprofen, and celecoxib in particular might reduce the gastrointestinal side effects associated with the other NSAIDs.

143. The answer is B (III).
Naprosyn (naproxen) is the only correct match. The generic name for Voltaren is diclofenac; the generic name for Lodine is etodolac.

144. The answer is E (I, II, III).
The onset of most of the DMARDs is prolonged; therefore, anti-inflammatory drugs are usually given concurrently as a bridge until therapeutic effects of the DMARD occur. The American College of Rheumatology recommends that DMARD therapy be initiated within 3 months of diagnosis, despite good control with nonsteroidal anti-inflammatory drugs (NSAIDs). The lowest effective dose should be used to minimize adverse effects.

145. The answer is B.
Patients with rheumatoid arthritis often have a normocytic, normochromic anemia, often referred to as an anemia of chronic disease. This anemia does not respond to drug therapy (i.e., iron therapy). Sometimes, this may produce a diagnostic dilemma because patients on nonsteroidal anti-inflammatory drugs (NSAIDs) may develop gastric irritation with chronic blood loss, which would lead to iron deficiency anemia. Other blood tests can help differentiate these two types of anemia—for example, serum iron to iron binding capacity and mean corpuscular volume (usually decreased in iron deficiency).

146. The answer is B (III).
Arthrotec is a combination of an nonsteroidal anti-inflammatory drug (NSAID; diclofenac sodium) and misoprostol. Misoprostol is a synthetic prostaglandin E_1 analog with mucosal protective properties and is given to patients at risk for developing NSAID-induced gastric or duodenal ulcers. Ms. Szymuniak is 60 years of age and is, therefore, at risk for NSAID-induced peptic ulcer disease. Diarrhea may be a side effect from misoprostol, but this medication would not be used to treat constipation. This combination is not a DMARD.

147. The answer is C (I, II).
In addition to the use of Arthrotec (see answer to question 146) and the use of selective cyclooxygenase 2 (COX-2) inhibitors (Celebrex), co-therapy using proton pump inhibitors or H_2-antagonists combined with nonselective NSAIDs have been shown to reduce the risk of NSAID-induced peptic ulcer disease. The use of two NSAIDs together would not be a rational alternative.

148. The answer is B.
Enbrel (etanercept) is a newer DMARD used to delay the progression of the disease. It binds to TNF-α and -β, inhibiting the inflammatory response mediated by immune cells. It is indicated as monotherapy or in conjunction with methotrexate. It is not a COX-2 inhibitor. All of the other statements are correct.

149. The answer is C.
Appropriate treatment measures are listed in choices A, B, D, and E. All bedrooms (where the concentration of pinworm eggs is likely to be the greatest) should be *vacuumed*—not swept—to remove the eggs.

150. The answer is C.
Tinea infections are superficial fungal dermatophyte infections of the skin. These infections are usually named based on the area of the skin involved: tinea cruris (groin), tinea capitis (head), tinea pedis (feet), tinea corporis (body), and tinea unguium (nails). Sally has tinea pedis.

151. The answer is D.
The antiseptic agent hexylresorcinol is not considered safe and effective for the treatment of tinea infections. The other four agents are all considered safe and effective for treating tinea pedis.

152. The answer is A.
Diphenhydramine and doxylamine are two ethanolamine antihistamines, generally considered the most sedating class of antihistamines. Brompheniramine, chlorpheniramine, dexbrompheniramine, and pheniramine are part of the alkylamine class of antihistamines, which are among the least sedating of the first-generation antihistamines. Thonzylamine, used very rarely today, is an ethylenediamine antihistamine; this class is between the other two classes in terms of sedation effects. Loratadine is a second-generation nonsedating antihistamine that recently was moved to OTC status.

153. The answer is B.
One of the second-generation nonsedating antihistamines, loratadine (e.g., Claritin), is now available over the counter. This patient's specific symptoms are related to histamine effects, so an antihistamine is warranted. Given his occupation, the pharmacist would not want to give this patient a sedating antihistamine, such as diphenhydramine. Even though loratadine is considered a nonsedating antihistamine, a small percentage of patients experience somnolence (8%) and fatigue (4%). Mr. Conway should certainly see how this agent affects him before he attempts to drive. He does not have nasal congestion, so the decongestant (pseudoephedrine) is not warranted at this time.

154. The answer is A.
Nonsalicylate nonsteroidal anti-inflammatory drugs (NSAIDs) (ibuprofen, naproxen, and ketoprofen) are the most effective over-the-counter (OTC) agents for primary dysmenorrhea. Aspirin and acetaminophen are generally less effective. Ketoprofen is the correct answer here because it should be used OTC only in patients 16 years of age and older.

155. The answer is C (I, II).
Pyrethrins with piperonyl butoxide (synergized pyrethrins) and permethrin are the two safe and effective OTC agents used to treat head lice. Patients should be warned to use these as directed because there is a growing trend of lice resistance to these products. Lindane is available only by prescription and has generally fallen into disfavor.

156. The answer is C.
Novolin is a trade name for human insulin that is a fixed-dose mixture of 70% NPH (intermediate action) and 30% regular insulin (short action).

157. The answer is C (I, II).
The Tambocor and Coumadin prescriptions would be filled because they would have no adverse effect on Ms. Urmeister's allergy to aspirin. Ecotrin is a brand name for enteric-coated aspirin, which may be less irritating to the gastrointestinal tract but would still be contraindicated in this patient because she has an aspirin allergy. Aspirin has been shown to be effective as an antiplatelet agent in patients after a myocardial infarction; but as with any drug therapy, the benefits of use must be weighed against the associated risks.

158. The answer is E (I, II, III).
Most antiarrhythmics fall into one of four classes, depending on their specific effects on the heart's electrical activity. Class I antiarrhythmic agents are divided into three groups based on their effects on depolarization rates and refractory period. Class I_A drugs include quinidine, procainamide, and disopyramide; class I_B drugs include lidocaine, tocainide, phenytoin, and mexiletine; class I_C drugs include flecainide, propafenone, and moricizine.

159. The answer is D (II, III).
Sustained-release drug products allow for less frequent dosing, resulting in better patient compliance. Sustained-release forms also provide smoother plasma drug concentrations, with smaller fluctuations between peak and trough concentrations compared with immediate-release dosage forms of the drug. Procan SR is a sustained-release or extended-release dosage form of procainamide hydrochloride. Pronestyl capsules are an immediate-release form of the drug; Pronestyl SR is the sustained-release product.

160. The answer is E (I, II, III).
Reteplase has been shown to be effective during the first several hours after a myocardial infarction to aid in the reperfusion of an infarcted coronary artery. Metoprolol, like other β-adrenergic receptor blocking agents administered shortly after an acute myocardial infarction, has been shown to be effective in reducing mortality and morbidity. In various studies, heparin has been shown to decrease the incidence of coronary reocclusion after the use of thrombolytic agents.

161. The answer is C (I, II).
Isosorbide dinitrate (Isordil) is used in both angina pectoris and heart failure. The development of angina pectoris centers around the balance between oxygen demand and oxygen supply to the myocardium. When the demand for oxygen exceeds the supply of oxygen, an angina attack occurs. Isosorbide dinitrate, like other nitrates, is a venous dilator resulting in reduced oxygen demand by the heart through a decrease in (venous return) preload. Isosorbide works in the heart failure patient by reducing venous return of blood to the heart, therefore, again, decreasing preload with a resultant decrease in fluid for the heart to pump. Clinical studies have demonstrated that the combination of isosorbide dinitrate with the arteriole dilator hydralazine has reduced mortality and morbidity in heart failure patients. Heart failure is a potential consequence of an acute myocardial infarction, and angina pectoris is a common underlying problem in many patients who have had a myocardial infarction. Both conditions are possible in Ms. Urmeister. Isosorbide dinitrate is not indicated in the acute treatment of hypertension.

162. The answer is C (I, II).
Isoproterenol is a sympathomimetic (β-adrenergic agonist) that increases oxygen demand by the heart through an increase in heart rate. Sympathomimetics, smoking, cold, and exercise all can increase oxygen demand, which may cause an acute angina attack or acute coronary syndrome in patients like Ms. Urmeister, who are at high risk. Acebutolol is a β-adrenergic receptor blocker that, like other β-blockers, reduces oxygen demand and is beneficial to patients with coronary artery disease.

163. The answer is A (I).
Bioavailability is a measurement of the rate and extent of systemic absorption of a drug or the speed and amount that reaches the systemic circulation. For drug products to be bioequivalent, they must contain the same amount of active ingredient, must use the same route of administration, and must have the same bioavailability. The parameters C_{max}, T_{max}, and AUC are used as a measurement of bioavailability of a drug. If these parameters are better than those for the parent product, the two products would not be considered equally bioavailable.

164. The answer is E.
Mexiletine (Mexitil) is an orally available drug that closely resembles lidocaine and is used to treat ventricular arrhythmias. As a class I_B antiarrhythmic, like lidocaine, it can be considered a first-line agent in the treatment of ventricular tachycardia. Lidocaine must be administered parenterally, making it unsuitable in the ambulatory setting. Flecainide (Tambocor) and encainide (Enkaid) are class I_C antiarrhythmics that are never indicated as first-line antiarrhythmics. Some physicians would argue that they should never be used; results of the Cardiac Arrhythmia Suppression Trial (CAST) study show that they can cause more harm than good. Encainide has already been removed from the market because of the major problems associated with its use. Dofetilide is a class I antiarrhythmic that is indicated in the treatment of atrial fibrillation and atrial flutter. Distribution in the United States is through a restricted access process and use requires inpatient treatment and close monitoring owing to safety concerns.

165. The answer is B (III).
Quinidine (Quinidex) has been reported to cause diarrhea in as many as 30% of patients who receive the drug. Although loperamide (Imodium) may be helpful in stopping the diarrhea, patients often must discontinue the quinidine to stop it. Both aluminum hydroxide gel and polygalacturonate salt (Cardioquin) have been effective in combating quinidine-induced diarrhea.

166. The answer is B.
Morphine sulfate is a narcotic analgesic with venous pooling properties that reduce preload. Preload reduction decreases the oxygen demand placed on the heart. For this reason, along with its ability to alleviate pain and reduce anxiety (anxiety and pain also increase oxygen demand), morphine is frequently used in the myocardial infarction patient.

167. The answer is D (II, III).
The β-adrenergic blockers timolol (Blocadren) and atenolol (Tenormin) have been shown effective in preventing sudden death after myocardial infarction. Patients do need to be monitored closely for signs and symptoms of myocardial depression because these drugs may have negative inotropic and chronotropic effects. Procainamide (Procan SR) is a class I_A antiarrhythmic agent used in the treatment of atrial and ventricular tachyarrhythmias.

168. The answer is C.
NicoDerm (nicotine) has been shown to be effective in helping patients stop smoking. Nitroglycerin patches are available in several brands (e.g., Nitro-Bid, Transderm-Nitro).

169. The answer is B.
Pseudoephedrine, a sympathomimetic amine, has central nervous system (CNS) stimulating properties and is the most likely agent to cause sleep disruption. Metamucil (psyllium) as a bulk laxative is not absorbed. Flonase (fluticasone) would be very unlikely. Benadryl (diphenhydramine) is one of the OTC agents used to treat insomnia and would more likely cause drowsiness. CNS stimulation from regular doses of aspirin is highly unlikely.

170. The answer is E.
Middle ear infection (otitis media) and external ear infection (swimmer's ear or otitis externa) require prescription antibiotics to treat. Water-clogged ears can be treated with an over-the-counter (OTC) product containing isopropyl alcohol and anhydrous glycerin. Impacted cerumen can be treated with carbamide peroxide.

171. The answer is A.
Oxymetazoline has a duration of action of 12 hr and should be used no more than twice daily. The other topical nasal decongestants listed are administered every 6 hr (naphazoline), every 4 hr (phenylephrine, ephedrine), or every 2 hr (propylhexedrine).

172. The answer is B.
The SPF is the minimal erythema dose (MED) of sunscreen-protected skin divided by the MED of unprotected skin. An SPF of 15 means that, if the sunscreen is applied properly, the user can stay out in the sun about 15 times longer to get a minimal sunburn compared to being in the sun with unprotected skin (i.e., with no sunscreen application): 15×10 min $= 150$ min $= 2\frac{1}{2}$ hr.

173. The answer is A.
If the patient misses a dose of Rogaine (minoxidil), he should just continue with the next dose. One should not make up missed doses. The other items noted are appropriate counseling points to cover.

174. The answer is C.
Sulfur, salicylic acid, and sulfur plus resorcinol are all considered safe and effective agents for the treatment of acne. Technically, benzoyl peroxide is currently classified as a Class III agent, meaning that more safety data are needed to determine that it does not have photocarcinogenic effects. Triclosan is an antibacterial agent with antigingivitis and antiplaque activity in the oral cavity and no proven efficacy against acne.

175. The answer is D.
Nonprescription treatment of acne is restricted to mild noninflammatory acne. It is clear that this young lady has more significant inflammatory acne. She has apparently had only a modest response to the OTC agents, and she needs to be referred to a physician for additional prescription therapy.

176. The answer is D.
This agent is generally considered the nonprescription drug of choice for the treatment of acne. It does have the twofold mechanism of action described in choice D.

177. The answer is C.
If topical nasal decongestants are used for more often than 3–5 days, rhinitis medicamentosa (rebound congestion) may occur in the nasal passages. Thus the patient ends up experiencing as a side effect what he sought to treat in the first place. For the common cold, a 3- to 5-day use of a topical nasal decongestant should be all that is needed.

178. The answer is D (II, III).
Tenuate Dospan is a controlled-release form of diethylpropion, a sympathomimetic agent. Many controlled-release drug products or modified dosage forms cannot be crushed because the integrity of the matrix would be destroyed and dangerous amounts of the active drug may be available for rapid absorption.

179. The answer is D (II, III).
First-order reactions are characterized by an exponential change in the drug amount or concentration with time, and these changes produce a straight line when plotted on a semilog graph. The half-life for a first-order reaction is a constant.

180. The answer is D (II, III).
FluMist is an inhaled influenza vaccine preparation approved for ages 5–49. The vaccine is viewed as unsafe in patients < 5 years owing to concerns about increased rates of asthma within 42 days of vaccination. Safety and efficacy in patients 50 years and older have not been adequately assessed.

181. The answer is A.
Calcium is available for oral administration in a salt form of lactate, gluconate, phosphate, and carbonate; it is not available for oral administration in a salt form of chloride. Calcium chloride is available for IV injection. Dosage regimens should be individualized because of differences in calcium content.

182. The answer is C.
Osteonecrosis, hyperglycemia, fluid retention, and cataracts are long-term complications of therapy with steroids, including prednisone. Steroids generally increase the white blood cell count.

183. The answer is C.
Cidofovir suppresses cytomegalovirus replication by selective inhibition of DNA synthesis. It is not a protease inhibitor and is not indicated for treatment of HIV infection. Saquinavir (Invirase), ritonavir (Norvir), and indinavir (Crixivan) are protease inhibitors used to treat HIV infection.

184. The answer is A (I).
A pyrogen test is a fever test in rabbits or an in vitro test using the limulus (horseshoe crab). A positive test shows the presence of fever-producing substances (pyrogens) in a sterile product; these substances may be dead microorganisms or extraneous proteins.

185. The answer is A (I).
Increases in BUN and serum creatinine generally indicate renal impairment. Levels of LDG, AST, and ALT rise with liver dysfunction and indicate liver damage.

186. The answer is D.
Nausea and vomiting are common adverse reactions to chemotherapy; therefore, antiemetic therapy should be initiated before administration of chemotherapeutic drugs. Common antiemetic agents include ondansetron (Zofran), metoclopramide (Reglan), droperidol (Inapsine), and tetrahydrocannabinol (Marinol). Cimetidine (Tagamet) has no value as an antiemetic.

187. The answer is A.
Laboratory findings in acute renal failure include hyperuricemia, hyperkalemia, hypocalcemia, and metabolic acidosis. In acute renal failure, phosphate excretion decreases, causing hyperphosphatemia, not hypophosphatemia.

188. The answer is E.
Iodine is a trace element essential to the synthesis of thyroxine (T_4) and triiodothyronine (T_3). Iodine also is needed for physical and mental development and metabolism. Iodine deficiency can cause cretinism in children and infants.

189. The answer is B.
Omalizumab (Xolair) must be administered subcutaneously every 2–4 weeks. Injection site reactions occur in nearly half of patients.

190. The answer is C.
Bentoquatam (Ivy-Block) is an organoclay that should be applied at least 15 min before poison ivy plant exposure and then every 4 hr for continued protection. Because the oleoresin (urushiol) can rapidly penetrate the skin, it should be washed off soon after exposure (within 10 min is ideal). Obviously, learning how to identify the poison ivy plant and avoiding it would be the best ways of preventing the dermatitis.

Test II

Use the patient profile below to answer questions 1–10.

PATIENT RECORD (INSTITUTION/NURSING HOME)

Patient Name: Thomas Anzalone

Address: 2098 West Central Ave.

Age: 31   Height: 5'11"

Sex: M   Race: white   Weight: 185 lb

Allergies: Penicillin

Social History: 20 pack-year history

DIAGNOSIS

Primary   (1)   Acute psychotic episode

           (2)   Schizophrenia

Secondary   (1)

           (2)

           (3)

LAB/DIAGNOSTIC TESTS

	Date	Test
(1)	8/14	Blood pressure 130/74 mm Hg; Na 140 mEq/L; K 4 mEq/L; Cl 95 mEq/L; CO_2 25 mEq/L; BUN 11 mg/dL; Cr 1.0 mg/dL; Hb 12.5 g/dL; HCT 39%

MEDICATION ORDERS (Including Parenteral Solutions)

	Date	Drug and Strength	Route	Sig
(1)	8/14	Haloperidol 5 mg	IM	stat
(2)	8/14	Haloperidol 5 mg	IM	q4h prn agitation
(3)	8/16	Diphenhydramine 50 mg	po	stat
(4)	8/17	Risperidone	po	2 mg bid
(5)	8/30	Risperidone	po	2 mg bid

ADDITIONAL ORDERS

	Date	Comments
(1)	8/14	Admit to security ward—chart notes previous positive response to Haldol per last hospitalization.
(2)	8/14	May restrain.
(3)	8/17	D.C. Haloperidol.
(4)	8/30	Discharge patient on risperidone.

DIETARY CONSIDERATIONS (Enteral and Parenteral)

	Date	Comments
(1)		
(2)		

PHARMACIST NOTES AND Other Patient Information

	Date	Comments
(1)	8/14	Smoker 2 packs/day for 10 years.
(2)	8/14	Positive family history for schizophrenia (mother).
(3)	8/14	Positive family history for alcoholism (father).
(4)	8/14	Medication history: includes haloperidol; may be compliance problem.
(5)		

1. Mr. Anzalone is hospitalized for an acute psychotic episode of his schizophrenia. The most common symptoms of schizophrenia are

   A. hallucinations and delusions.
   B. poor attention and apathy.
   C. insomnia and amotivation.
   D. combativeness and thought disorder.
   E. disorganized speech and asocial behavior.

2. The patient profile indicates that Mr. Anzalone responded to Haldol therapy the last time he was hospitalized for an acute psychotic episode. Antipsychotic therapy for this patient can be assessed by monitoring the target symptom of

   A. delusions.
   B. withdrawal.
   C. asocial behavior.
   D. apathy.
   E. poor judgment.

3. Extrapyramidal side effects can occur with all of the typical antipsychotics, especially high-potency ones like haloperidol. All of the following are extrapyramidal side effects *except*

   A. akasthisia.
   B. tardive dyskinesia.
   C. acute dystonia.
   D. pseudoparkinsonism.
   E. There is no exception; all of the above are extrapyramidal side effects.

4. Within 48 hr of initiating haloperidol, the patient experiences uncontrolled and involuntary neck twisting and a fixed upward gaze. The treatment of choice in this patient would be

   A. immediate haloperidol dose reduction by one half.
   B. immediate oral administration of bromocriptine 5 mg.
   C. immediate IM administration of diazepam 5 mg.
   D. immediate IM administration of diphenhydramine 50 mg.
   E. immediate change to an alternative antipsychotic agent, such as thioridazine.

5. In the medical record provided by Mr. Anzalone's primary-care provider, the physician recorded that at one patient visit "the patient was having difficulty keeping his legs and feet still." This movement abnormality most likely represented

   A. a dystonic reaction, which may be treated with oral diazepam.
   B. akathisia, which should respond to a dosage reduction in his haloperidol.
   C. drug-induced parkinsonism, which may respond to oral bromocriptine.
   D. a warning sign of reduced seizure threshold; low-dose antiseizure therapy should be initiated.
   E. tardive dyskinesia; the antipsychotic dose should be lowered.

6. During a discussion with Mr. Anzalone about his compliance with haloperidol therapy, the patient states that he did not like taking oral haloperidol because it made him "stiff." This apparent pseudoparkinsonism reaction can be treated by

   I. changing his therapy to an atypical antipsychotic agent (SGA).
   II. decreasing the dose of the haloperidol.
   III. adding an anticholinergic agent.

   A. I only
   B. III only
   C. I and II
   D. II and III
   E. I, II, and III

7. Mr. Anzalone was switched to risperidone, a second-generation antipsychotic, and discharged on this agent. In addition to this agent, all of the following are atypical antipsychotics *except*

   A. aripiprazole.
   B. olanzapine.
   C. ziprasidone.
   D. thioridazine.
   E. quetiapine.

8. Mr. Anzalone might be a candidate for a long-acting IM formulation of antipsychotic given the fact that he apparently had some compliance problems in the past. Which of the following agents are used as such?

   I. haloperidol decanoate
   II. fluphenazine decanoate
   III. long-acting risperidone

   A. I only
   B. III only
   C. I and II
   D. II and III
   E. I, II, and III

9. Second-generation antipsychotic agents (SGAs) would be preferred over first-generation agents (FGAs) because they

   I. have increased efficacy for negative symptoms (apathy, asocial behavior, etc.) compared to typical antipsychotics.
   II. have been associated with less extrapyramidal symptoms (EPSs)
   III. have been shown to be much more effective on positive symptoms (hallucinations, delusions, etc.) than the FGAs.

   A. I only
   B. III only
   C. I and II
   D. II and III
   E. I, II, and III

10. Clozapine (Clozaril) is a second-generation antipsychotic agent (SGA) that is reserved for use in patients who are refractory to treatment with other antipsychotics. Treatment plans for patients receiving this agent should include routine monitoring for

    A. renal failure.
    B. agranulocytosis.
    C. hair loss.
    D. severe diarrhea.
    E. excessive sodium loss.

End of this patient profile; continue with the examination

---

11. When counseling a parent with a 3-year-old on the administration of otic drops to this child, the pharmacist should instruct the parent to pull the ear

    A. backward and upward.
    B. backward and downward.
    C. 90° outward.
    D. straight forward.
    E. None of the above.

12. Which of the following agents is the only FDA-approved nonprescription cerumen-softening agent?

    A. carbamide peroxide
    B. mineral oil
    C. hydrogen peroxide
    D. sweet oil
    E. glycerin

13. Which of the following would be considered the most important counseling point for a patient taking mineral oil as a laxative?

    A. Remain in an upright position while taking this agent.
    B. Take with food.
    C. It may interfere with the absorption of water-soluble vitamins.
    D. An adult can take up to 3 ounces as a dose.
    E. Do not take if fluid compromised.

14. An older gentleman complains that his hemorrhoids are bothering him again. He has not had problems with them in quite some time. He is concerned because he has noticed that this time around he has had some bleeding into the toilet bowl. What product would you recommend to this elderly gentleman?

    A. Anusol suppositories
    B. Tucks pads
    C. Preparation H ointment
    D. hydrocortisone ointment
    E. none; he should be referred to a physician

15. A middle-aged woman explains that she has recently developed hemorrhoids and she wants something to stop the itching. Upon checking her profile in the computer, you find out that she is currently taking atenolol 20 mg/day for her hypertension and Lipitor 40 mg/day for her hyperlipidemia. Which of the following would *not* be appropriate for this woman?

    A. Anusol HC-1
    B. Tucks pads (witch hazel, glycerin)
    C. Anusol ointment
    D. Preparation H cream
    E. hydrocortisone 1% cream

Use the information below to answer questions 16–18.

A 49-year-old woman has recently been diagnosed with rheumatoid arthritis. Celebrex was initially prescribed for her condition. She was eventually prescribed Enbrel and a course of prednisone 5 mg/day was prescribed at the same time.

16. Which of the following apply to the drug celecoxib in the treatment of rheumatoid arthritis?

   I. This agent works by inhibiting prostaglandin synthesis by decreasing activity of the enzyme cyclooxygenase 2 (COX-2), which results in decreased formation of prostaglandin precursors.

   II. It does not alter the course of rheumatoid arthritis, nor does it prevent joint destruction.

   III. It may cause serious skin reactions.

   A. I only
   B. III only
   C. I and II
   D. II and III
   E. I, II, and III

17. The reason why prednisone is being used in this patient is best described by which of the following?

   I. as "bridge" therapy to allow the Enbrel to fully take effect

   II. to alter the course of the disease

   III. to minimize the side effects of nonsteroidal anti-inflammatory drugs (NSAIDs)

   A. I only
   B. III only
   C. I and II
   D. II and III
   E. I, II, and III

18. All of the following apply to the use of Enbrel in this patient *except* which one?

   A. This agent is used as one of a number of disease-modifying antirheumatic drugs (DMARDs).

   B. It is believed now that agents like Enbrel should be initiated in the rheumatoid arthritis patient within the first 3 months despite good control with NSAIDs.

   C. Inflammatory markers for the disease (e.g., erythrocyte sedimentation rate [ESR]) are reduced significantly by DMARDs (e.g., Enbrel) but not nonsteroidal anti-inflammatory drugs (NSAIDs).

   D. It binds to tumor necrosis factor α (TNF-α) and β, inhibiting the inflammatory response mediated by immune cells.

   E. There is no exception; all of the above apply to the use of Enbrel in this patient.

End of this patient profile; continue with the examination

19. When recommending an appropriate sun protectant for patients, it is important to recommend a product that protects against both ultraviolet A (UVA) and ultraviolet B (UVB) radiation wavelengths. Which agents and combination of agents would provide such protection?

    I. titanium dioxide
    II. octyl methoxycinnamate and avobenzone
    III. homosalate and padimate O

    A. I only
    B. III only
    C. I and II
    D. II and III
    E. I, II, and III

20. Which of the following vitamins and minerals would play a role in reducing the risk of neural tube defect birth abnormalities in an unborn child?

    A. micronutrients such as copper, manganese, and zinc
    B. niacin
    C. iodine
    D. folic acid
    E. vitamin B_{12}

Use the patient profile below to answer questions 21–31.

MEDICATION PROFILE (COMMUNITY)

Patient Name: John Smith

Address: 14 Francis St.

Age: 20   Height: 5'9"

Sex: M   Race: white   Weight: 196 lb

Allergies: Penicillin

DIAGNOSIS

Primary	(1)	Non-Hodgkin lymphoma
Secondary	(1)	Chemotherapy-induced nausea and vomiting

MEDICATION RECORD (Prescription and OTC)

	Date	Rx No.	Physician	Drug and Strength	Quan	Sig	Refills
(1)	6/1	432576	Golub	Cytoxan 1200 mg IV	1	administer in clinic	0
(2)	6/1	432577	Golub	Vincristine 2 mg IV	1	IV push × 2 min	0
(3)	6/1	432578	Golub	Procarbazine 50mg	56	IV caps qd × 14 days	0
(4)	6/1	432579	Golub	Prednisone 20 mg	56	40 mg/m^2 qd × 14 days	0
(5)	6/1	432580	Golub	Torecan 10 mg	10	q4h prn nausea	1
(6)	6/1	432581	Golub	Ativan 1 mg	10	q4h prn nausea	1
(7)	6/1	432582	Golub	Compazine suppositories 25 mg	6	i q6h prn	1
(8)	6/1	432583	Golub	Neupogen 300 µg	14	300 mg SQ q AM	0
(9)	6/1	432584	Ferrin	Peridex 16 oz	1	1\2 fl oz bid	1
(10)	6/1	432585	Ferrin	ACT Fluoride Rinse	1	swish and spit qd × 5 weeks	1
(11)	6/1	432586	Coleman	Hickman Line Kit	1	as directed	prn
(12)	6/1	432587	Golub	Kytril 1 mg IV over 5 min	1	30 min before chemo	

PHARMACIST NOTES AND Other Patient Information

	Date	Comments
(1)	6/1	Weight 89 kg; body surface area 2.0 m^2.
(2)	6/1	Treatment plan: C-MOPP q 28 days for 6 courses.
(3)	6/1	Return to clinic 6/8 for CBC and IV chemotherapy.
(4)	6/1	Cytoxan 600 mg/m^2; Oncovin (vincristine) 1 mg/m^2; procarbazine 100 mg/m^2.
(5)	6/1	Prednisone 40 mg/m^2 qd.
(6)	6/1	Daily Neupogen injections until absolute neutrophil count (ANC) = 10,000.
(7)		
(8)		
(9)		
(10)		
(11)		
(12)		
(13)		
(14)		
(15)		
(16)		
(17)		
(18)		
(19)		

21. All of the following statements about combination cancer chemotherapy regimens are true *except* which one?

    A. Combination cancer chemotherapy regimens are now used more commonly than single-agent regimens.
    B. Drugs in combination generally should have the same mechanisms of action.
    C. The drugs act during different cell cycle phases.
    D. The drugs should be associated with different adverse effects.
    E. Cell cycle–specific agents may be given with cell cycle–nonspecific agents.

22. Cyclophosphamide is classified as

    A. an alkylating agent.
    B. an antimetabolite.
    C. a natural alkaloid.
    D. a hormonal agent.
    E. a platinum derivative.

23. Which chemotherapy agents are associated with a low (10%) incidence of nausea and vomiting?

    I. cyclophosphamide
    II. procarbazine
    III. vincristine

    A. I only
    B. III only
    C. I and II
    D. II and III
    E. I, II, and III

24. Torecan is a phenothiazine derivative structurally related to

    I. Compazine.
    II. Tigan.
    III. Ativan.

    A. I only
    B. III only
    C. I and II
    D. II and III
    E. I, II, and III

25. To minimize the risk of neurotoxicity, vincristine should be given in doses only up to

    A. 100 mg.
    B. 1 mg.
    C. 2 mg.
    D. 200 mg.
    E. 200 mg.

26. What brand name product should be dispensed for ondansetron?

    A. Velban
    B. Zofran
    C. Kytril
    D. Emetrol
    E. Anzemet

27. All of the following drugs are adrenocorticosteroids *except*

    A. prednisone.
    B. Decadron.
    C. triamcinolone.
    D. Medrol.
    E. Provera.

28. Which statements describe chemotherapy-induced nausea and vomiting?

    I. Onset of nausea and vomiting usually occurs within 3–4 hr after drug administration.
    II. Severe nausea and vomiting may reduce patient tolerance to chemotherapy.
    III. Nausea and vomiting result from stimulation of the brain's chemoreceptor trigger zone (CTZ).

    A. I only
    B. III only
    C. I and II
    D. II and III
    E. I, II, and III

29. Mr. Smith develops a *Staphylococcus aureus* infection at his Hickman catheter site. Because of his history, he is hospitalized for treatment and evaluation. Based on Mr. Smith's profile, which antibiotics would be reasonable therapy choices?

    I. daptomycin
    II. dicloxacillin
    III. Unasyn

    A. I only
    B. III only
    C. I and II
    D. II and III
    E. I, II, and III

30. The microbiology laboratory reports Mr. Smith's cultures reveal the *S. aureus* to be vancomycin resistant. Which of the following is a reasonable choice for therapy?

    A. linezolid
    B. Rocephin
    C. Vancoled
    D. meropenem
    E. cefamandole

31. Filgrastim is used to

    I. reduce the risk of anemia and certain cancers of the blood.
    II. maintain cell membrane integrity, reduce cellular aging, and inhibit melanoma cell growth.
    III. reduce the risk of neutropenia, which can be life-threatening.

    A. I only
    B. III only
    C. I and II
    D. II and III
    E. I, II, and III

End of this patient profile; continue with the examination

Use the information below to answer questions 32–34.

Hydrophilic ointment USP has the following formula:
- Methylparaben 0.25 g
- Propylparaben 0.15 g
- Sodium lauryl sulfate 10 g
- Propylene glycol 120 g
- Stearyl alcohol 250 g
- White petrolatum 370 g
- Purified water to make approximately 1000 g

32. Preservatives in hydrophilic ointment include

    I. methylparaben and propylparaben
    II. propylene glycol
    III. stearyl alcohol

    A. I only
    B. III only
    C. I and II
    D. II and III
    E. I, II, and III

33. How much stearyl alcohol is needed to make 30 g of hydrophilic ointment?

    A. 0.3 g
    B. 1.2 g
    C. 3.7 g
    D. 7.5 g
    E. 8.3 g

34. Hydrophilic ointment is generally classified as

    A. a hydrocarbon base.
    B. an absorption base.
    C. a water-removable base.
    D. a water-soluble base.
    E. a water-insoluble base.

End of this section; continue with the examination

35. Which of the following sleep medications does *not* act on the benzodiazepine receptor?

    A. eszopiclone
    B. zaleplon
    C. zolpidem
    D. ramelteon
    E. triazolam

36. What patient counseling information should be provided when a patient is prescribed montelukast?

    A. Montelukast should be taken 1 hr before or 2 hr after a meal.
    B. Headache occurs more frequently than in placebo-treated patients.
    C. Asthma symptoms may improve on the first day of treatment.
    D. Worsened allergic rhinitis symptoms may be noted.
    E. Caution should be observed for increased anticoagulation when using montelukast and warfarin concurrently.

37. Which product is most likely to induce hypokalemia in an otherwise normal hypertensive patient?

    A. Dyazide
    B. Vasotec
    C. Aldactazide
    D. HydroDIURIL
    E. Moduretic

38. All of the following are potential advantages of low molecular weight heparin (LMWH) over unfractionated heparin *except* which one?

    A. increased plasma half-life
    B. lower incidence of heparin-induced thrombocytopenia
    C. less risk of osteoporosis
    D. uses the same monitoring process as for heparin (activated partial thromboplastin time [aPTT])
    E. more predictable dose response

39. Which dosages are available for Zestril tablets?

    I. 2.5 mg
    II. 5 mg
    III. 40 mg

    A. I only
    B. III only
    C. I and II
    D. II and III
    E. I, II, and III

40. Which agent has little value in treating acute inflammation?

    A. flurbiprofen
    B. choline salicylate
    C. acetaminophen
    D. Ecotrin
    E. Ascriptin

41. A theophylline drug interaction potentially exists with

    I. lansoprazole
    II. ciprofloxacin
    III. cimetidine

    A. I only
    B. III only
    C. I and II
    D. II and III
    E. I, II, and III

42. According to the Henderson-Hasselbalch equation, pH = pK_a + log ([base]/[salt]). When pK_a equals 9 and the ratio of the non-ionized species to the ionized species is 10:1, the pH equals

    A. 8.
    B. 9.
    C. 10.
    D. 11.
    E. 12.

43. Which substance should be used in a case of overdosage with methotrexate?

    A. brewer's yeast
    B. leucovorin
    C. *para*-aminobenzoic acid
    D. sulfisoxazole
    E. trimethoprim

44. 5-Fluorouracil is also known as:

    I. FUDR
    II. 5-FC
    III. 5-FU

    A. I only
    B. III only
    C. I and II
    D. II and III
    E. I, II, and III

Use the patient profile below to answer questions 45–59.

MEDICATION PROFILE (COMMUNITY)

Patient Name: Philip Green

Address: 2127 Sandra Ct.

Age: 47

Sex: M   Race: white

Height: 5'6"

Weight: 186 lb

Allergies: No known allergies

DIAGNOSIS

Primary   (1)   Hypertension

              (2)   Gouty arthritis

              (3)   Obesity

Secondary   (1)

              (2)

MEDICATION RECORD (Prescription and OTC)

	Date	Rx No.	Physician	Drug and Strength	Quan	Sig	Refills
(1)	11/21	15776	Melcher	Hydrochlorothiazide 25 mg	30	1 qd AM BP	5
(2)	11/21			Commit lozenge 2 mg	72	as directed	
(3)	12/4	15998	Melcher	Ionamin 30 mg	30	1 qd AM	0
(4)	1/7	16578	Melcher	Naprosyn 250 mg	20	3 stat, then1 tid	2
(5)	1/7	16579	Melcher	Lotensin 10 mg	30	1 qd AM	6
(6)	1/12			Tylenol 500 mg	100	1 – 2 prn HA	
(7)	6/22	20967	Melcher	Colchicine 0.5 mg	60	1 bid	2
(8)	7/30	21366	Melcher	Zyloprim 300 mg	30	1 qd AM	6

PHARMACIST NOTES AND Other Patient Information

	Date	Comments
(1)	1/6	Patient called and stated that he has severe pain and swelling in his right big toe that awakened him last night; referred him to his physician for evaluation.
(2)	1/7	Patient states that his MD told him that his serum uric acid was 11.5 mg/dL.
(3)	1/7	DC hydrochlorothiazide.
(4)	1/12	Patient brought aspirin to counter for purchase; advised to use Tylenol instead.
(5)		
(6)		
(7)		
(8)		
(9)		
(10)		
(11)		
(12)		
(13)		
(14)		
(15)		
(16)		
(17)		
(18)		
(19)		

45. Based on Mr. Green's height and weight, he has a BMI of ~ 30. Which of the following statements apply to his situation?

    I. BMI stands for basal metabolic index.
    II. His BMI value meets the definition of obesity.
    III. Gradual weight loss would likely lower his serum uric acid.

    A. I only
    B. III only
    C. I and II
    D. II and III
    E. I, II, and III

46. Ionamin should be used cautiously in this patient because

    I. he has gout.
    II. his BMI is not high enough.
    III. he has elevated blood pressure.

    A. I only
    B. III only
    C. I and II
    D. II and III
    E. I, II, and III

47. While he is waiting to see if his phentermine prescription can be filled, Mr. Green asks, "Is there any safe and effective over-the-counter medication that I can take to treat my obesity?" You reply, "The FDA has ruled that

    I. no over-the-counter agent is safe and effective."
    II. pseudoephedrine has taken the place of phenylpropanolamine as a safe and effective agent."
    III. benzocaine is effective."

    A. I only
    B. III only
    C. I and II
    D. II and III
    E. I, II, and III

48. Based on the information noted for 1/6 and 1/7, it appears that Mr. Green is suffering from an acute attack of gout. Which of the following *best* describes the usual pattern of the arthritis in gout?

    A. Morning stiffness for at least 30 min, usually lasting for 1 hr before maximal improvement.
    B. Periods of acute attacks with intense pain that completely resolve.
    C. Arthritis most commonly in the metacarpophalangeal and proximal interphalangeal joints of the hands.
    D. Gradual building of pain over a few days, then a sudden burst of intense pain that typically occurs in the late afternoon.
    E. Acute inflammation of two or more joints in a symmetrical pattern.

49. The Commit lozenges were recommended for Mr. Green for what purpose?

    I. to help treat his apparent sore throat
    II. as a treatment for an apparent cough
    III. as an aid to help him stop smoking

    A. I only
    B. III only
    C. I and II
    D. II and III
    E. I, II, and III

50. All of the following statements concerning Mr. Green's acute gouty arthritis attack are correct *except* which one?

    A. Corticosteroids should never be used to treat these attacks.
    B. A good response to colchicine therapy may help confirm the diagnosis of gouty arthritis, but some other forms of arthritis may respond to this agent.
    C. The first attack of gouty arthritis usually involves only one joint; when this is the first metatarsophalangeal joint of the foot, it is termed *podagra.*
    D. The patient will likely have an elevated serum uric acid level.
    E. Attacks most typically occur during the middle of the night.

51. Why did the pharmacist advise Mr. Green against taking the occasional aspirin for his headache?

    I. Because in low doses, aspirin can cause retention of uric acid in the body.
    II. Because milligram per milligram acetaminophen is much more effective than aspirin for pain from episodic tension-type headache.
    III. Because of his increased risk for Reye's syndrome.

    A. I only
    B. III only
    C. I and II
    D. II and III
    E. I, II, and III

52. All of the following statements concerning gout or uric acid excretion apply to Mr. Green *except* which one?

    A. As a man, Mr. Green is much more likely to develop gout compared to a woman.
    B. Most of Mr. Green's body uric acid is excreted through the gastrointestinal tract.
    C. Foods high in purine content may increase his serum uric acid level.
    D. If he were to take colchicine, it would have no effect on his serum uric acid level.
    E. Naproxen is a good choice over colchicine to treat his acute attack of gout because diarrhea secondary to colchicine therapy is common.

53. Mr. Green obtains refills on his Naprosyn for two additional episodes of gouty arthritis. Which of the following would be appropriate considerations in this patient?

    I. With his three attacks, Mr. Green is a candidate for uric acid–lowering therapy.
    II. Small daily doses of oral colchicine would likely benefit this patient by helping prevent additional attacks of acute gouty arthritis, especially if uric acid–lowering therapy is begun.
    III. It would be useful to consider switching him to another antihypertensive, as the current agent may be contributing to his hyperuricemia.

    A. I only
    B. III only
    C. I and II
    D. II and III
    E. I, II, and III

54. Which of the following apply to the Zyloprim prescription for Mr. Green?

    I. This drug is known as a xanthine oxidase inhibitor.
    II. He can take this just once daily because of the long half-life of the metabolite.
    III. He must drink plenty of fluids to prevent uric acid crystallization in the urine after starting this drug.

    A. I only
    B. III only
    C. I and II
    D. II and III
    E. I, II, and III

55. Cheryl Green, Philip's wife, comes up to the pharmacy counter and asks you to recommend a vaginal product for her yeast infection. Which of the following would apply to Mrs. Green?

    I. To use the over-the-counter (OTC) agents for this condition, she must have had at least one previous episode of vaginal candidiasis that was medically diagnosed.
    II. The OTC vaginal candidiasis products come in 1-, 3-, and 7-day treatment regimens.
    III. The characteristic symptoms of this condition are a vaginal discharge that is described as "cottage cheese–like" with no offensive odor, dysuria, or vulvar or vaginal redness.

    A. I only
    B. III only
    C. I and II
    D. II and III
    E. I, II, and III

56. One of Mr. Green's children, Megan (age 14), developed diarrhea. Which of the following agents are now considered by the FDA to be safe and effective over-the-counter (OTC) antidiarrheal agents?

    I. attapulgite
    II. kaolin
    III. bismuth subsalicylate

    A. I only
    B. III only
    C. I and II
    D. II and III
    E. I, II, and III

57. You decide to recommend Kaopectate liquid for the treatment of Megan's diarrhea. Which of the following apply to this agent?

    I. This product contains the same ingredient as Pepto-Bismol Original Liquid.
    II. This product should not be given to a teenager who has chickenpox.
    III. Harmless black-stained stools may occur with the administration of this product.

    A. I only
    B. III only
    C. I and II
    D. II and III
    E. I, II, and III

58. A further inquiry into the possible reason for Megan's diarrhea reveals that she seems to get it most often after eating ice cream or other dairy products. You decide against recommending Kaopectate in favor of another product called Lactaid Caplets. Which of the following can be stated about her condition and your product recommendation?

    I. She probably has lactose intolerance.
    II. Lactaid contains lactase, which would be the appropriate agent for treating her.
    III. The diarrhea is caused by the calcium in the dairy products.

    A. I only
    B. III only
    C. I and II
    D. II and III
    E. I, II, and III

59. Ryan (age 13) and Greg (age 15), Mr. Green's other children, are planning to go to the beach with some friends. Mr. Green's family has fair skin, and Mr. Green wants to make sure that his sons are protected from the sun. Which of the following would apply to the use of sunscreens for these two teens?

    I. A product with a sun protection factor (SPF) of 30 or 30 + would provide maximal protection against sunburn.
    II. An adequate amount should be applied, and then it should be reapplied frequently because of loss of sunscreen from sweating or swimming.
    III. The SPF indicates protection against both ultraviolet A (UVA) and UVB radiation.

    A. I only
    B. III only
    C. I and II
    D. II and III
    E. I, II, and III

End of this patient profile; continue with the examination

Use the patient profile below to answer questions 60–69.

MEDICATION PROFILE (COMMUNITY)

Patient Name: <u>Marilyn Fox</u>

Address: <u>48 Worthy Rd.</u>

Age: <u>22</u>

Sex: <u>F</u>   Race: <u>white</u>

Height: <u>5'5"</u>

Weight: <u>125 lb</u>

Allergies: <u>No known allergies</u>

DIAGNOSIS

Primary   (1) <u>Pelvic inflammatory disease</u>

           (2) <u>Anemia</u>

           (3) <u>Vaginal candidiasis</u>

Secondary (1) _____

           (2) _____

MEDICATION RECORD (Prescription and OTC)

	Date	Rx No.	Physician	Drug and Strength	Quan	Sig	Refills
(1)	9/3	617583	Tacs	Rocephin 250 mg	1	250 mg IM × 1	0
(2)	9/3	617584	Tacs	Benemid 500 mg	2	2 tabs stat	0
(3)	9/3	617585	Tacs	Tetracycline 500 mg	28	i q6h × 14 d	0
(4)	9/3	617586	Tacs	Tylenol with Codeine No. 3	20	i q4h prn	1
(5)	9/3			Feosol	100	i bid	
(6)	9/7	617843	Greene	Doxycycline 100 mg	30	i bid × 14 d	0
(7)	9/7	617967	Greene	Diflucan 150 mg	1	150 mg po × 1	0
(8)	10/1	618103	Greene	Triphasil	28	i qd	12

PHARMACIST NOTES AND Other Patient Information

	Date	Comments
(1)	9/7	D.C. tetracycline because of gastrointestinal intolerance; change to doxycycline with food (doxycycline is current CDC recommendation for PID, not tetracycline).
(2)	____	
(3)	____	
(4)	____	
(5)	____	
(6)	____	
(7)	____	
(8)	____	
(9)	____	
(10)	____	
(11)	____	
(12)	____	
(13)	____	
(14)	____	
(15)	____	
(16)	____	
(17)	____	
(18)	____	
(19)	____	

60. Ms. Fox has purchased some Feosol. All of the following statements about iron supplementation are correct *except* which one?

    A. Iron can cause dark discoloration of the stool.
    B. Taking iron with food can decrease absorption.
    C. The usual dose of elemental iron is 200 mg/day in divided doses.
    D. Ferrous gluconate has the highest percentage of elemental iron of all the oral iron salts.
    E. Non-enteric-coated preparations of iron supplements are preferred over enteric-coated products.

61. Ms. Fox's anemia is apparently the result of an iron deficiency. Which of the following would apply to this type of an anemia before treatment with iron supplementation?

    I. One would likely note a microcytic hypochromic blood smear.
    II. The serum hemoglobin (Hb) and the mean cell volume (MCV) would be low.
    III. The serum total iron-binding capacity (TIBC) would usually be high.

    A. I only
    B. III only
    C. I and II
    D. II and III
    E. I, II, and III

62. Which products in Ms. Fox's profile may interact adversely with Feosol?

    I. Rocephin
    II. codeine
    III. tetracycline

    A. I only
    B. III only
    C. I and II
    D. II and III
    E. I, II, and III

63. Ms. Fox's initial diagnosis is pelvic inflammatory disease (PID). Which of the following statements apply to this condition?

    I. PID is usually caused by the organisms *Neisseria gonorrhoeae* and *Chlamydia trachomatis.*
    II. An acceptable outpatient drug regimen for empiric treatment of this condition is ceftriaxone and doxycycline.
    III. The initial administration of Rocephin IM is a rational one.

    A. I only
    B. III only
    C. I and II
    D. II and III
    E. I, II, and III

64. Why did Ms. Fox receive the Benemid?

    I. She must have gout.
    II. Her serum uric acid level must be elevated.
    III. To prolong the serum levels of the Rocephin.

    A. I only
    B. III only
    C. I and II
    D. II and III
    E. I, II, and III

65. Which of the following drugs from Ms. Fox's profile is most likely responsible for her yeast infection (vaginal candidiasis)?

    A. tetracycline
    B. Feosol
    C. Triphasil-28
    D. Tylenol with Codeine No. 3
    E. None of the above is likely responsible.

66. All of the following statements about doxycycline are correct *except* which one?

    A. It is active against many gram-positive and gram-negative organisms, *Rickettsia, Mycoplasma,* and *Chlamydia.*
    B. It is mainly excreted in the feces.
    C. Its absorption is increased with concurrent use of antacids and milk.
    D. It commonly causes gastrointestinal distress.
    E. It may produce phototoxic reactions if the patient is exposed to sunlight.

67. Which of the following would most accurately describe the antibacterial activity of tetracycline antibiotics?

    I. They are mainly bacteriostatic at normal serum concentrations.
    II. They interfere with protein synthesis by binding to the 30S and possibly the 50S ribosomal subunit(s).
    III. They may cause alterations in the bacterial cytoplasmic membrane.

    A. I only
    B. III only
    C. I and II
    D. II and III
    E. I, II, and III

68. The selection of Diflucan to treat Ms. Fox's vulvovaginal candidiasis (VVC) is appropriate because

    I. it is less messy than vaginal creams.
    II. it is the only oral antifungal agent currently approved by the FDA for the treatment of VVC.
    III. It promotes patient compliance.

    A. I only
    B. III only
    C. I and II
    D. II and III
    E. I, II, and III

69. Based on Ms. Fox's profile, she has had only one occurrence of vulvovaginal candidiasis. Which of the following apply to recurrent vulvovaginal candidiasis?

    I. It would be diagnosed if she experienced at least four such infections in a 12-month period.
    II. If this is her diagnosis, she should not try to self-treat with any of the nonprescription products.
    III. It may be an early sign of HIV infection.

    A. I only
    B. III only
    C. I and II
    D. II and III
    E. I, II, and III

End of this patient profile; continue with the examination

70. Which of the following would be used to treat antibiotic-associated *Clostridium difficile* colitis?

    I. clindamycin
    II. metronidazole
    III. vancomycin

    A. I only
    B. III only
    C. I and II
    D. II and III
    E. I, II, and III

71. Which drug is a substituted imidazole for treating many systemic fungal infections and is an effective systemic agent when taken orally?

    A. butoconazole
    B. clotrimazole
    C. ketoconazole
    D. miconazole
    E. nystatin

Use the patient profile below to answer questions 72–83.

MEDICATION PROFILE (COMMUNITY)

Patient Name: _Phyllis Boch_

Address: _68 Ferris Dr._

Age: _34_   Height: _5'4"_

Sex: _F_   Race: _white_   Weight: _110 lb_

Allergies: _Amitriptyline, phenobarbital_

DIAGNOSIS

Primary	(1)	Epilepsy
	(2)	Mild hypertension
Secondary	(1)	Gastroesophageal reflux disease

MEDICATION RECORD (Prescription and OTC)

	Date	Rx No.	Physician	Drug and Strength	Quan	Sig	Refills
(1)	1/5	11238	Dunbar	Dilantin 100 mg	100	iii caps q AM	6
(2)	1/5	11239	Dunbar	Depakote 250 mg	200	ii tabs qid	6
(3)	1/5	11240	Dunbar	Tegretol 200 mg	100	i tab tid	6
(4)	1/30	11473	Huang	Folic acid 1 mg	100	i qd	2
(5)	1/30			Multivitamins	100	i qd	
(6)	1/30			Advil 200 mg	30	ii prn HA	
(7)	2/14	12372	Huang	Atacand HCT 16/12.5	90	i qd	3
(8)	2/14	12373	Huang	Ranitidine 150 mg	60	i qd	6

PHARMACIST NOTES AND Other Patient Information

	Date	Comments
(1)	1/10	Dilantin level 16 µg/mL.
(2)	2/4	Nystagmus observed at AM visit.
(3)	2/4	DC vaseretic previously ordered
(4)		
(5)		
(6)		
(7)		
(8)		
(9)		
(10)		
(11)		
(12)		
(13)		
(14)		
(15)		
(16)		
(17)		
(18)		
(19)		
(20)		
(21)		
(22)		

72. Which drugs should be avoided by this patient?

    I. phenytoin
    II. primidone
    III. carbamazepine

    A. I only
    B. III only
    C. I and II
    D. II and III
    E. I, II, and III

73. Ms. Boch has had difficulty swallowing various tablets and capsules. Which medications should she avoid crushing before administration?

    I. carbamazepine
    II. folic acid
    III. Depakote

    A. I only
    B. III only
    C. I and II
    D. II and III
    E. I, II, and III

74. Which of the following are common side effects of hormone-replacement therapy?

    I. irregular uterine bleeding
    II. weight gain
    III. breast tenderness

    A. I only
    B. III only
    C. I and II
    D. II and III
    E. I, II, and III

75. Therapeutic serum levels of phenytoin are generally considered to be in the range of

    A. 2–10 μg/mL.
    B. 10–20 μg/mL.
    C. 15–35 μg/mL.
    D. 20–40 μg/mL.
    E. 45–65 μg/mL.

76. Which drugs decrease hydantoin activity?

    I. Depakote
    II. folic acid
    III. Tegretol

    A. I only
    B. III only
    C. I and II
    D. II and III
    E. I, II, and III

77. Good oral hygiene is especially important for reducing adverse reactions related to

    I. Dilantin.
    II. Depakote.
    III. Tegretol.

    A. I only
    B. III only
    C. I and II
    D. II and III
    E. I, II, and III

78. The serum level of Tegretol is unaffected by

    A. erythromycin ethylsuccinate (EES).
    B. E-Mycin 333.
    C. amoxil.
    D. isoniazid.
    E. Tao.

79. Which drug is most likely responsible for Ms. Boch's nystagmus?

    A. Dilantin
    B. Depakote
    C. Tegretol
    D. folic acid
    E. Advil

80. Dilantin is available as

    I. a capsule.
    II. a tablet.
    III. an ampule.

    A. I only
    B. III only
    C. I and II
    D. II and III
    E. I, II, and III

81. In addition to hydrochlorothiazide 12.5 mg, Vaseretic 5-12.5 contains

    A. ramipril 5 mg.
    B. amlodipine 5mg.
    C. enalapril 5 mg.
    D. quinapril 5 mg.
    E. captopril 12.5 mg.

82. The most commonly reported dose-related side effects associated with carbamazepine are

    A. rash, renal failure, and decreased white blood cells.
    B. diplopia, nausea, and ataxia.
    C. liver toxicity, pulmonary fibrosis, and autoimmune disorders.
    D. angina, urticaria, and vomiting.
    E. headache, rash, and prolonged blood clotting.

83. True comparisons of Advil to Tylenol include which statements?

    I. Tylenol has less anti-inflammatory activity than does Advil.
    II. Tylenol is contraindicated in children because they are susceptible to Reye syndrome.
    III. Tylenol irritates the gastrointestinal tract more than does Advil.

    A. I only
    B. III only
    C. I and II
    D. II and III
    E. I, II, and III

End of this patient profile; continue with the examination

---

84. The brand name for fosphenytoin is

    A. Dilantin
    B. Cerebyx
    C. Valium
    D. Lamictal
    E. Topamax

85. What type of drug interaction is taking place when reduced blood levels of tetracycline result from taking the drug concurrently with a calcium-containing antacid?

    A. synergism
    B. complexation
    C. chemical antagonism
    D. electrostatic interaction
    E. enzyme inhibition

86. Which of the following adverse drug reactions has been reported with the use of quinupristin/dalfopristin?

    A. photosensitivity
    B. infusion site pain, erythema, or itching
    C. neutropenia
    D. cardiomyopathy
    E. renal failure

87. Naloxone is used in combination with Talwin Nx to

    I. decrease the first-pass effects of pentazocine when administered orally.
    II. produce additive analgesic effects with pentazocine when administered orally.
    III. provide narcotic antagonist activity when administered intravenously.

    A. I only
    B. III only
    C. I and II
    D. II and III
    E. I, II, and III

88. If co-trimoxazole oral suspension contains 40 mg trimethoprim and 200 mg sulfamethoxazole per 5 mL, how many milliliters of suspension are required to provide a dose equivalent to one Bactrim DS tablet?

    A. 5 mL
    B. 10 mL
    C. 15 mL
    D. 20 mL
    E. 25 mL

89. All of the following medications are classified as sustained-release theophylline products *except*

    A. Slo-Phyllin Gyrocaps.
    B. Sustaire.
    C. Aerolate JR.
    D. Accurbron.
    E. Theovent.

90. Based on a patient's malnutrition and symptoms such as fatigue, weight loss, and paresthesias, the physician suspects pernicious anemia. Which test is the most likely to diagnose this condition?

    A. Schilling test
    B. hematocrit
    C. hemoglobin
    D. serum folate
    E. Schlichter test

91. Which forms are available for potassium chloride?

    I. Oral solution
    II. powder in a packet
    III. liquid

    A. I only
    B. III only
    C. I and II
    D. II and III
    E. I, II, and III

92. What is the side effect most commonly associated with doxazosin?

    A. hyperkalemia
    B. postural hypotension
    C. cough
    D. taste disturbances
    E. angioedema

93. All of the following statements are true of Prilosec OTC *except* which one?

    A. It is available as a 20-mg dose.
    B. It is available as a purple capsule.
    C. It is indicated for treatment of frequent heartburn.
    D. The patient should not take it > 14 days without a physician's direction.
    E. The patient should not repeat a 14-day course more often than every 4 months, unless directed by a physician.

94. Which of the following is the proper treatment for syphilis?

    A. ceftriaxone 1g IM once
    B. metronidazole 500 mg three times a day for 10 days
    C. azithromycin 1 g by mouth once
    D. benzathine penicillin 2.4 million units once
    E. tetracycline 500 mg four times a day for 14 days

95. Potassium supplementation is contraindicated in patients using

    A. chlorthalidone
    B. hydrochlorothiazide (HCTZ).
    C. furosemide.
    D. triamterene.
    E. ethacrynic acid.

96. To determine the absolute bioavailability of a new controlled-release dosage form of quinidine gluconate, the extent of quinidine bioavailability after the new dosage form should be compared with

    I. the area under the curve (AUC) after an IV bolus dose of quinidine gluconate.
    II. the AUC after a reference standard controlled-release form of quinidine gluconate.
    III. the AUC after an oral solution of quinidine gluconate.

    A. I only
    B. III only
    C. I and II
    D. II and III
    E. I, II, and III

97. Which of the following is contraindicated in a patient with a history of anaphylaxis related to Thiosulfil Forte administration?

    A. carbamazepine
    B. Depakote
    C. Dilantin
    D. acetazolamide
    E. ethosuximide

Use the patient profile below to answer questions 98–108.

PATIENT RECORD (INSTITUTION/NURSING HOME)

Patient Name: Grace Wiley

Address: 57689 South Twenty-fourth St.

Age: 35   Height: 5′9″

Sex: F   Race: white   Weight: 126 lb

Allergies: No known allergies

DIAGNOSIS

Primary	(1)	Bleeding duodenal ulcer
	(2)	Hypotension
Secondary	(1)	
	(2)	

LAB/DIAGNOSTIC TESTS

	Date	Test
(1)	6/22	Hgb 9 g/dL; HCT 30%; Na 126 mEq/L; K 3.4 mEq/L; Cl 90 mEq/L; CO_2 24 mEq; BUN 25 mg/dL; Cr 0.8 mg/dL; guaiac positive

MEDICATION ORDERS (Including Parenteral Solutions)

	Date	Drug and Strength	Route	Sig
(1)	6/22	D5/0.45% NaCl 1000 mL	IV	125 mL/h
(2)	6/22	Al/Mg(OH)$_2$ 30 mL	per NG tube	q2h
(3)	6/22	Zantac 50 mg	IV	q6h
(4)	6/23	Esomeprazole 40 mg	per NG tube	qd × 10 days
(5)	6/23	Clarithromycin Suspension	per NG tube	500 mg bid × 10 days
(6)	6/23	Amoxicillin Suspension	per NG tube	1 g bid × 10 days

ADDITIONAL ORDERS

	Date	Comments
(1)	6/22	Endoscopy stat
(2)	6/22	Insert NG tube
(3)	6/22	Check *Helicobacter pylori* status (CLO test)

DIETARY CONSIDERATIONS (Enteral and Parenteral)

	Date	Comments
(1)		
(2)		

PHARMACIST NOTES AND Other Patient Information

	Date	Comments
(1)	6/22	Patient has 10 pack-years history of smoking.
(2)	6/22	Patient has recently completed a course of ibuprofen for sports injury.
(3)	6/22	Open Nexium capsule, administer esomeprazole beads in 50 cc water via NG tube.
(4)	6/23	Patient *H. pylori* positive.
(5)	6/23	D.C. antacids, Zantac.
(6)	6/23	Patient reports recent Entocort use (within last month)
(7)		

98. What is the primary reason for selecting an antacid containing both an aluminum salt and a magnesium salt as opposed to a single-ingredient antacid?

A. lower cost
B. a balance of untoward effects such as constipation and diarrhea
C. minimal potential for concomitant drug interactions
D. better palpability
E. decreased frequency of administration

99. Which of the following is FDA approved for treatment of Crohn disease?

A. Prednisone
B. Medrol
C. Entocort EC
D. Hydrocortisone
E. Celestone

100. Which of the following are true regarding *Helicobacter pylori*?

I. It is present in the majority of patients with duodenal ulcer.
II. *H. pylori* eradication can cure peptic ulcer disease and reduce ulcer recurrence.
III. An active duodenal ulcer is best managed with a combination of antisecretory therapy plus appropriate antibiotic(s).

A. I only
B. III only
C. I and II
D. II and III
E. I, II, and III

101. In the admission interview, the pharmacist records that the patient has recently completed a regimen of ibuprofen. This information is significant in the patient's history because

I. ibuprofen may cause ulcers even in *H. pylori*–negative individuals.
II. ibuprofen may injure the gastric mucosa directly.
III. ibuprofen inhibits synthesis of prostaglandins, thereby compromising the mucosal-protective effect of these substances.

A. I only
B. III only
C. I and II
D. II and III
E. I, II, and III

102. Adding clarithromycin and amoxicillin to omeprazole in this patient will

A. decrease time to symptom relief.
B. decrease time required to heal the ulcer.
C. stop bleeding in patients with a bleeding ulcer.
D. prevent ulcer recurrence.
E. prevent nonsteroidal anti-inflammatory drug (NSAID) induced ulcers.

103. The elimination half-life for ranitidine is approximately 2 hr. What percentage of this drug would be eliminated from the body 4 hr after an IV bolus dose?

A. 12.5%
B. 25%
C. 50%
D. 75%
E. 87.5%

104. The binding affinity of cimetidine to the cytochrome P450 mixed-function oxidase system of the liver may

A. enhance the therapeutic efficacy of cimetidine.
B. interfere with the metabolism of phenytoin, phenobarbital, diazepam, propranolol, and many other drugs.
C. decrease the healing rate of duodenal ulcers but not gastric ulcers.
D. increase the relapse rate of both duodenal and gastric ulcers.
E. allow for a decreased frequency of cimetidine dosing.

105. All of the following reduce acid secretion by inhibiting the proton pump of the parietal cell *except*

    A. Prevacid.
    B. Prilosec.
    C. Protonix.
    D. Nexium.
    E. Pepcid.

106. After leaving the hospital, the patient is given prescriptions for Nexium, amoxicillin, and Biaxin to complete the *H. pylori* eradication regimen. The pharmacist dispensed the remaining Biaxin Suspension to avoid waste and minimize the drug costs. You should counsel the patient regarding all of the following *except* which one?

    A. Continue Nexium 40 mg for a total of 10 days.
    B. Clarithromycin can be taken with food to minimize gastrointestinal side effects.
    C. Taste disturbances are common with Biaxin.
    D. Complete a full 10 days of antibiotic/antisecretory therapy for optimal eradication results.
    E. Refrigerate Biaxin and shake well before use.

107. All of the following are true regarding colloidal bismuth preparations for treatment of ulcer disease *except* which one?

    A. Bismuth is absorbed after oral administration but is quickly eliminated from the body.
    B. Bismuth products turn the stool black.
    C. The only commercial bismuth product available in the United States useful for ulcer disease is bismuth subsalicylate.
    D. In combination with metronidazole, tetracycline, and antisecretory therapy, they effectively eradicate *H. pylori*.
    E. Pepto-Bismol may cause salicylism when administered in high doses.

108. Which statements concerning the drug misoprostol are true?

    I. Misoprostol is effective for protecting patients from nonsteroidal anti-inflammatory drug (NSAID) induced gastric ulcer.
    II. Misoprostol frequently produces dose-related diarrhea.
    III. Misoprostol is contraindicated in women who are pregnant.

    A. I only
    B. III only
    C. I and II
    D. II and III
    E. I, II, and III

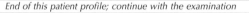

End of this patient profile; continue with the examination

Use the information below to answer questions 109–111.

- Hydrocortisone acetate 10 mg
- Bismuth subgallate 1.75%
- Bismuth resorcinol compound 1.2%
- Benzoyl benzoate 1.2%
- Peruvian balsam 1.8%
- Zinc oxide 11%
- Suppository base qs ad 2 g

109. The most appropriate suppository base in this preparation is

   A. glycerin.
   B. glycerinated gelatin.
   C. polyethylene glycol.
   D. theobroma oil.
   E. surfactant base.

110. Which of the following requires that patients be screened for tuberculosis infection before initiation of therapy?

   A. Celebrex
   B. Remicade
   C. sulfasalazine
   D. Colazal
   E. omeprazole

111. How many milligrams of Peruvian balsam are needed to prepare 12 suppositories?

   A. 180
   B. 216
   C. 288
   D. 420
   E. 432

End of this patient profile; continue with the examination
---

112. The following medication is prescribed:

   Pediazole suspension 400 mL
   Sig: 2 tsp q6h 3 10 d
   Which auxiliary labels should be affixed to the prescription bottle?

   I. Take with a full glass of water.
   II. Shake well.
   III. Take with food or milk.

   A. I only
   B. III only
   C. I and II
   D. II and III
   E. I, II, and III

113. Which medications should be labeled "Avoid Alcohol Consumption"?

   I. dideoxyinosine (DDI)
   II. metronidazole
   III. itraconazole

   A. I only
   B. III only
   C. I and II
   D. II and III
   E. I, II, and III

114. Which medications may discolor urine, sweat, and other body fluids and should be discussed as part of patient counseling?

    I. rifampin
    II. clofazimine
    III. atovaquone

    A. I only
    B. III only
    C. I and II
    D. II and III
    E. I, II, and III

115. Which medications are frequently in use when nephrotoxicity occurs?

    I. cisplatin
    II. foscarnet
    III. amphotericin B

    A. I only
    B. III only
    C. I and II
    D. II and III
    E. I, II, and III

116. Which conditions predispose a patient to toxicity from a highly protein-bound drug?

    I. hypoalbuminemia
    II. hepatic disease
    III. malnutrition

    A. I only
    B. III only
    C. I and II
    D. II and III
    E. I, II, and III

PATIENT RECORD (INSTITUTION/NURSING HOME)

Patient Name: Robert Smith

Address: Sharon View Nursing Home, 98 Colling Rd.

Age: 81   Height: 5'8"

Sex: M   Race: white   Weight: 175 lb

Allergies: No known allergies

DIAGNOSIS

Primary	(1)	Pneumonia
	(2)	Asthma
Secondary	(1)	Alzheimer disease
	(2)	Hypercholesterolemia
	(3)	Hypertension

LAB/DIAGNOSTIC TESTS

	Date	Test
(1)	10/2	Total cholesterol 242 mg/dL
(2)	10/14	WBC $9.2 \times 10^3/mm^3$; Cr 1.4 mg/dL

MEDICATION ORDERS (Including Parenteral Solutions)

	Date	Drug and Strength	Route	Sig
(1)	10/1	Advair Diskus	inhalation	ii puffs bid
(2)	10/1	Zafirlukast 20 mg	po	i bid
(3)	10/1	Rosuvastatin 20 mg	po	qd
(4)	10/1	Felodipine 5 mg	po	qd
(5)	10/12	Terbutaline 5 mg	po	i tab tid
(6)	10/15	Cefuroxime 1.5 g	IV	q8h
(7)	10/21	Amoxil 500 mg	po	q8h
(8)	10/22	Ciprofloxacin 750 mg	po	bid
(9)	10/22	Theo-24 300 mg	po	iii qd AM

ADDITIONAL ORDERS

	Date	Comments
(1)	10/15	Encourage fluids.
(2)	10/15	Rinse mouth with water after Advair dosing.

DIETARY CONSIDERATIONS (Enteral and Parenteral)

	Date	Comments
(1)	10/1	Low-fat diet.

PHARMACIST NOTES AND Other Patient Information

	Date	Comments
(1)	10/14	Fever to 102.4°F.
(2)	10/18	Temperature 98.6°F.
(3)	10/22	D.C. Amoxil because rash occurred.
(4)		
(5)		

117. What is the generic name for Accolate?

    A. metaproterenol
    B. albuterol
    C. ipratropium bromide
    D. zafirlukast
    E. cromolyn sodium

118. Which drug is most likely to cause tremor?

    A. Atrovent
    B. terbutaline
    C. Mandol
    D. nicotinic acid
    E. Amoxil

119. Which statements concerning cefuroxime are true?

    I. It is a first-generation cephalosporin.
    II. It may produce a disulfiram-type reaction if this patient receives alcohol-containing products concurrently.
    III. It is commonly used in patients with community-acquired pneumonia.

    A. I only
    B. III only
    C. I and II
    D. II and III
    E. I, II, and III

120. Which of the following should *not* be used to provide acute relief of bronchospasm?

    A. albuterol
    B. pirbuterol
    C. Atrovent
    D. bitolterol
    E. Proventil

121. All of the following statements concerning amoxicillin are true *except* which one?

    A. It has an antimicrobial spectrum of activity similar to that of ampicillin.
    B. It is appropriately dosed every 6 hr.
    C. It may cause a generalized erythematous, maculopapular rash in addition to urticarial hypersensitivity.
    D. It produces diarrhea less frequently than does ampicillin.
    E. It is contraindicated in patients with a history of hypersensitivity to cyclacillin.

122. Which agents should Mr. Smith avoid?

    I. ampicillin
    II. ciprofloxacin
    III. erythromycin

    A. I only
    B. III only
    C. I and II
    D. II and III
    E. I, II, and III

123. When using an inhaler a patient should

    A. wait 5 min between puffs.
    B. rinse mouth with water between puffs.
    C. check peak flow readings before and after puffs.
    D. wait 1 min between puffs.
    E. lie down for 10 min after dose has been administered.

124. Which agents are suitable for this patient's infection?

    I. cinoxacin
    II. norfloxacin
    III. ofloxacin

    A. I only
    B. III only
    C. I and II
    D. II and III
    E. I, II, and III

125. Which statements concerning fever are true?

    I. When treating a fever, either acetaminophen or aspirin would be acceptable antipyretic therapy.
    II. Fever is a useful assessment tool; treat only if the fever is dangerously high or the patient experiences chills.
    III. Fever should be treated aggressively; antipyretic therapy should begin on day 1 of antibiotic therapy.

    A. I only
    B. III only
    C. I and II
    D. II and III
    E. I, II, and III

126. Which drugs require that serum levels be measured and recorded in the patient's medication profile?

    I. theophylline
    II. cefuroxime
    III. terbutaline

    A. I only
    B. III only
    C. I and II
    D. II and III
    E. I, II, and III

127. Crestor is available as tablets in all of the following strengths *except*

    A. 5 mg.
    B. 10 mg.
    C. 20 mg.
    D. 40 mg.
    E. 80 mg.

128. The physician would like the patient to use a generic drug product equivalent to Slo-Phyllin. For a generic drug product to be bioequivalent

    I. both the generic and the brand-name drug products must be pharmaceutical equivalents.
    II. both the generic and brand-name drug products must have the same bioavailability.
    III. both the generic and brand-name drug products must have the same excipients.

    A. I only
    B. III only
    C. I and II
    D. II and III
    E. I, II, and III

End of this patient profile; continue with the examination

---

129. Which of the following are thought to shorten the activity of theophylline?

    I. smoking
    II. phenobarbital
    III. cimetidine

    A. I only
    B. III only
    C. I and II
    D. II and III
    E. I, II, and III

130. Procrit is used in chronic renal failure to treat

    A. peripheral neuropathy.
    B. anemia.
    C. hyperphosphatemia.
    D. metabolic alkalosis.
    E. hyperuricemia.

131. The most common adverse effect of raloxifene is

    A. irregular uterine bleeding.
    B. rash and allergic reactions.
    C. hot flashes and leg cramps.
    D. nausea and gastrointestinal upset.
    E. breast tenderness.

132. Emulsifying agents can be described as

    I. compounds that lower interfacial tension.
    II. molecules that contain a hydrophobic and a hydrophilic functional group.
    III. compounds that have surfactant properties.

    A. I only
    B. III only
    C. I and II
    D. II and III
    E. I, II, and III

133. Amitiza is indicated for treatment of

    A. acute diarrhea.
    B. migraine headache.
    C. chronic idiopathic constipation.
    D. gastroesophageal reflux disease (GERD).
    E. insomnia.

134. Which agents interfere with folic acid metabolism?

    I. trimethoprim
    II. methotrexate
    III. pyrimethamine

    A. I only
    B. III only
    C. I and II
    D. II and III
    E. I, II, and III

135. In the preparation shown below, salicylic acid is used for which property?

Salicylic acid 13.9%

Zinc chloride 2.7%

Flexible collodion base qs ad 30 mL

    A. analgesic
    B. antipyretic
    C. astringent
    D. keratolytic
    E. rubefacient

136. All of the following agents represent an approved over-the-counter (OTC) treatment for acne vulgaris *except*

    A. PROPApH
    B. Liquimat
    C. Rezamid
    D. Carmol-HC
    E. Fostex

137. Which statements about type 1, or insulin-dependent, diabetes mellitus are true?

    I. The disease is more common in obese patients > 40 years of age.
    II. The cause of the disease is decreased insulin secretion and peripheral tissue insensitivity to insulin.
    III. Increased serum glucose levels can cause ketoacidosis in these patients.

    A. I only
    B. III only
    C. I and II
    D. II and III
    E. I, II, and III

138. Which type of hormone is represented in the structure below?

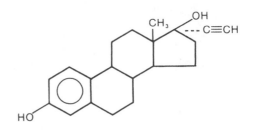

    A. androgen
    B. estrogen
    C. glucocorticoid
    D. mineralocorticoid
    E. progestin

139. All of the following situations are thought to contribute to the development of Parkinson disease *except*

    A. dopamine deficiency.
    B. norepinephrine deficiency.
    C. γ-aminobutyric acid (GABA) deficiency.
    D. acetylcholine deficiency.
    E. serotonin deficiency.

140. Which combination of antipsychotic agents provides the lowest risk of extrapyramidal side effects?

    A. Tindal and Trilafon
    B. Serentil and Mellaril
    C. Navane and Taractan
    D. Haldol and Moban
    E. Stelazine and Prolixin

PATIENT RECORD (INSTITUTION/NURSING HOME)

Patient Name: _Florence Backs_

Address: _2325 Prospect Blvd._

Age: _72_   Height: _5′5″_

Sex: _F_   Race: _white_   Weight: _158 lb_

Allergies: _Penicillin_

DIAGNOSIS

Primary   (1)   Acute pneumonia

            (2)   Chronic obstructive pulmonary disease

Secondary   (1)   History of recurrent pneumonia

LAB/DIAGNOSTIC TESTS

LAB/DIAGNOSTIC TESTS

	Date	Test
(1)	2/28	Chest x-ray (bilateral lower lobe infiltrate)
(2)	2/28	WBC 18,000/mm³; differential: segs 80%, bands 10%
(3)	2/28	Na 140 mEq/L; K 4.0 mEq/L; Cl 96 mEq/L; bicarbonate 24 mEq/L; BUN 32 mg/dL; Cr 1.4 mg/dL; glucose 124 mg/dL; albumin 2.5 g/dL
(4)	2/28	Arterial blood gases: pH 7.4, P_{O_2} 70 mm Hg, P_{CO_2} 45 mm Hg, O_2 saturation 90%
(5)	2/28	Temperature 102°F (oral); sputum culture and sensitivity; theophylline level stat = 7.5 mg/mL

MEDICATION ORDERS (Including Parenteral Solutions)

	Date	Drug and Strength	Route	Sig
(1)	2/28	Aminophylline 250 mg	IVPB	stat
(2)	2/28	Aminophylline infusion	IV drip	40 mg/h
(3)	2/28	Acetaminophen 650 mg	po or rectal	q4h prn
(4)	2/28	Ceftazidime 1 g	IVPB	q8h
(5)	2/28	Gentamicin 140 mg	IVPB, loading dose	stat
(6)	2/28	Gentamicin 100 mg	IVPB	q12h
(7)	2/28	Albuterol 5% nebulizer solution	inhalation	q4h prn

ADDITIONAL ORDERS

	Date	Comments
(1)	3/1	Gentamicin peak and trough after third dose.
(2)	3/1	Theophylline level (steady state).
(3)	3/2	Cimetidine 300 mg IVPB q8h.
(4)	3/4	Theophylline level.

DIETARY CONSIDERATIONS (Enteral and Parenteral)

	Date	Comments
(1)		
(2)		

PHARMACIST NOTES AND Other Patient Information

	Date	Comments
(1)		Check influenza vaccination status.
(2)		

141. Based on a volume of distribution of 0.5 L/kg theophylline in Ms.Backs, the IV bolus dose of aminophylline would be expected to achieve an initial *total* theophylline serum concentration of

    A. 3.2 μg/mL.
    B. 6.9 μg/mL.
    C. 10.7 μg/mL.
    D. 13.1 μg/mL.
    E. 14.4 μg/mL.

142. After IV bolus administration, theophylline follows the pharmacokinetics of a two-compartment model. Drugs that exhibit the characteristics of two-compartment pharmacokinetics have

    I. an initial rapid distribution followed by a slower elimination phase.
    II. a rapid distribution and equilibration into highly perfused tissues (central compartment) followed by a slower distribution and equilibration into the peripheral tissues (tissue compartment).
    III. a plasma drug concentration that is the sum of two first-order processes.

    A. I only
    B. III only
    C. I and II
    D. II and III
    E. I, II, and III

143. Results of the theophylline level on 3/1 indicate a serum level of 14 μg/mL. Without any change in the theophylline infusion and without any interruption in therapy, the theophylline level on 3/4 was reported as 17.5 μg/mL. Which statement most likely represents the reason for this increase?

    A. The blood drawn for the theophylline level was not timed at steady state.
    B. The blood taken for the theophylline level was drawn from the same arm in which theophylline was infusing.
    C. The presence of ceftazidime in the blood sample caused a falsely elevated theophylline level.
    D. The co-administration of cimetidine competitively blocked the metabolism of theophylline, resulting in a decreased elimination of theophylline.
    E. The patient had a larger than usual volume of distribution for theophylline.

144. After the third dose of gentamicin, levels of the drug were reported as follows:

    Peak—drawn half hour after ending a half-hour infusion, was 6.2 μg/mL.
    Trough—drawn half hour before the next dose, was 1.2 μg/mL.
    Gentamicin follows first-order elimination kinetics. Which statements concerning gentamicin pharmacokinetics are correct?

    I. The elimination rate constant cannot be calculated.
    II. The elimination half-life can be calculated as 4.65 hr.
    III. If C_{max} is 7.2 μg/mL, the volume of distribution can be calculated as 16.6 L (0.23 L/kg).

    A. I only
    B. III only
    C. I and II
    D. II and III
    E. I, II, and III

145. The culture and sensitivity report for the sputum specimen indicates the following minimum inhibitory concentrations (MICs):

    Ceftazidime < 8 μg/mL
    Mezlocillin < 8 μg/mL
    Gentamicin = 4 μg/mL
    Tobramycin < 0.5 μg/mL
    Ciprofloxacin = 8 μg/mL
    Based on these results, a rational therapeutic decision would be to

    A. continue existing regimens without change.
    B. continue ceftazidime only.
    C. continue gentamicin; change ceftazidime to mezlocillin.
    D. change gentamicin to tobramycin; continue ceftazidime.
    E. change ceftazidime to mezlocillin; discontinue gentamicin.

146. Ms. Backs has reported a penicillin allergy. The incidence of cephalosporin–penicillin cross-hypersensitivity is reported to be approximately

    A. 0%.
    B. 10%.
    C. 25%.
    D. 75%.
    E. 95%.

147. Ms. Backs has been stabilized on an IV infusion of aminophylline equivalent to 32 mg theophylline per hour. The physician would like to convert her to an oral controlled-release theophylline product such as Theo-Dur. Which dosage of Theo-Dur would the pharmacist recommend?

    A. 100 mg q12h
    B. 200 mg q12h
    C. 300 mg q12h
    D. 400 mg q12h
    E. 500 mg q12h

148. Which statements about converting Ms. Backs from IV to oral sustained-release theophylline therapy are true?

    I. Considering the theophylline infusion rate of 40 mg/h, conversion to a sustained-release product at 300 mg q8h is appropriate.
    II. Administration with meals will not significantly decrease the amount of theophylline absorbed.
    III. Subsequent theophylline levels should be determined when no doses have been missed in the preceding 48 hr, and the sample should be drawn 3–7 hr after the last dose.

    A. I only
    B. III only
    C. I and II
    D. II and III
    E. I, II, and III

149. The patient would like to receive a generic equivalent of Theo-Dur. In the process of selecting a generic theophylline product, the pharmacist obtains the following information on the generic theophylline product from the pharmaceutical manufacturer:

Eighteen healthy men received either a single oral dose of 300 mg theophylline in controlled-release tablet form or an equal daily dose of 100 mg theophylline elixir given tid. A two-way crossover design was used for this study. In this study, no significant difference was observed in the AUC (0 h–24 h) for serum theophylline concentrations from the tablet compared with the elixir dosage forms. A graph of the plasma drug concentrations versus time was included.

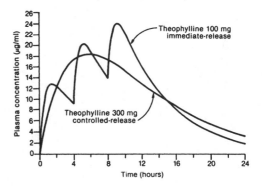

From this study, the pharmacist concludes that the

    I. theophylline tablet demonstrates controlled-release characteristics compared with those of the theophylline elixir.
    II. extent of theophylline bioavailability from both the tablet and the elixir is the same.
    III. theophylline elixir is bioequivalent to the theophylline tablet.

    A. I only
    B. III only
    C. I and II
    D. II and III
    E. I, II, and III

End of this patient profile; continue with the examination

150. Influenza vaccine use in chronic obstructive pulmonary disease (COPD) patients

    A. has no demonstrated benefit.
    B. is recommended for asthma but not COPD.
    C. is recommended annually, usually in the fall, for COPD patients.
    D. is too risky for COPD patients owing to drug interaction potential.
    E. is effective for 5 years after immunization; no need for more frequent administration.

151. Ingredients with antitussive action that may be found in over-the-counter (OTC) cough preparations include

    I. dextromethorphan.
    II. diphenhydramine.
    III. dihydrocodeinone.

    A. I only
    B. III only
    C. I and II
    D. II and III
    E. I, II, and III

152. Which of the following statements about antithyroid agents iare true?

    I. Propylthiouracil (PTU) and methimazole may help attain remission through direct interference with thyroid hormone synthesis.
    II. PTU or methimazole may be used preoperatively to establish and maintain a euthyroid state until definitive surgery can be performed.
    III. PTU has been associated with serious blood dyscrasias such as agranulocytosis.

    A. I only
    B. III only
    C. I and II
    D. II and III
    E. I, II, and III

153. The belladonna alkaloids are

    I. Oncovin.
    II. Velban.
    III. atropine.

    A. I only
    B. III only
    C. I and II
    D. II and III
    E. I, II, and III

154. Spiriva may aggravate

    A. narrow angle glaucoma.
    B. asthma.
    C. chronic obstructive pulmonary disease (COPD).
    D. irritable bowel syndrome.
    E. excessive salivation.

155. Which statements describe potential problems with drug substances packaged in ampules?

    I. Ampules are made of glass, which can break on opening or during transport.
    II. Drug substances packaged in ampules must be filtered to prevent broken particles of glass from being infused.
    II. Once the ampule is broken open, it must be used; therefore, it cannot be a multiple-dose product.

    A. I only
    B. III only
    C. I and II
    D. II and III
    E. I, II, and III

156. The hypotonic parenteral product is

    A. normal saline solution.
    B. half-normal saline solution.
    C. 0.9% sodium chloride.
    D. dextrose 40% total parenteral nutrition (TPN) solution.
    E. 3% sodium chloride solution.

157. Which infusion methods allow reliable administration of a medication with a narrow therapeutic index?

    I. continuous IV infusion
    II. intermittent IV infusion
    III. IV bolus with intermittent infusion

    A. I only
    B. III only
    C. I and II
    D. II and III
    E. I, II, and III

Use the patient profile below to answer questions 158–166.

PATIENT RECORD (INSTITUTION/NURSING HOME)

Patient Name: John Stevens

Address: Shady Grove Nursing Home

Age: 81   Height: 5'9"

Sex: M   Race: black   Weight: 150 lb

Allergies: No known allergies

DIAGNOSIS

Primary	(1)	Chronic renal failure	
	(2)	Dementia	
Secondary	(1)	Anemia	

LAB/DIAGNOSTIC TESTS

	Date	Test
(1)	5/4	BUN 75 mg/dL; Cr 6.0 mg/dL; K 7.5 mEq/L; HCT 24%; Hb 7.8 g/dL; phosphate 7.6 mg/dL
(2)	5/7	K 7.5 mEq/L

MEDICATION ORDERS (Including Parenteral Solutions)

	Date	Drug and Strength	Route	Sig
(1)	5/4	Mylanta 30 mL	po	prn
(2)	5/4	Kayexalate 30 g	po	qid prn
(3)	5/4	Calcitriol 1 mg	po	i qd
(4)	5/4	Calcium carbonate 1 g	po	ii qid
(5)	5/4	Colace 100 mg	po	bid
(6)	5/7	Haloperidol 1 mg	po	bid
(7)	5/9	Amphojel 30 mL	po	qid pc
(8)	5/9	Ferrous sulfate 300 mg	po	qid pc

ADDITIONAL ORDERS

	Date	Comments
(1)		
(2)		

DIETARY CONSIDERATIONS (Enteral and Parenteral)

	Date	Comments
(1)	5/4	Protein-restricted diet.

PHARMACIST NOTES AND Other Patient Information

	Date	Comments
(1)	5/9	D.C. Mylanta.
(2)		
(3)		
(4)		
(5)		
(6)		
(7)		
(8)		

158. Which mechanism describes how Amphojel achieves its therapeutic effect in Mr. Stevens?

    A. potassium binding
    B. phosphate binding
    C. acid neutralizing
    D. base neutralizing
    E. ion exchange

159. Kayexalate achieves its therapeutic effect by acting as an exchange resin. Which ion is exchanged with sodium?

    A. potassium
    B. phosphorus
    C. calcium
    D. nitrogen
    E. magnesium

160. Which type of anemia is most likely to occur in chronic renal failure?

    A. normochromic, normocytic
    B. hypochromic, normocytic
    C. hypochromic, microcytic
    D. normochromic, macrocytic
    E. hypochromic, macrocytic

161. Which medications would need a dosage reduction in renal failure?

    I. haloperidol
    II. digoxin
    III. tobramycin

    A. I only
    B. III only
    C. I and II
    D. II and III
    E. I, II, and III

162. Calcitriol is the same substance as

    A. calcium carbonate.
    B. calcium gluconate.
    C. 1,25-dihydroxycholecalciferol.
    D. calcium leucovorin.
    E. dihydrotachysterol.

163. Which drugs in Mr. Stevens's therapeutic regimen are likely to cause constipation?

    I. Amphojel
    II. Kayexalate
    III. calcitriol

    A. I only
    B. III only
    C. I and II
    D. II and III
    E. I, II, and III

164. Life-threatening cardiac arrhythmias owing to hyperkalemia should be treated with

    I. calcium chloride or calcium gluconate intravenously.
    II. loop diuretics to rapidly eliminate potassium.
    III. sodium polystyrene sulfonate.

    A. I only
    B. III only
    C. I and II
    D. II and III
    E. I, II, and III

165. Which adverse effect of haloperidol is most likely to occur in Mr. Stevens?

    A. neuroleptic malignant syndrome
    B. extrapyramidal symptoms
    C. urinary retention
    D. cardiovascular effects
    E. decreased seizure threshold

166. When Mr. Stevens complained of gastrointestinal discomfort, the physician prescribed cimetidine. The nurse should be alerted that cimetidine interacts with

    I. Amphojel.
    II. Colace.
    III. ferrous sulfate.

    A. I only
    B. III only
    C. I and II
    D. II and III
    E. I, II, and III

End of this patient profile; continue with the examination

Use the patient profile below to answer questions 167–176.

PATIENT RECORD (INSTITUTION/NURSING HOME)

Patient Name: __Mina Peterson__

Address: __1422 Arlington St.__

Age: __31__   Height: __5'6"__

Sex: __F__   Race: __white__   Weight: __130 lb__

Allergies: __Penicillin (rash)__

DIAGNOSIS

Primary	(1)	Acute nonlymphocytic leukemia
Secondary	(1)	Drug-induced congestive heart failure

LAB/DIAGNOSTIC TESTS

	Date	Test
(1)		
(2)		

MEDICATION ORDERS (Including Parenteral Solutions)

	Date	Drug and Strength	Route	Sig
(1)	3/5	Cytarabine 200 mg/m^2	IV	qd × 7 days
(2)	3/5	Daunorubicin 45 mg/m^2	IV	qd × 3 days
(3)	3/6	Lorazepam 1 mg	IV	30 min prechemotherapy
(4)	3/6	Dolasetron 1.8 mg/kg	IV	30 min prechemotherapy
(5)	3/6	Dexamethasone 20 mg	IV	30 min prechemotherapy
(6)	3/6	Ortho-Novum 1/50	po	i qd
(7)	3/7	Nystatin Suspension	po	5 mL swish and swallow
(8)	3/7	Cetacaine Spray	to throat	prn
(9)	3/7	Colace 100 mg	po	i tid
(10)	3/7	Gentamicin 100 mL in D$_5$W	IV	i tid
(11)				

ADDITIONAL ORDERS

	Date	Comments
(1)	3/7	Serum creatinine before gentamicin dosing.

DIETARY CONSIDERATIONS (Enteral and Parenteral)

	Date	Comments
(1)		
(2)		

PHARMACIST NOTES AND Other Patient Information

	Date	Comments
(1)	3/5	Patient has had 3 previous courses of chemotherapy.
(2)	3/5	Family requests antidepressant therapy be reinstituted (previously received SSRI); patient asks for OTC Ranitidine
(3)		
(4)		
(5)		
(6)		
(7)		

167. Which drug in Ms. Peterson's profile is most likely to cause congestive heart failure?

    A. cytarabine
    B. metoclopramide
    C. dexamethasone
    D. lorazepam
    E. daunorubicin

168. The most likely complications seen with Ms. Peterson's chemotherapy include

    I. renal failure.
    II. peripheral neuropathy.
    III. alopecia.

    A. I only
    B. III only
    C. I and II
    D. II and III
    E. I, II, and III

169. When the second dose of chemotherapy is administered, extravasation occurs. Management of this condition includes all of the following measures *except*

    A. leaving the needle in place.
    B. administering potassium chloride.
    C. applying ice.
    D. administering a corticosteroid.
    E. injecting sodium bicarbonate.

170. The probable reason for administration of Ortho-Novum 1/50 in this patient is

    A. birth control.
    B. estrogen stimulation of white blood cell production.
    C. discontinuation of menstrual bleeding.
    D. progestin stimulation of white blood cell production.
    E. chemotherapy for acute nonlymphocytic leukemia.

171. Approximately 10 days after chemotherapy, the cells most commonly affected include

    I. granulocytes.
    II. platelets.
    III. erythrocytes.

    A. I only
    B. III only
    C. I and II
    D. II and III
    E. I, II, and III

172. In preparing Ms. Peterson's chemotherapy, the pharmacist should take all of the following precautions *except*

    A. a horizontal laminar flow hood.
    B. a surgical gown.
    C. latex gloves.
    D. negative-pressure technique for vials.
    E. syringes with Luer-Lok fittings.

173. A patient who is taking an antihypertensive medication

    A. should avoid the serotonin and norepinephrine reuptake inhibitor (SNRI) venlafaxine.
    B. can safely take a tricyclic antidepressant.
    C. should reduce the dosage of antihypertensive when initiating antidepressant therapy.
    D. should not take any antidepressant medication.
    E. can take duloxetine without risk of increased blood pressure.

174. Ms. Peterson develops a hospital-acquired pneumonia and requires an antibiotic. Which drug should be administered with caution to this patient?

    A. clindamycin
    B. tetracycline
    C. vancomycin
    D. ceftazidime
    E. tobramycin

175. Gentamicin is also ordered for Ms. Peterson's infection. The major toxicityies of gentamicin include

    I. hepatotoxicity.
    II. neurotoxicity.
    III. nephrotoxicity.

    A. I only
    B. III only
    C. I and II
    D. II and III
    E. I, II, and III

176. The FDA-recommended dose of ranitidine to treat gastroesophageal reflux disease (GERD) is

    A. 75 mg.
    B. 150 mg twice a day.
    C. 300 mg at bedtime.
    D. 150 mg four times a day.
    E. 300 mg four times a day.

End of this patient profile; continue with the examination

---

177. Which sign or symptom reflects a vitamin K deficiency?

    A. dementia
    B. bleeding
    C. depression
    D. dermatitis
    E. diarrhea

178. Body surface area (BSA) is used in calculating chemotherapy doses because

    A. it is an indicator of tumor cell mass.
    B. it correlates with cardiac output.
    C. it correlates with gastrointestinal transit time.
    D. the National Cancer Institute requires that it be used.
    E. the FDA requires that it be used.

179. Aspirin in high doses has been shown to extend the activity of methenamine in the treatment of urinary tract infections. What mechanism is responsible for this drug interaction?

    A. Urinary alkalinization reduces methenamine elimination.
    B. Urinary acidification reduces methenamine elimination.
    C. Urinary alkalinization promotes methenamine elimination.
    D. Urinary acidification promotes methenamine elimination.
    E. Acidification of the gastric contents decreases methenamine absorption.

180. All of the following agents are available as over-the-counter (OTC) products for the treatment of hemorrhoids *except*

    A. steroid-containing products such as full-strength Anusol-HC.
    B. astringent-containing products such as witch hazel and zinc oxide.
    C. local anesthetic-containing products such as Medicone rectal ointment.
    D. vasoconstrictor-containing products such as Pazo or Wyanoids.
    E. aerosol foam products such as Procto-Foam.

181. Which of the following narcotics has the longest duration of effect?

    A. methadone
    B. controlled-release morphine
    C. levorphanol
    D. transdermal fentanyl
    E. dihydromorphone

182. What is the principal ingredient in Burow's solution?

    A. acetic acid
    B. aluminum acetate
    C. boric acid
    D. sodium hypochlorite
    E. aluminum hydroxide

183. Which therapeutic agents have been developed from recombinant DNA technology?

    I. Activase
    II. Neupogen
    III. Epogen

    A. I only
    B. III only
    C. I and II
    D. II and III
    E. I, II, and III

184. Effects of the gastrointestinal anticholinergic agent Pro-Banthine include

    I. dry mouth, blurred vision, and urinary retention.
    II. increased secretions, diarrhea, and pupillary constriction.
    III. acceleration of gastric emptying time.

    A. I only
    B. III only
    C. I and II
    D. II and III
    E. I, II, and III

185. Coumadin should be given with caution to patients in end-stage liver disease because

    I. Coumadin binding to albumin decreases.
    II. plasma albumin concentrations decrease.
    III. prothrombin clotting time increases.

    A. I only
    B. III only
    C. I and II
    D. II and III
    E. I, II, and III

186. A woman has a prescription for 32 mEq KCl by mouth. The pharmacy has 600-mg KCl controlled-release tablets. How many tablets does she need to take each day to provide this dose (molecular weight of KCl is 74.5)?

    A. 2 tablets
    B. 3 tablets
    C. 4 tablets
    D. 5 tablets
    E. 6 tablets

Use the information below to answer questions 187–188.

A woman brings the following prescription to the pharmacy after visiting her oncologist:

Carafate 1 g   8 tablets
Sorbitol 70%   40 mL
Vari-Flavors   2 packets
Water qs ad   120 mL
Sig: swish and expectorate 10 mL q4h

187. What is the percentage of sucralfate in the final suspension?

   A. 1.0%
   B. 6.7%
   C. 12.4%
   D. 8.0%
   E. 15%

188. How much sucralfate is in 10 mL of this product?

   A. 1.0 g
   B. 500 mg
   C. 66.7 mg
   D. 0.667 g
   E. 6.7 g

End of this patient profile; continue with the examination

189. Passive diffusion of a drug molecule across a cell membrane depends on the

   I. lipid solubility of the drug.
   II. extent of ionization of the drug.
   III. concentration difference on either side of the cell membrane.

   A. I only
   B. III only
   C. I and II
   D. II and III
   E. I, II, and III

190. Which type of laxative includes the agent psyllium?

   A. stimulant
   B. bulk-forming
   C. emollient
   D. saline
   E. lubricant

TEST II ANSWERS AND EXPLANATIONS

1. The answer is A.
All of the symptom pairs listed are possible symptoms of schizophrenia. The most common are hallucinations (perception disturbances in sensory experiences of the environment) and delusions (incorrect or false beliefs).

2. The answer is A.
Treatment of schizophrenia is primarily symptomatic. Target symptoms of schizophrenia have been categorized as "positive" and "negative" and may be used as a guide in evaluation of therapy. Positive symptoms (e.g., hallucinations, delusions, combativeness, insomnia) are more likely to respond to first-generation (typical) antipsychotic therapy (i.e., a drug like haloperidol [Haldol]). Negative symptoms (e.g., poor judgment, apathy, asocial behavior, withdrawal) are less likely to respond to treatment with first-generation antipsychotic agents.

3. The answer is E.
Each of the choices (A through D) is an extrapyramidal side effect of the first-generation (typical) antipsychotics.

4. The answer is D.
An acute dystonic reaction is characterized by involuntary tonic contractions of skeletal muscles of virtually any striated muscle group. The greatest period of risk for such a reaction usually is within the first 24–48 hr of initiating an antipsychotic agent; 95% of dystonic reactions have occurred within 96 hr of antipsychotic initiation or dosage increase. Mr. Anzalone is experiencing torticollis (muscle spasm of the neck causing the head to be twisted to the side) and oculogyric crisis (a spasm of the eye muscles causing one or both eyes to become fixed in an upward gaze). Dystonic reactions occur more often with first-generation agents (FGAs) and are more common among patients < 40 years of age; they occur approximately twice as often among men as among women. The reaction is treated initially with an anticholinergic agent such as diphenhydramine or benztropine, given intramuscularly or intravenously. Relief is usually seen within 15–20 min. The antipsychotic may be continued along with a short course of anticholinergic agent. Alternative agents include the benzodiazepines diazepam, and lorazepam.

5. The answer is B.
Akathisia is a subjective experience of motor restlessness, and patients usually complain of an inability to sit still. This adverse symptom occurs in 20–40% of patients receiving high-potency first-generation agents (FGAs). Onset of akathisia occurs within the first few weeks or months of therapy, and treatment may include dosage reduction, lipophilic β-blockers, benzodiazepines, or anticholinergic agents.

6. The answer is E (I, II, III).
All three approaches would be useful in helping this patient. Given the option of using equally effective second-generation antipsychotic agents, with which these reactions are rare, and the previously noted reactions that Mr. Anzalone has experienced with the haloperidol, it seems prudent that the best option would be to discontinue the haloperidol and switch him to a second-generation agent.

7. The answer is D.
Thioridazine (Mellaril) is a first-generation antipsychotic. The other agents —aripiprazole (Abilify), olanzapine (Zyprexa), ziprasidone (Geodon), and quetiapine (Seroquel)—are all second-generation agents. Risperidone (Risperdal) and clozapine (Clozaril) are the other second-generation agents.

8. The answer is E (I, II III).
Haloperidol decanoate is given IM every 3–4 weeks. Fluphenazine decanoate is administered every 2–3 weeks. Long-acting risperidone is administered IM every 2 weeks and was the first of the second-generation agents to be available in this dosage form.

9. The answer is C (I, II).
With the exception of clozapine, all antipsychotics (FGAs and SGAs) are thought be have similar efficacy for positive symptoms. Clozapine has demonstrated efficacy for treatment-refractory schizophrenia.

10. The answer is B.
Agranulocytosis, defined as a granulocyte count $< 500/mm^3$, occurs in association with clozapine use at a cumulative incidence at 1 year of approximately 1.3%. This reaction could prove fatal if it is not detected early and therapy is not interrupted. Patients should have a white blood cell (WBC) count before therapy begins and a clear plan for frequent (weekly), routine WBC assessment throughout therapy.

11. The answer is B.
The objective is to straighten the ear canal so that the drops are easily instilled. In a child, this is accomplished by pulling the ear backward and downward. In an adult patient, the ear canal is straightened by pulling it backward and upward.

12. The answer is A.
Carbamide peroxide is effective in softening, loosening, and helping remove cerumen from the ear canal. Although the other agents have been used in practice for years, there are no data to support their efficacy above carbamide peroxide in anhydrous glycerin. Sweet oil is another name for olive oil.

13. The answer is A.
Mineral oil (liquid petrolatum) is the only over-the-counter (OTC) lubricant laxative available. It may rarely be recommended in situations in which a soft stool is warranted, to avoid the patient from straining. In most of these cases, a stool softener would be preferable (e.g., docusate sodium). Lipid pneumonia may result if the patient takes this medication while lying down. It should not be given to bedridden patients or before bedtime for ambulatory patients. It should be taken on an empty stomach because taking it with meals will delay gastric emptying. Although the clinical effect is uncertain, mineral oil may decrease the absorption of fat-soluble vitamins A, D, E, and K. The usual dose is 15–45 mL (1–3 tablespoons). Patients will not lose fluid with this lubricant laxative as they would with a saline laxative.

14. The answer is E.
Symptoms of hemorrhoids such as burning, discomfort, irritation, inflammation, itching, pain, and swelling can all be treated safely and effectively with various over-the-counter (OTC) agents. Patients with bleeding, seepage, prolapse, thrombosis, and severe pain should be referred to a physician to rule out a cause other than a hemorrhoid.

15. The answer is D.
All of the agents would be effective for treating itching from hemorrhoids. Anusol HC-1 contains hydrocortisone, and Anusol ointment contains pramoxine (over-the-counter topical anesthetic). Preparation H cream contains phenylephrine in addition to shark liver oil, petrolatum, and glycerin. Because drugs absorbed in the anal area go directly into the systemic circulation, this agent might increase the blood pressure in this patient. An appropriate warning label against its use in hypertensive patients is on the product.

16. The answer is E (I, II, III).
Celecoxib (Celebrex) is a COX-2 inhibitor used for pain and inflammation of rheumatoid arthritis. These agents do not alter the course of the disease, nor do they prevent joint destruction. Warnings concerning postmarketing reports of serious skin reactions and hypersensitivity reactions in patients receiving this drug were issued in November 2002. Patients experiencing a rash while receiving this medication are advised to discontinue the drug immediately.

17. The answer is A (I).
Low-dose systemic corticosteroids can work well either orally or parenterally for anti-inflammatory and immunosuppressant activity. They do not alter the course of the disease, but they are often used to bridge therapy as patients are started on disease-modifying antirheumatic drugs (DMARDs). Corticosteroids will not counteract the side effects of the NSAIDs.

18. The answer is E.
All of the statements (A through D) apply to the use of Enbrel.

19. The answer is C (I, II).
Titanium dioxide is a physical sunscreen agent that blocks ultraviolet radiation over both the UVA and UVB spectrum (actually over the entire solar spectrum). Octyl methoxycinnamate blocks UVB radiation and avobenzone blocks UVA radiation, so both spectra are blocked if combined into one product. Homosalate and padimate O block only UVB radiation.

20. The answer is D.
Increased amounts of folic acid are needed during pregnancy to prevent neural tube defects of the newborn.

21. The answer is B.
Combination cancer chemotherapy regimens are now used more commonly than single-agent therapy and usually involve three or more agents. Combination regimens may have a dramatically higher response rate than single-agent therapy. Drugs given in combination generally should have different mechanisms of action, should act during different cell cycle phases, should have known activity as single agents, and should be associated with different adverse effects. Cell cycle–specific drugs may be given in combination with cell cycle–nonspecific agents.

22. The answer is A.
Cyclophosphamide is an alkylating agent. These agents affix an alkyl group to cellular DNA, causing cross-linking of DNA strands, which triggers cell death. Cell cycle–nonspecific agents kill nondividing as well as dividing cells.

23. The answer is B (III).
Only vincristine is associated with a low incidence of nausea and vomiting. Both cyclophosphamide and procarbazine are associated with relatively high incidences of nausea and vomiting (60–90%), which are caused largely by stimulation of the chemoreceptor trigger zone in the brain.

24. The answer is A (I).
Prochlorperazine (Compazine) is a phenothiazine derivative that is structurally related to thiethylperazine (Torecan). Lorazepam (Ativan) is a benzodiazepine derivative, and Tigan (trimethobenzamide) is structurally unrelated to either.

25. The answer is C.
Administration of vincristine may lead to toxic neurologic effects (e.g., peripheral neuropathy, paresthesias, ataxia). To minimize the risk of neurotoxicity, vincristine should be given in doses up to 2 mg only.

26. The answer is B.
Ondansetron is the generic name for Zofran. The brand names for the other products are Velban (vinblastine), Kytril (granisetron), Emetrol (phosphorated carbohydrate solution), and Anzemet (dolasetron).

27. The answer is E.
Prednisone (Deltasone), dexamethasone (Decadron), triamcinolone (Aristocort), and methylprednisolone (Medrol) are all adrenocorticosteroids. Medroxyprogesterone (Provera) is a progesterone derivative.

28. The answer is E (I, II, III).
Nausea and vomiting, common occurrences with many chemotherapeutic drugs, result from stimulation of the brain's CTZ. Onset of nausea and vomiting usually occurs within 3–4 hr after drug administration. In many cases, symptoms subside in < 24 hr. A few drugs (e.g., cisplatin) may cause prolonged distress. Severe nausea and vomiting may reduce patient tolerance to treatment regimens. Effective use of antiemetic drug regimens is an important adjunct to successful chemotherapy.

29. The answer is A (I).
Although all three drugs are reliable antistaphylococcal therapy, Mr. Smith's history of penicillin allergy is a contraindication for the use of penicillin derivatives such as dicloxacillin and Unasyn (ampicillin and sulbactam). Daptomycin (Cubicin) is not a penicillin derivative and is a valuable alternative for penicillin-sensitive patients. It has excellent activity against *Staphylococcus aureus* (including most methicillin-resistant strains).

30. The answer is A.
Linezolid (Zyvox) is effective treatment for vancomycin-resistant *S. aureus.* Vancoled is a brand of vancomycin, to which the organism has demonstrated resistance. Rocephin, meropenem, and cefamandole are generally ineffective for vancomycin-resistant *S. aureus.*

31. The answer is B (III).
Filgrastim (Neupogen) is used to reduce the risks of neutropenic complications in patients with cancer who are receiving myelosuppressive chemotherapy. Potential benefits include a decreased incidence of febrile neutropenia, hospitalization, and antibiotic treatment.

32. The answer is A (I).
Methylparaben and propylparaben are esters of *para*-hydroxybenzoic acid and are common preservatives for both pharmaceutical and cosmetic preparations. Sodium lauryl sulfate is an emulsifier, and the stearyl alcohol acts as an adjuvant emulsifier and adds to the hardness of the ointment. Propylene glycol is hygroscopic and acts as a humectant and co-solvent for water-soluble drugs.

33. The answer is D.

$$\frac{250 \text{ g}}{1000 \text{ g}} = \frac{X \text{ g stearyl alcohol}}{30 \text{ g total}}$$
$$X = 7.5 \text{ g stearyl alcohol}$$

34. The answer is C.
The USP lists four general classes of ointments that are used as vehicles: (1) hydrocarbon bases, represented by white petrolatum and white ointment; (2) absorption bases, represented by hydrophilic petrolatum and cold cream; (3) water-removable bases, represented by hydrophilic ointment; and (4) water-soluble bases, represented by polyethylene glycol ointment. Ophthalmic ointments are listed separately by the USP as ointments for application to the eye.

35. The answer is D.
Ramelteon (Rozerem) is the first agent that acts on the melatonin system, binding to the melatonin 1 and melatonin 2 receptors in the brain. Eszopiclone (Lunesta), zaleplon (Sonata), and zolpidem (Ambien) are benzodiazepine agonists that bind to the γ-aminobutyric acid 1 (GABA-1) receptor and the benzodiazepine receptor, but they are not benzodiazepine in structure. Triazolam (Halcion) is structurally a benzodiazepine that binds to the benzodiazepine receptor on the GABA-A receptor complex.

36. The answer is C.
Clinical studies have shown that many patients experience an early response to montelukast. Although food may increase absorption of montelukast, the drug may be administered without regard to meal times because it has a wide margin of safety and there are no dose-response effects at doses < 10 mg/day. Headache occurs at about the same frequency as observed in patients receiving placebo, and allergic rhinitis symptoms are not increased. No interaction has been demonstrated with concurrent warfarin administration.

37. The answer is D.
Triamterene-hydrochlorothiazide(Dyazide), spironolactone-hydrochlorothiazide (Aldactazide), hydrochlorothiazide (HydroDIURIL), and amiloride-hydrochlorothiazide (Moduretic) contain the thiazide diuretic hydrochlorothiazide (HCTZ), which can cause hypokalemia. However, Dyazide, Aldactazide, and Moduretic also contain a potassium-sparing diuretic, which helps prevent potassium losses. Enalapril (Vasotec) is an angiotensin-converting enzyme inhibitor that inhibits potassium loss from the kidney by inhibiting angiotensin effects.

38. The answer is D.
LMWHs (ardeparin, dalteparin, enoxaparin) can be given without anticoagulation monitoring because they have a more predictable dose-response relationship. LMWHs have longer half-lives than unfractionated heparin and can be administered subcutaneously with greater bioavailability. LMWHs are also associated with a lower risk of adverse effects typical of heparin, such as thrombocytopenia and osteoporosis.

39. The answer is E (I, II, III).
Zestril and Prinivil, brands of lisinopril, are available as 2.5-, 5-, 10-, 20-, and 40-mg tablets.

40. The answer is C.
Acetaminophen, a *para*-aminophenol derivative, interferes with prostaglandin synthesis in a manner similar to that of salicylates. However, unlike salicylates, *para*-aminophenols have little value in reducing inflammation. Flurbiprofen is a phenylpropionic acid derivative with analgesic, antipyretic, and anti-inflammatory actions. It may be beneficial in patients with contraindications for salicylates but must be used cautiously in patients with peptic ulcer disease.

41. The answer is E (I, II, III).
Cimetidine, lansoprazole, and ciprofloxacin all have demonstrated an ability to decrease the clearance of theophylline.

42. The answer is C.
Substitution in the Henderson-Hasselbalch equation gives pH = $9 + \log (10/1) = 9 + 1 = 10$. When pH is equal to pK_a, the ratio of nonionized to ionized species is 1. When the pK_a is 1 unit above or below the pH, the ratio of nonionized to ionized species is 10:1 or 1:10, respectively. For weak acid drugs, the reverse is true.

43. The answer is B.
Methotrexate (amethopterin, or MTX) is a competitive inhibitor of dihydrofolic acid reductase. Leucovorin (citrovorum factor) is used to neutralize the effects of MTX.

44. The answer is B (III).
5-Fluorouracil is commonly referred to as 5-FU. FUDR is floxuridine; 5-FC is flucytosine.

45. The answer is D (II, III).
BMI stands for body mass index. BMI = [weight (lb)/height (in^2)] $\times$ 703; $(186/66^2) \times 703 \approx 30$. It is the most commonly used indicator for obesity. Height and weight charts are available to quickly determine this number. A BMI $\geq$ 30 defines obesity. Gradual weight loss does result in a decrease in serum uric acid.

46. The answer is B (III).
Ionamin (phentermine) is structurally similar to amphetamine, but it has less severe central nervous system stimulation. Because it can cause significant increases in blood pressure, its use in hypertensive patients is not advisable. His body mass index (BMI) of 30 justifies the use of pharmacotherapy-facilitated weight loss (a BMI of 27 justifies the use of drug therapy if other risk factors such as hypertension are present); however, another agent without the adverse effect on blood pressure should probably be selected. There is no contraindication to the use of phentermine in a patient with gout.

47. The answer is A (I).
The sympathomimetic agent phenylpropanolamine and the topical anesthetic benzocaine were originally ruled as safe and effective over-the-counter (OTC) weight loss drugs. Because of safety issues (hemorrhagic stroke), phenylpropanolamine was removed from the OTC drug market. Pseudoephedrine, an oral decongestant that remains on the market for that indication, has not been shown to be an effective weight loss agent. Because of insufficient evidence of efficacy, the FDA advised manufacturers of benzocaine-containing products to remove these from the market. The manufacturers have complied, so there are no safe and effective OTC weight loss agents on the market.

48. The answer is B.
Gouty arthritis attacks occur acutely with complete resolution after a few days. The morning stiffness described in choice A is typical of rheumatoid arthritis. Metacarpophalangeal and proximal interphalangeal joint involvement is classic for rheumatoid arthritis. Gouty arthritis most commonly affects the first metatarsophalangeal joint of the big toe. Gouty arthritis attacks typically occur suddenly in the middle of the night. This scenario matches the pharmacist's note in the profile. Joint inflammation with simultaneous involvement of the same joint areas on both sides of the body may be characteristic of rheumatoid arthritis.

49. The answer is B (III).
Commit lozenges contain nicotine polacrilex (the same ingredient as nicotine gum), which is one of the newer dosage forms for nicotine replacement. Patients are instructed to use the 2-mg or 4-mg strength based on the amount of time after awakening when the urge to smoke occurs. Patients who have this urge within 30 min should use the 4-mg product.

50. The answer is A.
Although not generally given as first-line agents, corticosteroids (e.g., oral prednisone) may be used to treat acute gouty arthritis. Nonsteroidal anti-inflammatory drugs (NSAIDs) and oral colchicine are the usual first-line agents. A positive response to colchicine may help confirm the diagnosis of acute gouty arthritis, but other causes of acute arthritis may respond positively to this agent. Choices C, D, and E are "classic" components of gout. Mr. Green's presentation per his phone call to the pharmacy matches the descriptions in choices C and E. The serum uric acid reported in Mr. Green's profile (11.5mg/dL) is elevated.

51. The answer is A (I).
Aspirin in low doses (< 2 g/day) inhibits the tubular secretion of uric acid, causing uric acid to be retained. For the treatment of minor pain such as headache, dosages for both aspirin and acetaminophen are essentially the same. Reye's syndrome, an acute and potentially fatal illness, occurs with rare exceptions in children < 15 years. Fatty liver with encephalopathy develops with this syndrome. The onset most often follows an influenza or chickenpox infection. The risk for this syndrome increases with salicylate ingestion. Because of Mr. Green's age, he is not at risk for this condition.

52. The answer is B.
By almost a 10:1 margin, gout affects more males than females. Most (about two thirds) of the uric acid excreted by the body is through the kidneys, and this is helpful in using drugs such as probenecid, which aids in the excretion of uric acid through the kidneys. High-purine foods (i.e., organ meats) should be avoided because these may increase serum uric acid levels. Colchicine has no effect on serum uric acid levels. Most clinicians now select nonsteroidal anti-inflammatory drugs (NSAIDs) over colchicine because of the high incidence of diarrhea from colchicine.

53. The answer is E (I, II, III).
Initially, acute gouty arthritis attacks resolve completely, usually with no residual effects. The repeated attacks of gouty arthritis and the fact that his serum uric acid level is elevated would indicate the need for uric acid-lowering therapy. Prophylactic low doses of colchicine (usually 0.5–1.0 mg/day) may help prevent acute attacks of gouty arthritis, especially during the initiation of uric acid-lowering therapy. Thiazide diuretics (hydrochlorothiazide) may cause hyperuricemia, and switching this patient to a different antihypertensive agent would be appropriate. The use of this agent probably was what initiated his first attack on 1/6.

54. The answer is C (I, II).
Zyloprim (allopurinol) is a xanthine oxidase inhibitor that works to prevent uric acid formation from xanthine. The long half-life of the main active metabolite (oxypurinol) permits the drug to be dosed just once daily. Unlike uricosuric agents (probenecid and sulfinpyrazone), which block tubular absorption of uric acid resulting in increased amounts of uric acid in the urine, allopurinol actually decreases uric acid formation. Therefore, increased fluid intake is not required as it is with the uricosurics.

55. The answer is E (I, II, III).
To use the OTC agents, a woman must have had this condition once before, must have had it diagnosed by a physician previously, and must experience the same type of symptoms. These agents are available in 1-, 3-, and 7-day regimens. These are all "azole" antifungal agents. The characteristic symptoms are noted in choice III. Other vaginal conditions that are not amenable to OTC treatment will produce symptoms that require medical referral, such as a malodorous discharge and dysuria. Patients who experience recurrent vulvovaginal candidiasis infections (four or more over 12 months) should be referred to a physician. The FDA now requires this warning: "If your symptoms return within 2 months or if you have infections that do not clear up easily with proper treatment, consult your doctor. You could be pregnant or there could be a serious underlying medical cause for your infections, such as diabetes or a damaged immune system (including damage from infection with HIV, the virus that causes AIDS).

56. The answer is D (II, III).
Kaolin by itself (without pectin), bismuth subsalicylate, and loperamide are now considered safe and effective by the FDA for OTC use for diarrhea. Also lactase products are specifically indicated for lactase-intolerant patients. Attapulgite and calcium polycarbophil, which were previously considered safe and effective, were reclassified in April 2003 as Class III agents owing to insufficient effectiveness data. Even though the FDA has granted kaolin monograph status, no single-ingredient kaolin products are currently available in the United States.

57. The answer is E (I, II, III).
The trade name product Kaopectate was changed to contain bismuth subsalicylate, which is the same active ingredient in Pepto-Bismol original liquid. As with other salicylates, these should not be given to children or teenagers with the flu or chickenpox because of the increased risk of Reye's syndrome. A black-stained stool, which is harmless, may occur and should not be confused with melena, which is blood in the stool. Harmless darkening of the tongue can also occur with bismuth subsalicylate use.

58. The answer is C (I, II).
Lactose intolerance is relatively common. Disaccharides, like lactose and sucrose, are normally hydrolyzed by lactase. If lactase is not present, these disaccharides may produce an osmotic diarrhea. Products such as Lactaid, which contain lactase, can be administered before eating dairy products to relieve this problem. Also, lactose-free milk products can be used in place of regular milk. Calcium, although probably not in the doses present in various dairy products, will eventually cause constipation, not diarrhea.

59. The answer is C (I, II).
An SPF of 30 blocks about 97% of UVB radiation and would certainly provide maximal protection against sunburn. Any benefit from using SPFs above 30 would be negligible. All sun-exposed surfaces should be covered liberally and evenly. An average-size adult in a swimsuit would require about 1 oz per application. Perspiration, swimming, and toweling off all contribute to the need for reapplication. The SPF is a measure of only UVB protection. UVA radiation, which is relatively constant throughout the day, is not blocked by sunscreen agents that are limited to the UVB spectrum. The sunscreen agent avobenzone blocks most of the UVA rays.

60. The answer is D.
Ferrous sulfate and fumarate have higher percentages of elemental iron than the gluconate salt. Enteric-coated formulations do not dissolve until they enter the small intestine, which causes a reduction in iron absorption. The other statements concerning iron supplementation are correct.

61. The answer is E (I, II, III).
Iron-deficiency anemia usually produces a microcytic hypochromic type of anemia. The red blood cells are smaller and lighter in color than normal. The hemoglobin level in the blood will be low. Red blood cell indices such as MCV and the mean cell hemoglobin concentration (MCHC) will both be low, reflecting the microcytic and hypochromic nature of the red cells. Total iron-binding capacity will be high.

62. The answer is B (III).

Iron preparations form a chelate with tetracycline, inhibiting its absorption; therefore, iron preparations should not be administered with oral tetracyclines. If a patient needs both types of therapy, the iron product should be administered 3 hr before or 2 hr after the tetracycline to minimize the adverse interaction.

63. The answer is E (I, II, III).

Common organisms that can cause PID include *Neisseria gonorrhoeae* and *Chlamydia trachomatis.* Empiric treatment is, therefore, directed toward eradicating these organisms. One of the options for empiric outpatient treatment uses a combination regimen of ceftriaxone (Rocephin) given intramuscularly once followed by doxycycline given for 14 days.

64. The answer is B (III).

The patient does not have any symptoms of gout or any notation of an elevated uric acid level. Benemid (probenecid) could be used for long-term management of those two conditions, but she received only one dose. Probenecid competes with the tubular secretion of β-lactam antibiotics, resulting in prolongation of serum levels. The Centers for Disease Control and Prevention (CDC) recommendations for pelvic inflammatory disease include probenecid as part of the regimen.

65. The answer is A.

Tetracycline and other broad-spectrum antibiotics are a common cause for vulvovaginal candidiasis. Estrogen-containing oral contraceptives (e.g., Triphasil-28) might cause this problem, but it was started after the candida infection. The other agents, ferrous sulfate and Tylenol with Codeine, are not associated with the development of this infection.

66. The answer is C.

Tetracyclines are broad-spectrum agents effective against gram-negative and gram-positive organisms, spirochetes, *Mycoplasma* and *Chlamydia* organisms, rickettsial species, and certain protozoa. Phototoxic reactions (enhanced sunburn) can develop with exposure to sunlight. Doxycycline has the least binding affinity for calcium ions of any of the tetracyclines, but the net effect is a slight decrease in absorption, not an increase. Unlike other tetracycline derivatives, food and/or antacids do not significantly inhibit absorption of doxycycline. Gastrointestinal distress is a common adverse effect of all tetracyclines; it may be minimized by concurrent administration with food.

67. The answer is E (I, II, III).

Tetracyclines are mainly bacteriostatic, but at high concentrations they can be bactericidal. They inhibit bacterial protein synthesis by binding to the 30S and possibly the 50S ribosomal subunit(s), thus interfering with the transfer of genetic information. They may also inhibit the bacterial cytoplasmic membrane, reducing membrane stability and thus causing bacterial cell lysis.

68. The answer is E (I, II, III).

Single-dose oral fluconazole has been shown to have clinical efficacy as good as or better than topical antifungal products. Because it can be given as a single oral tablet, it is considered cleaner than topical agents, many of which need to be dosed three or more times to reach the efficacy afforded by one oral dose of fluconazole. These factors have led to improved patient compliance.

69. The answer is E (I, II, III).

Patients who experience these recurrent vulvovaginal candidiasis infections may be experiencing a mixed infection or a strain of candidal infection other than *C. albicans.* These infections might be resistant to standard therapy. All of the statements are correct.

70. The answer is D (II, III).

Clindamycin is commonly associated with the development of pseudomembranous colitis or *Clostridium difficile* colitis as a side effect. Vancomycin and metronidazole are commonly used to treat antibiotic-associated *C. difficile* colitis when discontinuation of the offending antibiotic does not fully resolve the condition.

71. The answer is C.
Ketoconazole is an oral agent effective for treating systemic fungal infections. Butoconazole, clotrimazole, and miconazole are administered topically or vaginally for local infection. Nystatin is a polyene antifungal antibiotic, not a substituted imidazole derivative. It is available for topical and vaginal administration to treat local infections. Nystatin oral tablets are not absorbed and are, therefore, therapeutic only for infections of the gastrointestinal tract, especially oral and esophageal *Candida* infections.

72. The answer is D (II, III).
Phenytoin, primidone, and carbamazepine are all agents indicated for treatment of generalized tonic–clonic seizures. Primidone metabolizes to phenobarbital; therefore, patients who are allergic to phenobarbital should not receive primidone. Carbamazepine is contraindicated in patients with hypersensitivity to tricyclic antidepressants, such as amitriptyline.

73. The answer is B (III).
Depakote is an enteric-coated preparation of valproic acid and should not be crushed. All enteric-coated products must remain intact to prevent dissolution in the stomach.

74. The answer is E (I, II, III).
As many as 54–86% of women receiving hormone-replacement therapy (estrogen–progestin replacement therapy) will experience irregular uterine bleeding. Other adverse effects include breast tenderness, headache, nausea, and weight gain.

75. The answer is B.
The normal therapeutic range for phenytoin serum levels is 10–20 mg/mL. Nystagmus, ataxia, and slurred speech have been reported with serum levels of 20–30 mg/mL, with coma reported when the level reaches 40 mg/mL.

76. The answer is D (II, III).
Folic acid enhances phenytoin (hydantoin) clearance, which can result in reduced phenytoin serum levels and loss of efficacy. Carbamazepine (Tegretol) may also enhance phenytoin metabolism and thus reduce plasma phenytoin levels and therapeutic efficacy. Phenytoin has the same effect on carbamazepine.

77. The answer is A (I).
Good oral hygiene, including gum massage, frequent brushing and flossing, and appropriate dental care, may decrease gingival hyperplasia related to phenytoin (Dilantin) use.

78. The answer is C.
Penicillins such as Amoxil have not been shown to affect carbamazepine (Tegretol) levels. Erythromycin (EES or E-Mycin 333), isoniazid (Laniazid), and troleandomycin (Tao) all have reportedly increased Tegretol levels.

79. The answer is A.
Nystagmus is an early sign of phenytoin (Dilantin) intoxication. Other reactions common with phenytoin use are confusion, slurred speech, drowsiness, and ataxia. All are dose-related adverse effects involving the central nervous system.

80. The answer is E (I, II, III).
Phenytoin sodium (Dilantin) is available as a capsule, as a tablet, and as an ampule for IV administration.

81. The answer is C.
Vaseretic 5-12.5 contains enalapril 5 mg and hydrochlorothiazide (HCTZ) 12.5 mg.

82. The answer is B.
Diplopia, nausea and ataxia are the most common dose-related side effects associated with carbamazepine.

83. The answer is A (I).
Acetaminophen (Tylenol) has analgesic and antipyretic activity but very little anti-inflammatory activity. Aspirin, not acetaminophen, is contraindicated in small children with fever caused by a viral infection because they are susceptible to Reye syndrome.

84. The answer is B.
The brand name for fosphenytoin is Cerebyx. The generic name for Dilantin is phenytoin, for Valium is diazepam, for Lamictal is lamotrigine, and for Topamax is topiramate.

85. The answer is B.
When tetracycline is administered with a calcium-containing antacid, a complex is formed that reduces the absorption of tetracycline. Synergism is an example of potentiation of one drug's interaction with another—for example, when aminoglycosides are combined with agents such as mezlocillin, their combined effect is greater than the addition of each individual effect. Competitive antagonism results when two agents compete for the same receptor site, such as when atropine sulfate competes with acetylcholine for the cholinergic receptor site.

86. The answer is B.
Reported adverse drug reactions with quinupristin/dalfopristin (Synercid) are generally mild and infusion-related: pain, erythema, or itching at the infusion site, increases in pulse and diastolic blood pressure, headache, nausea or vomiting, and diarrhea. Synercid does not alter hematologic or renal indices, but it may increase liver function tests slightly.

87. The answer is B (III).
Naloxone, which is a pure opioid antagonist, reverses or prevents the effects of opioids but has no opioid-receptor agonist activity. Naloxone is not absorbed after oral administration; however, after IV administration, it blocks the pharmacologic effects of pentazocine (Talwin), producing withdrawal symptoms in opioid-dependent persons.

88. The answer is D.
Bactrim DS contains 160 mg trimethoprim and 800 mg sulfamethoxazole; thus 20 mL of co-trimoxazole suspension would be required to provide an equivalent dose.

89. The answer is D.
Accurbron is the brand name for a theophylline liquid preparation. Slo-Phyllin Gyrocaps, Sustaire, Aerolate JR, and Theovent are theophylline sustained-release preparations.

90. The answer is A.
The Schilling test is used to diagnose pernicious anemia, or vitamin B_{12} deficiency. Hematocrit, hemoglobin, and serum folate measurements are not specific for B_{12} deficiency. The Schlichter test is used in bacterial endocarditis to ensure adequate antibiotic concentration in the blood.

91. The answer is E (I, II, III).
Potassium chloride is available as an oral solution, as a powder, and as a liquid to be given by IV injection. For ambulatory use, potassium chloride is available as an oral solution or as a powder in a packet to be mixed with water or juice. The injection form is for rapid IV potassium repletion or as an addition to total parenteral nutrition (TPN).

92. The answer is B.
Postural hypotension is commonly experienced with α_1-blockers, including doxazosin, because of the direct action.

93. The answer is B.
Prilosec OTC is available as salmon-colored tablets; prescription Prilosec 20 mg is available as purple capsules.

94. The answer is D.
Benzathine penicillin 2.4 million units once is the preferred therapy for syphilis. All other choices (ceftriaxone, metronidazole, azithromycin, or tetracycline regimens) are inappropriate.

95. The answer is D.
Hyperkalemia is a major risk with potassium-sparing diuretics, and potassium supplementation is, therefore, contraindicated. To reduce the risk of hyperkalemia, the patient may use a combination of diuretic products such as Dyazide (triamterene with HCTZ), Aldactazide (spironolactone with HCTZ), or other combinations.

96. The answer is A (I).
Absolute bioavailability is a measurement of the fraction of the dose that is systemically absorbed. To estimate absolute bioavailability, the AUC after the drug product is given orally is compared with the AUC after an IV bolus dose, because only the IV bolus dose is known to be 100% absorbed. Relative bioavailability compares the AUC of one dosage form with that of another dosage form, usually a drug solution or reference drug product given by the same route of administration.

97. The answer is D.
Acetazolamide (Diamox) is a carbonic anhydrase inhibitor and a nonbacteriostatic sulfonamide derivative. Sulfamethizole (Thiosulfil Forte) is a sulfonamide antibiotic. Therefore, cross-sensitivity may exist between these drugs.

98. The answer is B.
Antacids, which act to neutralize gastric acids, are available primarily as magnesium, aluminum, calcium, or sodium salts. A product that is a combination of magnesium and aluminum salts permits a lower dosage of each compound. In addition, with such a combination, the constipating effect of the aluminum salt counteracts the laxative effect of the magnesium salt, thereby minimizing the consequences of each compound.

99. The answer is C.
Only Entocort EC is FDA approved for treatment of Crohn disease. Although frequently used to treat patients with Crohn disease, other corticosteroids have not been approved for such indication by the FDA.

100. The answer is E (I, II, III).
Helicobacter pylori infection is present in the majority of duodenal ulcer patients. The major benefit to eradication of the infection is prevention of recurrent ulcer disease. Ulcers recur in > 80% of *H. pylori*–positive patients whose duodenal ulcers are healed within 1 year. Eradication prevents recurrence in most patients and may eliminate the need for maintenance antisecretory therapy. Treatment of active duodenal ulcers is best managed with a combination of antisecretory agents to relieve symptoms and heal the ulcer, and appropriate antibiotics to eradicate the infection and prevent recurrence.

101. The answer is E (I, II, III).
Nonsteroidal anti-inflammatory drugs (NSAIDs) such as ibuprofen are inhibitors of prostaglandin synthesis. Although the inhibition is an important mechanism for anti-inflammatory therapy, it also compromises the protective effects that prostaglandins exert on the gastric mucosa. NSAIDs can also injure the gastric mucosa directly by allowing back-diffusion of hydrogen ions into the mucosa. NSAIDs are independent risk factors for peptic ulcer disease and can cause ulcers in *Helicobacter pylori*–negative patients. In fact, NSAIDs are the principal cause of ulcers in patients who are not infected.

102. The answer is D.
The addition of clarithromycin to this patient's regimen is intended to prevent ulcer recurrence and rebleeding. Symptom resolution and ulcer healing are produced by the antisecretory therapy (omeprazole), and efficacy for these outcomes is not changed by addition of the antibiotic. Neither drug seems to stop bleeding, although it is believed that increasing intragastric pH with antisecretory agents may improve clotting. NSAIDs are independent risk factors for ulcers, and eradication of the infection does not prevent ulcers caused by NSAIDs.

103. The answer is D.
For any first-order process, 50% of the initial amount of drug is eliminated at the end of the first half-life, and 50% of the remaining amount of drug (i.e., 75% of the original amount) is eliminated at the end of the second half-life. The half-life for ranitidine is about 2 hr; therefore, in 2 hr 50% of the drug is eliminated, and in 4 hr 75% of the drug is eliminated.

104. The answer is B.
Cimetidine is known to bind to the cytochrome P450 mixed-function oxidative pathway of the liver. This binding affinity may interfere with the metabolism of other agents dependent on this route of clearance. These agents include phenytoin, theophylline, phenobarbital, lidocaine, warfarin, imipramine, diazepam, and propranolol.

105. The answer is E.
Prevacid (lansoprazole), Prilosec (omeprazole), Protonix (pantoprazole), and Nexium (esomeprazole) are proton pump inhibitors. Pepcid (famotidine) is an H_2-receptor antagonist.

106. The answer is E.
Biaxin Suspension should be stored at room temperature. It should be shaken well before use. Appropriate advice for the patient should include recommendations to take the complete 10 days of antibiotics required for eradication, together with Nexium 40 mg daily. Finally, administration of clarithromycin with food may minimize gastrointestinal complaints.

107. The answer is A.
Bismuth is not well absorbed after administration of bismuth subsalicylate or bismuth subcitrate. Only bismuth subsalicylate (Pepto-Bismol) is available in the United States. Bismuth compounds discolor the stool black; this may alarm patients because black stools may also be a sign of blood (gastrointestinal bleeding). Bismuth compounds have been effectively combined with antibiotics and antisecretory compounds to eradicate *Helicobacter pylori*. Large doses of bismuth subsalicylate may cause salicylism.

108. The answer is E (I, II, III).
Misoprostol is the only agent approved to protect patients from NSAID-induced gastric ulcers. Misoprostol is a synthetic prostaglandin that appears to suppress gastric acid secretion and may provide a mucosal protective effect. It is used in patients taking NSAID therapy to counter the undesired effect that these compounds exert on prostaglandin activity in the parietal cell of the gastric mucosa. Misoprostol is contraindicated in pregnant women because it may induce spontaneous uterine contractions.

109. The answer is D.
Theobroma oil (cocoa butter) is a mixed triglyceride suppository base that melts at 34°–35°C. Its emollient and nonirritating characteristics allow its use as a base for hemorrhoidal suppositories. Glycerinated gelatin suppositories are used as vaginal suppositories for the local application of antibacterial agents. Glycerin or soap suppositories contain sodium stearate, which is used for its laxative effect. Polyethylene glycol bases are water-miscible suppository bases used with various drugs for systemic absorption.

110. The answer is B.
Remicade (infliximab) prescribing information contains a warning that tuberculosis (frequently disseminated or extrapulmonary at clinical presentation) and other opportunistic infections have been observed in patients receiving the drug. Some of these infections have been fatal. It is recommended that patients be evaluated for latent tuberculosis with a tuberculin skin test and that therapy of latent tuberculosis be initiated before therapy with infliximab.

111. The answer is E.
The amount of Peruvian balsam in one suppository (2 g) is equal to 0.018 × 2000 mg; therefore, for 12 suppositories

$$0.018 \times \left(\frac{2000 \text{ mg}}{\text{suppositories}}\right) \times 12 \text{ suppositories} = 432 \text{ mg}$$

112. The answer is C (I, II).
Pediazole suspension (erythromycin and sulfisoxazole) requires proper shaking before each dose. As with other sulfonamides, a full glass of water is recommended with each dose to ensure adequate hydration to minimize the risk of crystalluria.

113. The answer is C (I, II).
Patients receiving metronidazole may experience a disulfiram-type reaction if they consume alcohol concurrently with the drug. Tachycardia and flushing may occur if alcohol is consumed during DDI therapy. The use of DDI and alcohol should be avoided because of the potential for drug-induced pancreatitis. These reactions have not been reported in patients receiving itraconazole.

114. The answer is C (I, II).
Rifampin colors urine, sweat, tears, saliva, and feces orange-red. Clofazimine may discolor urine, sweat, and other body fluids pink to brownish. Clofazimine produces pink to brownish skin pigmentation in 75–100% of patients within a few weeks. The skin discoloration has led to severe depression in some patients. Atovaquone produces no body fluid discoloration or skin pigmentation.

115. The answer is E (I, II, III).
Cisplatin, foscarnet, and amphotericin B can cause nephrotoxicity. Renal function tests should be performed and serum creatinine levels and blood urea nitrogen (BUN) should be monitored when these medications are administered.

116. The answer is E (I, II, III).
Although the theory is controversial, it is thought that drugs that are highly bound to albumin will have higher concentrations of free drug circulating in the blood if albumin levels are reduced. Hypoalbuminemia, liver (hepatic) disease, malnutrition, and cancer are several of the more common conditions that result in decreased albumin levels, which necessitate alterations in dosage in highly albumin-bound drugs.

117. The answer is D.
The generic name for Accolate is zafirlukast. It is a leukotriene receptor antagonist used for the prophylaxis and treatment of asthma.

118. The answer is B.
Tremor is often the dose-limiting side effect related to terbutaline use. Tremor also has been reported to occur with other sympathomimetic drugs.

119. The answer is B (III).
Cefuroxime (Ceftin, Kefurox, Zinacef) is a second-generation cephalosporin. Alcohol consumption can result in a disulfiram-type reaction in patients receiving cefamandole (or the third-generation agents moxalactam and cefoperazone), but this does not occur with cefuroxime. Cefuroxime often is prescribed as an alternative to ampicillin (as is cefamandole) to treat community-acquired pneumonia and is administered in a dosage of 2.25–4.5 g per day, which is divided and given every 8 hr. All cephalosporins should be used cautiously in penicillin-allergic patients.

120. The answer is C.
Atrovent (ipratropium) should not be used for symptom relief or for exacerbations of bronchospasm. The onset of action is within 15 min, and the agent is useful mainly for maintenance regimens in patients with chronic obstructive pulmonary disease (COPD) and some patients with asthma. The other agents listed have more rapid onsets (within 5 min) and are useful to relieve acute bronchospasm.

121. The answer is B.
Amoxicillin has a spectrum of antimicrobial activity similar to that of ampicillin. It has a longer half-life, which allows less frequent dosing (250–500 mg every 8 hr, as opposed to ampicillin, which is given in a dosage of 250 mg–2 g every 4–6 hr). Both drugs may produce an erythematous, maculopapular rash not seen with other penicillins. Amoxicillin has more complete oral absorption than ampicillin—a characteristic that may explain the lower frequency of diarrhea as a side effect. It is contraindicated in patients with a history of hypersensitivity to other penicillins.

122. The answer is A (I).

With this patient's recent history of rash caused by amoxicillin, ampicillin should be avoided because an erythematous, maculopapular rash or an urticarial hypersensitivity is seen with other penicillins. Ciprofloxacin and erythromycin are both reasonable alternatives in terms of the potential interaction of these agents with theophylline (Slo-Phyllin).

123. The answer is D.

For optimal dose retention, patients should be instructed to wait 1 min between each puff. Longer waits between puffs are unnecessary and may contribute to nonadherence to the prescribed regimen. Patients using steroid inhalers, especially, should be instructed to rinse well after completing their dosing. If the immediate response to an inhaled β-agonist needs to be documented, patients should wait until all of their puffs have been administered before checking their peak flows. Lying down is unnecessary following administration of inhaled agents.

124. The answer is B (III).

Only ofloxacin (Floxin) is suitable for systemic infections such as pneumonia. Cinoxacin and norfloxacin are indicated for only urinary tract infections.

125. The answer is C (I, II).

Fever is an important monitoring parameter in infectious diseases; however, administration of antipyretics masks fever. Subsidence of a fever (defervescence) usually indicates a favorable response to therapy. Fever should be treated only if the patient has chills or if the fever is dangerously high. If needed, acetaminophen or aspirin is acceptable. Because fever sometimes stems from noninfectious conditions that do not respond to antibiotics (e.g., metabolic disorders, drug reactions, and neoplasms), fever should not be treated with anti-infective agents unless infection has been identified as the cause.

126. The answer is A (I).

Of the medications that this patient is receiving, only theophylline levels are commonly measured. These tests are available through commercial clinical laboratories.

127. The answer is E.

Crestor is currently available as 5-, 10-, 20-, and 40-mg tablets. There is currently no 80-mg tablet.

128. The answer is C (I, II).

Bioequivalent drug products must contain the same active ingredient in the same chemical form and in the same amount (i.e., they must be pharmaceutical equivalents), and they must have the same rate and extent of systemic drug absorption (i.e., the same bioavailability). The inactive ingredients or excipients may be different.

129. The answer is C (I, II).

Theophylline is an agent that depends on the cytochrome P450 microsomal enzyme for its metabolism. Tobacco tars and phenobarbital are both considered to be enzyme inducers of the cytochrome P450 microsomal enzyme system; consequently, theophylline metabolism may be increased in patients taking these agents concurrently. The H_2-receptor antagonists cimetidine and ranitidine have both been shown to inhibit the P450 enzyme system and thus reduce theophylline metabolism.

130. The answer is B.

Anemia is a common complication of chronic renal failure caused by a decrease in production of erythropoietin and endocrine product in the kidney. Erythropoietin, or epoetin α (Epogen, Procrit), stimulates red blood cell production in the bone marrow. This production is reflected by an increase in hematocrit and hemoglobin and a decrease in the need for blood transfusions. Recently, erythropoietin has been approved for the treatment of anemia in HIV-positive patients or for the prevention of anemia owing to zidovudine (AZT).

131. The answer is C.
The most frequently reported adverse effects of raloxifene include hot flashes (up to 28% of women) and leg cramps (5.9%). Raloxifene has not been associated with irregular uterine bleeding or breast tenderness. Gastrointestinal complaints and allergic manifestations occur less frequently.

132. The answer is E (I, II, III).
Emulsifying agents, also known as wetting agents, surfactants, or surface-active agents (e.g., soaps, sodium lauryl sulfate, and dioctyl sodium sulfosuccinate), lower the surface and interfacial tension. These agents permit more intimate contact between an aqueous (water) phase and a lipid phase.

133. The answer is C.
Amitiza (lubiprostone) is indicated for treatment of chronic idiopathic constipation in adults.

134. The answer is E (I, II, III).
Pyrimethamine, trimethoprim, and methotrexate act on the folic acid pathway to inhibit reduction of dihydrofolic acid to tetrahydrofolic acid by the enzyme dihydrofolate reductase.

135. The answer is D.
Salicylic acid is commonly used externally as a keratolytic in corn and wart preparations (e.g., Wart-Off and Freezone) to remove the horny layers of the skin in a process known as desquamation.

136. The answer is D.
Products containing benzoyl peroxide, sulfur, salicylic acid (3–6%), and resorcinol (1–2%) have been shown to be effective agents in the treatment of acne vulgaris. Benzoyl peroxide (Fostex), salicylic acid (PROPApH), sulfur (Liquimat and Fostex Medicated Cover-Up), and resorcinol and sulfur (Rezamid Lotion) are available OTC anti-acne products. Carmol-HC, a urea-containing product that also contains hydrocortisone, is effective in treating dry skin.

137. The answer is B (III).
Patients with type 1, or insulin-dependent, diabetes, are normally younger, are not obese, have an absolute lack of insulin in the pancreas, and are predisposed to ketoacidosis if they do not receive insulin.

138. The answer is B.
The choices are all steroids. Estrogenic steroids have an aromatic A ring. Progesterone and other progestins are derivatives of pregnane.

139. The answer is D.
Any disturbance in the balance between dopaminergic receptors and cholinergic receptors seems to result in various movement disorders. Increases in acetylcholine and decreases in dopamine, norepinephrine, serotonin, or GABA have been linked to the development of various forms of Parkinson disease. These alterations may occur because of the aging process, infection, drug consumption, or trauma.

140. The answer is B.
Aliphatic phenothiazine derivatives such as chlorpromazine and the piperidine derivatives mesoridazine (Serentil) and thioridazine (Mellaril) have the lowest risk for extrapyramidal side effects. Piperazine derivatives such as acetophenazine (Tindal), perphenazine (Trilafon), trifluoperazine (Stelazine), and fluphenazine (Prolixin), along with the thioxanthene derivatives thiothixene (Navane) and chlorprothixene (Taractan), have the highest likelihood of causing extrapyramidal side effects among the phenothiazines. The butyrophenone derivative haloperidol (Haldol) and the dihydroindolone derivative molindone (Moban) are also highly capable of inducing extrapyramidal side effects.

141. The answer is D.
Aminophylline, the parenteral form of theophylline, is commonly available as the dihydrate salt and contains approximately 80% theophylline. Enter this information into the calculation of the final serum concentration by first converting the aminophylline dose into the equivalent theophylline dose. The expected serum concentration then can be calculated by dividing the corrected theophylline dose by the volume of distribution and adding that to the initial level of 7.5 mg/mL in this patient. The calculations are as follows:

$$250 \text{ mg aminophylline bolus} = 200 \text{ mg theophylline}$$
$$250 \times 0.80 = 200$$
$$C = \frac{\text{Dose}}{V_D} = \frac{200 \text{ mg}}{0.5 \text{L/kg}} = \frac{200 \text{ mg}}{0.5 \text{ L/kg} \times 71.8 \text{ kg}} = \frac{200 \text{ mg}}{36 \text{ L}} = 5.55 \text{ } \mu\text{g/mL}$$
$$5.55 + 7.5 = 13.05 = 13.1 \text{ } \mu\text{g/mL}$$

142. The answer is E (I, II, III).
Drugs that follow two-compartment pharmacokinetics have a rapid distribution phase, followed by a slower elimination phase representing the elimination of the drug after equilibration with the body. The plasma drug concentration at any time is the sum of two first-order processes. The slope of the terminal elimination phase, b, is generally used in the calculation of a dosage regimen.

143. The answer is D.
Competitive binding of cimetidine (and ranitidine) to the cytochrome P450 mixed-function oxidase metabolic pathway of the liver acts to interfere with the metabolism of other drugs dependent on this pathway. Phenytoin, theophylline, phenobarbital, lidocaine, warfarin, imipramine, diazepam, and propranolol may be cleared more slowly and their effects may be accentuated if they are administered concomitantly with cimetidine or ranitidine.

144. The answer is D (II, III).
First-order elimination kinetics is expressed as $C = C_0 e^{-kt}$, where $C = 1.2$ mg/mL, $C_0 = 6.2$ mg/mL, and $t = 11$ hr. By substitution, $1.2 = 6.2 e^{-k(11)}$; $k = 0.149$ hr^{-1}. The $t_{1/2}$ is estimated by the relationship, $t_{1/2} = 0.693/k$. Therefore, $t_{1/2} = 0.693/0.149 = 4.65$ hr. The dose and serum concentration must be known to determine the volume of distribution for this patient. A dose of 100 mg is reported to achieve a C_{max} of 7.2 μg/mL based on a trough value of 1.2 μg/mL, or an increase of 6.0 μg/mL.

$$V_D = \frac{100 \text{ mg}}{6.0 \text{ } \mu\text{g/mL}} = 16.6 \text{ L or } 0.23 \text{ L/kg}$$

145. The answer is D.
The MIC for an antibiotic indicates the lowest concentration of antibiotic that prevents microbial growth after 18–24 hr of incubation. Typically, the peak antibiotic concentration at the site of infection must be four to five times the MIC to be considered therapeutic and effective.

146. The answer is B.
True cross-reactivity between cephalosporin antibiotics and penicillin is considered rare. Commonly, the rate of cross-reactivity is approximately 10%.

147. The answer is D.
If the patient is receiving 32 mg theophylline per hour by IV infusion, then the patient should receive the oral dose of theophylline at the same approximate dosing rate:
Theophylline dose = 32 mg × 12 hr = 384 mg
Therefore, the patient should be given 400 mg of theophylline controlled-release product every 12 hr.

148. The answer is E (I, II, III).
Conversion from IV to oral theophylline dosing should be accomplished using a sustained-release theophylline preparation designed to deliver a daily dose of theophylline comparable to the dose from the IV infusion. Although food may delay the achievement of a "peak" theophylline level, the amount absorbed is not compromised. A steady-state theophylline level is achievable if no doses are missed within the preceding 48-hr period. Reasonable sampling time should be within 3–7 hr of dosing.

149. The answer is C (I, II).
To demonstrate bioequivalency of two products, both must be the same dosage form (e.g., both must be controlled-release tablets), both must contain the same amount of the same active ingredient, and both must be given in the same dose and via the same route of administration. This manufacturer's study is, instead, a bioavailability study to demonstrate the controlled-release characteristics of the tablet.

150. The answer is C.
It is recommended that COPD patients receive influenza vaccine annually, usually in the fall. Frequent viral mutations require administration of the most current vaccine each year to ensure protection from the current virus strain(s) causing infections.

151. The answer is C (I, II).
Dextromethorphan is a dextro-isomer of levorphanol, and many clinicians consider it equivalent to codeine as an antitussive. It depresses the cough center in the medulla. Diphenhydramine has both antitussive and antihistamine properties. Its antitussive effect results from direct medullary action. Dihydrocodeinone (hydrocodone) is a narcotic antitussive available only in prescription products.

152. The answer is E (I, II, III).
PTU and methimazole may help attain remission in hyperthyroid patients. Both agents inhibit iodide oxidation and iodotyrosyl coupling. PTU (but not methimazole) also diminishes peripheral deiodination of thyroxine (T_4) to triiodothyronine (T_3). These drugs can be used to induce remission by themselves or as adjunctive therapy with radioiodine. They can be used for preoperative preparation of hyperthyroid patients to establish and maintain a euthyroid state until definitive surgery can be performed. Dermatologic reactions (e.g., rash, urticaria, pruritus, hair loss, and skin pigmentation) are the most troublesome. Patients receiving either PTU or methimazole are at increased risk for developing agranulocytosis.

153. The answer is B (III).
Atropine is a belladonna alkaloid that possesses anticholinergic properties. Vincristine (Oncovin) and vinblastine (Velban) are vinca alkaloids used in the treatment of various malignancies.

154. The answer is A.
Spiriva (tiotropium bromide) is an anticholinergic agent used to treat bronchospasm associated with chronic obstructive pulmonary disease (COPD) that may aggravate narrow angle glaucoma.

155. The answer is E (I, II, III).
Ampules, the oldest form of parenteral vehicle, are composed entirely of glass, which may break during transport. Because the ampule is cut open on use, glass particles may be mixed with the drug substance. Therefore, all drugs supplied in ampules must be filtered before use to remove any glass particles from the solution. Once broken open, the solution must be used to avoid contamination, and it is thus not a multiple-dose product.

156. The answer is B.
Half-normal saline solution (0.45% sodium chloride) has an osmotic pressure less than that of blood and is referred to as a hypotonic solution. Isotonic and isosmotic solutions have osmotic pressures that are equal to blood. Normal saline solution, 0.9% sodium chloride, usually is given as an example of an isotonic solution. Hypertonic solutions have osmotic pressures greater than blood (e.g., high concentrations of dextrose used in total parenteral therapy).

157. The answer is A (I).
Drug substances that have narrow therapeutic indexes (i.e., for which the difference between a therapeutic effect and a toxic effect is small, such as with heparin) may be given via the continuous infusion route. This method allows less fluctuation in blood levels of such drugs. Intermittent infusions, although used extensively in medicine, provide for greater differences between peak effects and trough effects compared to agents with narrow therapeutic indexes. Agents such as norepinephrine, nitroprusside, and dopamine, which have very short half-lives, are routinely given by continuous infusion to provide a continuous therapeutic effect, which would not be available from intermittent dosing.

158. The answer is B.
Aluminum hydroxide (Amphojel) is used in patients with renal failure because it binds excess phosphate in the intestine, thereby reducing the serum phosphate concentration. The aluminum hydroxide can be in liquid or tablet form and is administered three or four times daily with meals.

159. The answer is A.
Kayexalate, or sodium polystyrene sulfonate (SPS), is an ion-exchange resin that exchanges sodium ion for potassium in the intestines. SPS, with its potassium content, is excreted in the feces. The result is a decrease in potassium levels in the serum and other body fluids.

160. The answer is A.
Chronic renal failure causes a normochromic, normocytic anemia, usually reflected in a decreased hemoglobin and decreased hematocrit. In most patients, the hematocrit is between 20% and 30%.

161. The answer is D (II, III).
The major route of elimination for both digoxin and tobramycin (an aminoglycoside) is the kidney. Both medications require dosage adjustment in patients with acute or chronic renal failure. Haloperidol is mainly metabolized by the liver and, therefore, would not need dosage adjustment.

162. The answer is C.
Calcitriol is 1,25-dihydroxycholecalciferol, the active form of vitamin D_2. Because of its increased efficacy, calcitriol is the preferred form of vitamin D therapy used in patients with renal failure. Vitamin D enhances calcium absorption from the gut and is used to treat the hypocalcemia that occurs in renal failure.

163. The answer is C (I, II).
Aluminum hydroxide gel (Amphojel), which is used to treat the patient's hyperphosphatemia, and sodium polystyrene sulfonate (SPS; Kayexalate), which is used to treat his hyperkalemia, are both major causes of constipation.

164. The answer is A (I).
Calcium chloride or gluconate is used to treat potassium-induced arrhythmias. Loop diuretics and sodium polystyrene sulfonate (SPS) do not have a significant effect on potassium in a short period to treat life-threatening arrhythmia. SPS and loop diuretics, along with dialysis, may be considered to remove potassium in the short term, preventing recurrence of arrhythmias.

165. The answer is B.
The most common adverse reaction to haloperidol is extrapyramidal effects, which include dystonic reactions, akinesia, drug-induced parkinsonism, and tardive dyskinesia. Cardiovascular and anticholinergic side effects occur less frequently. Neuroleptic malignant syndrome is rare. A decreased seizure threshold is uncommon, except in patients with a history of seizures.

166. The answer is A (I).
Antacids, when given at the same time as cimetidine, decrease the absorption of cimetidine from the stomach. No interaction occurs between cimetidine and Colace or ferrous sulfate.

167. The answer is E.
Chemotherapeutic agents may cause dysfunction of many organ systems. Patients treated with daunorubicin, doxorubicin, and mitoxantrone are at greater risk for developing cardiotoxicity, ranging from electrocardiogram changes to cardiomyopathy. The risk is dose-related and cumulative. Total dose for daunorubicin should not exceed 550 mg/m^2.

168. The answer is B (III).
Alopecia occurs 1–2 weeks after treatment with most chemotherapeutic agents. Neither cytarabine nor daunorubicin causes renal dysfunction or peripheral neuropathy.

169. The answer is B.
When extravasation takes place, the needle is left in place and excess drug is drawn off with a syringe. A corticosteroid is injected to reduce local inflammation. Ice can also be applied. Sodium bicarbonate can be injected when the extravasation involves doxorubicin and other anthracyclines. Local anesthetics (e.g., potassium chloride) are not recommended and can cause local tissue damage.

170. The answer is C.
Ortho-Novum 1/50 contains 50 mg estrogen. When it is continuously administered, the monthly menstrual period will be suppressed. After chemotherapy, thrombocytopenia and neutropenia can occur, and Ms. Peterson will be at risk for increased bleeding owing to thrombocytopenia.

171. The answer is C (I, II).
The chemotherapeutic agents used to treat Ms. Peterson cause myelosuppression, with attendant infection and bleeding, usually 10–14 days after chemotherapy. White blood cell lines, leukocytes, granulocytes, and platelets are affected because of their shorter life span.

172. The answer is A.
Chemotherapeutic agents may be toxic to the pharmacist if handled improperly; therefore, many organizations have developed special guidelines. A vertical (rather than horizontal) laminar flow hood should be used to prevent airborne particles from contaminating room air. Special techniques, equipment, and protective gowns and gloves are recommended.

173. The answer is A.
Patients with hypertension should avoid the SNRIs venlafaxine and duloxetine because of the risk of increased blood pressure. Tricyclic antidepressants may interact with antihypertensive agents to either intensify or counteract their effect.

174. The answer is D.
Ms. Peterson is allergic to penicillin. Cross-sensitivity between cephalosporins and penicillins is currently approximately 10%. The literature still recommends caution when cephalosporins are administered to patients with acute nonlymphocytic leukemia and an allergy to penicillin.

175. The answer is B (III).
Gentamicin, an aminoglycoside, is excreted unchanged in the urine. The drug accumulates in the proximal tubule, causing renal damage in up to 25% of patients. The aminoglycosides do not cause hepatotoxicity or neurotoxicity.

176. The answer is D.
The approved dosage of ranitidine for management of GERD is 150 mg four times a day. GERD treatment requires aggressive acid inhibition that will maintain the esophageal pH at 4 or greater around the clock. Higher doses of ranitidine have not been proven to improve outcomes in GERD patients; lower doses may provide some improvement in heartburn symptoms but are less effective in eliminating symptoms or healing erosive esophagitis.

177. The answer is B.
Bleeding abnormalities result from vitamin K deficiency because of reduced formation of clotting factors II, VII, IX, and X.

178. The answer is B.
BSA correlates with cardiac output, which determines renal and hepatic blood flow and thus affects drug elimination.

179. The answer is B.
When weak acids are presented to the kidney for elimination, drugs that increase the ionization of these agents also increase their elimination. However, weak acids (e.g., methenamine) have their elimination delayed when agents such as aspirin decrease their ionization. This relative increase in un-ionized methenamine results in greater reabsorption of methenamine and, therefore, an increase in activity.

180. The answer is A.
Numerous hemorrhoid preparations are available OTC to treat the discomforts associated with hemorrhoids. These products contain steroids, astringents, anesthetics, and vasoconstrictors. However, Anusol-HC contains a local anesthetic combined with a concentration of hydrocortisone, which makes it a prescription item. Anusol is available OTC as a single-entity anesthetic product for the treatment of hemorrhoids. A low-strength form of Anusol-HC has been released OTC.

181. The answer is D.
Transdermal fentanyl is a controlled-release dosage form that is effective for a 72-hr period. All of the other drugs listed are effective for periods of 1–8 hr.

182. The answer is B.
Burow's solution is an aluminum acetate solution commonly used as an astringent solution and as an astringent mouthwash and gargle. Aluminum acetate is found in products that treat diaper rash, athlete's foot, and poison ivy.

183. The answer is E (I, II, III).
Activase (recombinant tissue plasminogen activator) is a thrombolytic agent. Neupogen (granulocyte colony-stimulating factor [G-CSF]) is a cytokine that regulates the proliferation and differentiation of white blood cells. Epogen (recombinant erythropoietin) stimulates the production of red blood cells.

184. The answer is A (I).
Although anticholinergic agents have no proven value in ulcer healing, they have been used in conjunction with antacids for relief of refractory duodenal ulcer pain. An anticholinergic, Pro-Banthine (propantheline) can cause dry mouth, blurred vision, urinary retention, constipation, and pupillary dilation.

185. The answer is E (I, II, III).
The liver is the main organ for the synthesis of plasma proteins. During end-stage liver disease, a decrease in plasma albumin concentrations leads to less drug protein binding and more free Coumadin drug concentrations, causing a more intense pharmacodynamic effect and, therefore, an increase in prothrombin time.

186. The answer is C.
To calculate the number of mEq KCl per tablet, divide the tablet strength (600 mg) by the molecular weight (74.5). Each tablet contains 8 mEq KCl. The woman needs to take four tablets to provide a dose of 32 mEq KCl.

187. The answer is B.
The final suspension contains 8 g in 120 mL, which is 6.7% sucralfate (8/120 = 0.067 = 6.7%).

188. The answer is D.
The amount of sucralfate in 10 ml of this product is 0.667 g (8 g sucralfate/120 mL = 10 ml = 0.667 g sucralfate).

189. The answer is E (I, II, III).
Passive diffusion follows Fick's principle of diffusion, in which the rate of diffusion depends on the concentration gradient, the partition coefficient (e.g., lipid solubility to water solubility ratio), and the surface area of the cell membrane. The extent of ionization relates the ratio of the nonionized or nonpolar species to the ionized or more water-soluble species.

190. The answer is B.
Psyllium is one of the bulk-forming laxatives. These agents absorb intestinal water and swell, increasing the bulk and moisture content of the stool to promote peristalsis. They act in both the small and large intestines.

PRESCRIPTION DISPENSING INFORMATION AND METROLOGY

Prescriptions

PARTS OF THE PRESCRIPTION

A prescription is an order for medication for use by a patient that is issued by a physician, dentist, veterinarian, or other licensed practitioner who is authorized to prescribe medication or by their agent via a collaborative practice agreement. A prescription is usually written on a single sheet of paper that is commonly imprinted with the prescriber's name, address, and telephone number. A medication order is similar to a prescription, but it is written on the patient chart and intended for use by a patient in an institutional setting.

All prescriptions should contain accurate and appropriate information about the patient and the medication that is being prescribed. In addition, a prescription order for a **controlled substance** must contain the following information:

1. Date of issue
2. Full name and address of the patient
3. Drug name, strength, dosage form, and quantity prescribed
4. Directions for use
5. Name, address, and Drug Enforcement Agency (DEA) number of the prescriber
6. Signature of the prescriber

A written prescription order is required for substances listed in **Schedule II.** Prescriptions for controlled substances listed in **Schedule II** are **never** refillable. Any other prescription that has no indication of refills is not refillable.

Prescriptions for medications that are listed in Schedules III, IV, and V may be issued either in writing or orally to the pharmacist. If authorized by the prescriber, these prescriptions may be refilled up to five times within 6 months of the date of issue. If the prescriber wishes the patient to continue to take the medication after 6 months or five refills, a new prescription order is required.

THE PRESCRIPTION LABEL

In addition to the name of the patient, the pharmacy, and the prescriber, the prescription label should accurately identify the medication and provide directions for its use.

The label for a prescription order for a controlled substance must contain the following information:

1. Name and address of the pharmacy
2. Serial number assigned to the prescription by the pharmacy
3. Date of the initial filling
4. Name of the patient
5. Name of the prescriber
6. Directions for use
7. Cautionary statements as required by law*

AUXILIARY LABELS

Auxiliary, or cautionary, labels provide additional important information about the proper use of the medication. Examples include "Shake Well" for suspensions or emulsions; "For External Use Only" for

---

*The label of any drug that is listed as a controlled substance in Schedule II, III, or IV of the Controlled Substances Act must contain the following warning: **CAUTION: Federal law prohibits the transfer of this drug to any person other than the patient for whom it was prescribed.**

topical lotions, solutions, or creams; and "May Cause Drowsiness" for medications that depress the central nervous system. The information contained on auxiliary labels should be brought to the attention of the patient when the medication is dispensed. The pharmacist should place only appropriate auxiliary labels on the prescription container because too many labels may confuse the patient.

BEFORE DISPENSING THE PRESCRIPTION

Double-check the accuracy of the prescription.
Provide undivided attention when filling the prescription.

1. Check the patient information (e.g., name, address, date of birth, telephone number).
2. Check the patient profile (e.g., allergies, medical conditions, other drugs, including over-the-counter medications).
3. Check the drug (e.g., correct drug name, correct spelling, appropriate drug for the patient's condition), and verify that there are no known drug interactions. **Always verify the name of the drug. Beware of drug names that look alike (see table).**
4. Check the dosage, including the drug strength, the dosage form (e.g., capsule, liquid, modified release), the individual dose, the total daily dose, the duration of treatment, and the units (e.g., mg, mL, tsp, tbsp).
5. Check the label. Compare the drug dispensed with the prescription. Verify the National Drug Code (NDC) number. Ensure that the information is accurate, that the patient directions are accurate and easily understood, and that the auxiliary labels are appropriate.
6. **Provide patient counseling. Be sure that the patient fully understands the drug treatment as well as any precautions.**

Examples of Drugs with Similar Names

Brand name	Celebrex	Cerebyx	Celexa
Generic name	Celecoxib capsules	Fosphenytoin sodium injection	Citalopram HCl
Manufacturer	Searle	Parke-Davis	Forest
Indication	Osteoarthritis and rheumatoid arthritis	Prevention and treatment of seizures	Major depression

Dangerous or Confusing Abbreviations

Numerous common abbreviations and symbols have been associated with errors. Detailed lists of these can be found at the websites of the Institute for Safe Medication Practices (ISMP) and Joint Commission for the Accreditation of Healthcare Organizations (JCAHO) at :

http://www.ismp.org/Tools/abbreviationslist.pdf.
http://www.jcaho.org/accredited + organizations/patient + safety/06_dnu_list.pdf.

The JCAHO has created a "Do Not Use" list of abbreviations that its accredited organizations should not allow to be used.

➤**"U" or "IU" for units**: the "U" has been misinterpreted as various numbers such as zero, four; serious harm has occurred with insulin and heparin as a result of confusion. For example, a patient received 66 units of insulin instead of 6 units. The order was written for "6u" of regular insulin but was misinterpreted. The word "units" should be written out in full.
➤**"QD, Q.D, qd, q.d."**: common abbreviations for daily have been misinterpreted as "QID" or "qid" and overdoses have occurred. "Daily" should be written out in full.
➤**"Q.O.D, QOD, qod"**: common abbreviations for every other day have been misinterpreted as QID (four times daily). This should be written out completely as "every other day."

➤**Trailing zero**: when a dose is ordered and followed with a decimal point and a zero, such as 2.0 mg. or 25.0 mg., errors can occur. The decimal point may be missed and an overdose can occur. For example, Warfarin 2.0 mg may be misinterpreted as 20 mg. Trailing zeros should be avoided and the dose written without the additional zero, for example Warfarin 2 mg. rather than 2.0 mg.

➤**Lack of leading zero**: a drug's dose may be less than 1 mg., such as Digoxin. Often the dose may be written without a leading zero, such as Digoxin .25 mg., rather than as Digoxin 0.25 mg. Errors have occurred because the decimal point is missed. For example, Warfarin .5 mg may be interpreted as Warfarin 5 mg. Leading zeroes should be included, so the dose is written as "Digoxin 0.25 mg. or Warfarin 0.5 mg."

➤**MS, MSO4, MgSO$_4$: Abbreviations for morphine sulfate (MS, MSO$_4$) have been confused with Magnesium sulfate (MgSO$_4$). It is recommend to write out each name in full rather than using abbreviations: morphine sulfate or magnesium sulfate.**

In addition to the above abbreviations, there are numerous other hazardous symbols and abbreviations which should be reviewed with caution when used on prescriptions. Examples include:

➤**"cc"** : Often used instead of "mL." This has been misinterpreted as a "0" (zero). Use "mL."

➤**"µg"**: Used for "micrograms," for example, Levothyroxine 250 µg. daily. The symbol has been mistaken for "mg." and overdoses have occurred. Best to use "mcg." Or write out "micrograms."

➤**"<" or " >"** : Symbols for " less than" (<) or "greater than" (>) have been mistaken for each other or misinterpreted as numbers. Best to write out as "less than" or "greater than."

➤**"HCT"** : An abbreviation for "hydrocortisone" has been misinterpreted as "hydrochlorothiazide. " Best to write name out completely.

➤**"HCl"**: An abbreviation for "hydrochloric acid" has been misinterpreted as "KCl" (potassium chloride). Best to write out name completely.

Common Abbreviations

Considerable variation occurs in the use of capitalization, italicization, and punctuation in abbreviations. The following list shows the abbreviations that are most often encountered by pharmacists.

A, aa., or aa	of each	mcg, mcg., or μg	microgram
a.c.	before meals	mEq	milliequivalent
ad	to, up to	mg or mg.	milligram
a.d.	right ear	ml or mL	milliliter
ad lib.	at pleasure, freely	μl or μL	microliter
a.m.	morning	ℳ	minim
amp.	ampule	N&V	nausea and vomiting
ante	before	Na	sodium
aq.	water	N.F.	National Formulary
a.s.	left ear	No.	number
asa	aspirin	noct.	night, in the night
a.u.	each ear, both ears	non rep.	do not repeat
b.i.d.	twice a day	NPO	nothing by mouth
BP	British Pharmacopoeia	N.S., NS, or N/S	normal saline
BSA	body surface area	1/2 NS	half-strength normal saline
c. or c	with	O	pint
cap. or caps.	capsule	o.d.	right eye, every day
cp	chest pain	o.l. or o.s.	left eye
D.A.W.	dispense as written	OTC	over the counter
cc or cc.	cubic centimeter	o.u.	each eye, both eyes
comp.	compound, compounded	oz.	ounce
dil.	dilute	p.c.	after meals
D.C., dc, or disc.	discontinue	PDR	*Physicians' Desk Reference*
disp.	dispense	p.m.	afternoon, evening
div.	divide, to be divided	p.o.	by mouth
dl or dL	deciliter	Ppt	precipitated
d.t.d.	give of such doses	pr	for the rectum
DW	distilled water	prn or p.r.n.	as needed
D5W	dextrose 5% in water	pt.	pint
elix.	elixir	pulv.	powder
e.m.p.	as directed	pv	for vaginal use
et	and	q.	every
ex aq.	in water	q.d.	every day
fl or fld	fluid	q.h.	every hour
fl oz	fluid ounce	q. 4 hr.	every four hours
ft.	make	q.i.d.	four times a day
g or Gm	gram	q.o.d.	every other day
gal.	gallon	q.s.	a sufficient quantity
GI	gastrointestinal	q.s. ad	a sufficient quantity to make
gr or gr.	grain	R	rectal
gtt or gtt.	drop, drops	R.L. or R/L	Ringer's lactate
H	hypodermic	℞	prescription
h. or hr.	hour	s. or s	without
h.s.	at bedtime	Sig.	write on label
IM	intramuscular	sol.	solution
inj.	injection	S.O.B.	shortness of breath
IV	intravenous	s.o.s.	if there is need (once only)
IVP	intravenous push	ss. or ss	one-half
IVPB	intravenous piggyback	stat.	immediately
K	potassium	subc, subq, or s.c.	subcutaneously
l or L	liter	sup. or supp	suppository
lb.	pound	susp.	suspension
μ	Greek mu	syr.	syrup
M	mix	tab.	tablet
m² or M²	square meter	tal.	such, such a one

tal. dos.	such doses	**U or u.**	unit
tbsp. or T	tablespoonful	**u.d. or ut dict.**	as directed
t.i.d.	three times a day	**ung.**	ointment
tr. or tinct.	tincture	**U.S.P. or USP**	United States Pharmacopoeia
tsp. or t.	teaspoonful	**w/v**	weight/volume
TT	tablet triturates		

Metrology

THE METRIC, APOTHECARY, AND AVOIRDUPOIS SYSTEMS

Metric system

1. Basic units

Mass = g or gram
Length = m or meter
Volume = L or liter
1 cc (cubic centimeter) of water is approximately equal to 1 mL and weighs 1 g.

2. Prefixes

kilo- 10^3, or 1000 times the basic unit
hekto- 10^2, or 100 times the basic unit
deka- 10^1, or 10 times the basic unit
deci- 10^{-1}, or 0.1 times the basic unit
centi- 10^{-2}, or 0.01 times the basic unit
milli- 10^{-3}, or 0.001 times the basic unit
micro- 10^{-6}, or one-millionth of the basic unit
nano- 10^{-9}, or one-billionth of the basic unit
pico- 10^{-12}, or one-trillionth of the basic unit

Examples of these prefixes include milligram (mg), which equals one-thousandth of a gram, and deciliter (dL), which equals 100 mL, or 0.1 L.

Apothecary system

1. Volume (fluids or liquid)

60 minims (♍) = 1 fluidrachm or fluidram (f ʒ) or (ʒ)
8 fluidrachms (480 minims) = 1 fluidounce (f ℥ or ℥)
16 fluidounces = 1 pint (pt or 0)
2 pints (32 fluidounces) = 1 quart (qt)
4 quarts (8 pints) = 1 gallon (gal or C)

2. Mass (weight)

20 grains (gr) = 1 scruple (℈)
3 scruples (60 grains) = 1 drachm or dram (ʒ)
8 drachms (480 grains) = 1 ounce (℥)
12 ounces (5760 grains) = 1 pound (lb)

Avoirdupois system

1. Volume

1 fluidrachm = 60 min.
1 fluid ounce = 8 fl. dr.
　　　　　　 = 480 min.
1 pint = 16 fl. oz.
　　　 = 7680 min.

1 quart = 2 pt.
        = 32 fl. oz.
1 gallon = 4 qt.
        = 128 fl. oz.

2. Mass (weight)

The grain is common to both the apothecary and the avoirdupois systems.

437.5 grains (gr) = 1 ounce (oz)
16 ounces (7000 grains) = 1 pound (lb)

CONVERSION

Exact equivalents

Exact equivalents are used for the conversion of specific quantities in pharmaceutical formulas and prescription compounding.

1. Length

1 meter (m) = 39.37 in.
1 inch (in) = 2.54 cm.

2. Volume

1 ml = 16.23 minims (℥)
1 ℥ = 0.06 mL
1 f ʒ = 3.69 mL
1 f ʒ = 29.57 mL
1 pt = 473 mL
1 gal (U.S.) = 3785 mL

3. Mass

1 g = 15.432 gr
1 kg = 2.20 lb (avoir.)
1 gr = 0.065 g or 65 mg
1 oz (avoir.) = 28.35 g
1 ʒ (apoth.) = 31.1 g
1 lb (avoir.) = 454 g
1 lb (apoth.) = 373.2 g

4. Other equivalents

1 oz (avoir.) = 437.5 gr
1 ʒ (apoth.) = 480 gr
1 gal (U.S.) = 128 fl ʒ
1 fl ʒ (water) = 455 gr
1 gr (apoth.) = 1 gr (avoir.)

Approximate equivalents

Physicians may use approximate equivalents to prescribe the dose quantities using the metric and apothecary systems of weights and measures, respectively. Household units are often used to inform the patient of the size of the dose. In view of the almost universal practice of using an ordinary household teaspoon to administer medication, a teaspoon may be considered 5 mL. However, when accurate measurement of a liquid dose is required, the USP recommends the use of a calibrated oral syringe or dropper.

1 fluid dram = 1 teaspoonful
             = 5 mL
4 fluidounces = 120 mL
8 fluidounces = 1 cup
             = 240 mL
1 grain = 65 mg
1 kg = 2.2 pounds (lb)

COMMON PRESCRIPTION DRUGS AND OVER-THE-COUNTER PRODUCTS

The FDA Approved Drug Products With Therapeutic Equivalence Evaluation: The *Orange Book*

The United States Food and Drug Administration (FDA) publishes the book, *Approved Drug Products With Therapeutic Equivalence Evaluation,* often known as the *Orange Book.* An electronic version of the *Orange Book* is available on the Internet at http://www.fda.gov/cder/ob/. This book is also reproduced by the United States Pharmacopeial Convention, Inc., in the publication, USP DI, Volume III, *Approved Drug Products and Legal Requirements.*

The texts, which are published annually, identify the prescription and nonprescription products that are formally approved by the FDA on the basis of safety and effectiveness. They also provide the FDA's therapeutic equivalence evaluations for approved multiple-source prescription drug products.

The *Orange Book* is a drug product selection guide for pharmacists to use when dispensing a generic drug product as a substitute for the brand-name equivalent. A few drug products that were on the market before 1938 received a "grandfathered" FDA approval. These products are assumed to be safe and effective because of their long usage (e.g., digoxin tablets, phenobarbital tablets). These older products do not have therapeutic equivalence ratings at this time.

The *Orange Book* uses various codes to indicate therapeutic equivalence. The first letter "A" designates drug products that the FDA considers therapeutically equivalent to a pharmaceutically equivalent drug product. These products can be safely substituted. The first letter "B" designates drug products that, for various reasons, the FDA does not consider bioequivalent to the pharmaceutically equivalent drug product.

Therapeutic Equivalence Evaluation Codes

A Codes

Drug products that the FDA considers therapeutically equivalent to other pharmaceutically equivalent products

AA Products in conventional dosage forms that do not present bioequivalence problems
AB Products that meet necessary bioequivalence requirements
AN Solutions and powders for aerosolization
AO Injectable oil solutions
AO Injectable aqueous solutions, and in certain instances, intravenous nonaqueous solutions
AT Topical products

B Codes

Drug products that the FDA does not consider therapeutically equivalent to other pharmaceutically equivalent products at this time

B* Drug products that require further FDA investigation and review to determine therapeutic equivalence
BC Extended-release dosage forms (capsules, injectables, and tablets)
BD Active ingredients and dosage forms that have documented problems with bioequivalence
BE Delayed-release oral dosage forms
BN Products in aerosol-nebulizer drug-delivery systems

BP Active ingredients and dosage forms that have potential problems with bioequivalence
BR Suppositories or enemas that deliver drugs for systemic absorption
BS Drug products that have drug standard deficiencies
BT Topical products that have bioequivalence issues
BX Drug products for which the data are sufficient to determine therapeutic equivalence

Top 200 Prescription Drugs by Trade Name and Generic Name[a]

Rank	Trade Name	Generic Name
1	Lipitor	Atorvastatin
2	Synthroid	Levothyroxine
3	Lortab	Hydrocodone/acetaminophen
4	Toprol-XL™	Metoprolol succinate
5	Hydrochlorothiazide	Hydrochlorothiazide
6	Norvasc	Amlodipine
7	Zithromax	Azithromycin
8	Proventil	Albuterol
9	Tenormin	Atenolol
10	Zoloft	Sertraline
11	Lasix	Furosemide
12	Lexapro	Escitalopram
13	Amoxil	Amoxicillin
14	Coumadin	Warfarin
15	Singulair	Montelukast
16	Fosamax	Alendronate
17	Zestril	Lisinopril
18	Prevacid	Lansoprazole
19	Potassium Chloride	Potassium chloride
20	Allegra	Fexofenadine
21	Advair	Fluticasone/salmeterol
22	Effexor (XR)	Venlafaxine
23	Zyrtec	Cetirizine
24	Nexium	Esomeprazole
25	Ambien	Zolpidem
26	Wellbutrin (SR, XL)	Bupropion
27	Maxzide™	Triamterene/hydrochlorothiazide
28	Premarin	Conjugated estrogens
29	Flonase™	Fluticasone
30	Plavix	Clopidogrel
31	Levaquin	Levofloxacin
32	Keflex & Keflet	Cephalexin
33	Lanoxin	Digoxin
34	Celebrex	Celecoxib
35	Xanax	Alprazolam
36	Protonix	Pantoprazole
37	Glucophage (XR)	Metformin ER
38	Darvocet–N	Propoxyphene/acetaminophen
39	Diovan	Valsartan
40	Lotrel	Amlodipine/benazepril
41	Zetia	Ezetimibe
42	Prilosec	Omeprazole
43	Lopressor	Metoprolol tartrate
44	Ortho-Novum 7/7/7	Ethinyl estradiol/norethindrone
45	Avandia	Rosiglitazone
46	Zocor	Simvastatin
47	Actos	Pioglitazone
48	Motrin	Ibuprofen
49	Tylenol with Codeine	Acetaminophen/codeine
50	Zantac	Ranitidine

Continued.

Rank	Trade Name	Generic Name
51	Lantus	Insulin glargine
52	Actonel	Risedronate
53	Altace	Ramipril
54	Ortho Tri-Cyclen	Ethinyl estradiol/norgestimate
55	Seroquel	Quetiapine
56	Amitriptyline	Amitriptyline
57	Diovan-HCT	Valsartan/hydrochlorothiazide
58	Adderall (XR)	Dextroamphetamine/amphetamine
59	TriCor	Fenofibrate
60	Ativan	Lorazepam
61	Paxil (CR)	Paroxetine
62	Viagra	Sildenafil
63	Pravachol	Pravastatin
64	Coreg	Carvedilol
65	Flomax	Tamsulosin
66	Humulin	Insulin
67	Augmentin (XR)	Amoxicillin/clavulanate
68	Crestor	Rosuvastatin
69	Nasonex	Mometasone
70	Concerta	Methylphenidate
71	Glucotrol (XL)	Glipizide ER
72	Yasmin	Ethinyl estradiol/drospirenone
73	Ortho Evra	Ethinyl estradiol/norelgestromin
74	Allegra-D	Fexofenadine/pseudoephedrine
75	Depakote (ER)	Divalproex
76	Amaryl	Glimepiride
77	Folic Acid	Folic Acid
78	Isoptin (SR)	Verapamil SR
79	Percocet	Oxycodone/acetaminophen
80	Combivent	Ipratropium/albuterol
81	Risperdal	Risperidone
82	Xalatan™	Latanoprost
83	Prozac	Fluoxetine
84	Zyloprim	Allopurinol
85	Flexeril	Cyclobenzaprine
86	Neurontin	Gabapentin
87	AcipHex	Rabeprazole
88	Vytorin	Simvastatin/ezetimibe
89	Detrol (LA)	Tolterodine
90	Mobic	Meloxicam
91	Evista	Raloxifene
92	Deltasone	Prednisone
93	Dyazide	Triamterene/hydrochlorothiazide
94	Celexa	Citalopram
95	Humalog	Insulin lispro
96	Catapres	Clonidine
97	Ultram	Tramadol
98	Dilantin	Phenytoin
99	Imdur	Isosorbide mononitrate
100	Inderal (LA)	Propranolol LA
101	Aricept™	Donepezil
102	Desyrel	Trazodone
103	Omnicef	Cefdinir
104	Anaprox (DS)	Naproxen sodium
105	Veetids	Penicillin V K
106	Bactrim™ (DS)	Trimethoprim/sulfamethoxazole
107	Klonopin	Clonazepam

(*Continued on next page*)

Continued.

Rank	Trade Name	Generic Name
108	Valtrex	Valacyclovir
109	Zyprexa	Olanzapine
110	Topamax	Topiramate
111	OxyContin	Oxycodone ER
112	Strattera	Atomoxetine
113	Cozaar	Losartan
114	Hyzaar	Losartan/hydrochlorothiazide
115	Valium	Diazepam
116	Niaspan	Niacin SR
117	Biaxin (XL)	Clarithromycin ER
118	Benicar	Olmesartan
119	Cymbalta	Duloxetine
120	Patanol	Olopatadine
121	Relafen	Nabumetone
122	MiraLax™	Polyethylene glycol
123	Avapro	Irbesartan
124	Cardizem (CD)	Diltiazem
125	Ultracet	Tramadol/acetaminophen
126	Flovent	Fluticasone
127	Clarinex	Desloratadine
128	Imitrex™	Sumatriptan
129	Accupril	Quinapril
130	Avalide	Irbesartan/hydrochlorothiazide
131	Lopid	Gemfibrozil
132	Lamictal	Lamotrigine
133	Antivert	Meclizine
134	Zyrtec-D	Cetirizine
135	Ditropan(XL)	Oxybutynin
136	Mytussin AC	Guaifenesin/codeine
137	Mircette	Ethinyl estradiol/desogestrel
138	Micronase	Glyburide
139	Hytrin	Terazosin
140	Rhinocort AQ	Budesonide
141	Nitrostat	Nitroglycerin
142	Prempro™	Estrogens: conjugated/equine, medroxyprogesterone
143	Benicar-HCT	Olmesartan/hydrochlorothiazide
144	Cipro (XR)	Ciprofloxacin
145	Lescol (XL)	Fluvastatin
146	Alesse™	Ethinyl estradiol/levonorgestrel
147	Vasotec	Enalapril
148	Lotrisone	Betamethasone/clotrimazole
149	Ortho-Cept	Ethinyl estradiol/desogestrel
150	Pulmicort	Budesonide
151	Skelaxin	Metaxalone
152	Remeron	Mirtazapine
153	Ketek	Telithromycin
154	Methotrexate	Methotrexate
155	Cosopt	Dorzolamide/timolol
156	Abilify™	Aripiprazole
157	Zestoretic	Lisinopril/hydrochlorothiazide
158	Spiriva	Tiotropium
159	Procardia (XL)	Nifedipine
160	Kenalog	Triamcinolone
161	Miacalcin	Calcitonin
162	Namenda	Memantine
163	Tessalon	Benzonatate

Continued.

Rank	Trade Name	Generic Name
164	Estrace	Estradiol
165	Vigamox	Moxifloxacin
166	Cialis	Tadalafil
167	Phenergan with Codeine	Promethazine/codeine
168	Reglan	Metoclopramide
169	Ortho-Cyclen	Ethinyl estradiol/norgestimate
170	Medrol	Methylprednisolone
171	Alphagan P	Brimonidine
172	Ceftin	Cefuroxime
173	Lumigan	Bimatoprost
174	Macrodantin & Macrobid	Nitrofurantoin
175	Histinex HC	Phenylephrine/hydrocodone/chlorpheniramine
176	Feldene	Piroxicam
177	Sinemet	Carbidopa/levodopa
178	Lo/Ovral	Ethinyl estradiol/norgestrel
179	Restoril	Temazepam
180	Sumycin	Tetracycline
181	Ritalin	Methylphenidate
182	Travatan	Travoprost
183	Naprosyn & EC-Naprosyn™	Naproxen
184	Lamisil	Terbinafine
185	Necon 1/35	Ethinyl estradiol/norethindrone
186	Cardura	Doxazosin
187	Atacand	Candesartan
188	Voltaren	Diclofenac
189	Mirapex	Pramipexole
190	Prometrium	Progesterone
191	Pamelor	Nortriptyline
192	Triphasil	Ethinyl estradiol/levonorgestrel
193	Xopenex Inhalation Solution	Levalbuterol
194	Serevent	Salmeterol
195	Timoptic	Timolol
196	DuoNeb	Albuterol/ipratropium
197	BenzaClin	Clindamycin/benzoyl peroxide
198	Ciprodex	Ciprofloxacin/dexamethasone
199	Vibramycin & Vibra-Tabs	Doxycycline
200	Mevacor	Lovastatin

[a]This table contains the top 200 prescription drugs dispensed through independent, chain, food store, mass merchandiser, and deep discount pharmacies. All forms of the same generic equivalent drug are grouped together and listed under the brand name when appropriate. Rankings are based on total number of prescriptions for August 2004 to August 2005, as measured by SFI's Prescription Drug Audit. Insulin products are included in the tally.
Adapted with permission from Prescription Drug Cards, 21st ed. SFI Medical Publishing, 2005.

Top Over-the-Counter (OTC) Drugs[a]

Trade Name	Drug Use
Abreva	Cold sore medication
Actifed	Allergy and cold relief
Advil	Analgesic
Afrin	Nasal decongestant
Aleve	Analgesic
ALternaGEL	Antacid
Anbesol	Oral cavity analgesic
Anusol	Hemorrhoidal agent
Azo Standard	UTI analgesic
Bayer Aspirin	Analgesic
Benadryl Oral	Allergy and cold relief
BEN-GAY	Topical analgesic
Betadine	Antiseptic
Bonine	Motion sickness medication
Bufferin	Analgesic
Caladryl	Topical antipruritic
Campho-Phenique	Topical antiseptic/antibiotic
Capastat	Oral cavity analgesic
Chlor-Trimeton	Allergy and cold relief
Chloraseptic	Oral cavity analgesic
Citrucel	Laxative
Claritin	Allergy and cold relief
Claritin-D	Allergy and cold relief
Colace	Stool softener
COLD-EEZE	Cold relief
Compound W	Keratolytic
Comtrex	Cough and cold relief
Cortaid	Topical antipruritic
Debrox	Ear wax removal aid
Delsym	Cough suppressant
Dramamine & Dramamine II	Motion sickness medication
Dulcolax	Laxative
Duofilm	Keratolytic
Emetrol	Antiemetic
Estroven	Menopause support
Excedrin	Analgesic
FiberCon	Laxative
Fungi-Nail	Topical antifungal
Gas-X	Antiflatulent
Gyne-Lotrimin	Vaginal antifungal
Imodium A-D	Antidiarrheal
Kank-A	Oral cavity analgesic
Kaopectate	Antidiarrheal
Lactaid	Digestive aid
Lactinex	Antidiarrheal
Lamisil AT	Antifungal
Listerine	Oral cavity antiseptic
Lotrimin AF	Topical antifungal
Maalox & Maalox Plus	Antacid
Metamucil	Laxative
Midol & Midol PMS	Analgesic
Monistat Vaginal	Vaginal antifungal
Motrin IB	Analgesic
Mucinex	Expectorant
Mylanta	Antacid
Mylicon Drops	Antiflatulence
Myoflex	Topical analgesic

Continued.

Trade Name	Drug Use
Naphcon A	Ophthalmic anti-allergy
NasalCrom	Allergy and cold relief
Neo-Synephrine	Nasal decongestant
Neosporin	Topical anti-infective
NicoDerm CQ	Smoking cessation aid
Nicorette	Smoking cessation aid
Nix	Pediculicide
Nizoral Shampoo	Topical antifungal
NoDoz	Analeptic
NyQuil	Cough and cold relief
Ocean	Nasal decongestant
Opcon-A	Ophthalmic anti-allergy
Orabase	Oral cavity analgesic
OralBalance	Oral moisturizer
Os-Cal	Essential mineral
Pamprin	Analgesic
PediaCare	Cough and cold relief
Pepcid Complete	Acid reducer
Pepcid-AC	Acid reducer
Pepto Bismol	Antidiarrheal
Peri-Colace	Stool softener plus laxative
Phillips' MOM	Laxative/antacid
Pin-X	Anthelmintic
Preparation H	Hemorrhoidal agent
Prilosec OTC	Acid reducer
RID	Pediculicide
Robitussin (Adult)	Cough relief
Rogaine	Hair growth stimulant
Salivart	Saliva substitute
Senokot	Laxative
Similasan Earache Relief	Earache relief
Slow-Mag	Essential mineral
Sominex	Sleeping aid
Sudafed	Allergy and cold relief
Tagamet HB 200	Acid reducer
Tavist	Allergy and cold relief
Tears Naturale	Artificial tears
Triaminic Oral	Cough and cold relief
Tums	Antacid
Tylenol	Analgesic
Tylenol Allergy & Sinus	Allergy and cold relief
Tylenol Cold & Flu (Adult)	Allergy and cold relief
Tylenol PM	Analgesic
Unisom	Sleeping aid
Zantac 75	Acid reducer
Zicam Cold Remedy	Cold relief
Zostrix	Topical analgesic

[a]This table contains the top OTC drugs by pharmacist recommendation in specific therapeutic classes.
Adapted with permission from Nonprescription Drug Cards, 4th ed. SFI Medical Publishing, 2003.

REFERENCE CHARTS FOR PATIENT COUNSELING

Drugs That Should Not Be Crushed

Listed below are various slow-release as well as enteric-coated products that should not be crushed or chewed. Slow-release (sr) represents products that are controlled-release, extended-release, long-acting, or timed-release. Enteric-coated (ec) represents products that are delayed-release.

In general, capsules containing slow-release or enteric-coated particles may be opened and their contents administered on a spoonful of soft food. Instruct patients not to chew the particles, though. (Patients should, in fact, be discouraged from chewing any medication unless it is specifically formulated for that purpose.)

This list should not be considered all-inclusive. Generic and alternate brands of some products may exist. Tablets intended for sublingual or buccal administration (not included in this list) should also be administered only as intended, in an intact form.

Drug	Manufacturer	Form
Aciphex	Eisai	ec
Adalat CC	Schering Plough	sr
Adderall XR	Shire US	sr
Advicor	KOS	sr
Aerohist	Aero	sr
Aerohist Plus	Aero	sr
Afeditab CR	Watson	sr
Aggrenox	Boehr, Ingelheim	sr
Aldex	Zyber	sr
Aldex-G	Zyber	sr
Aleve Cold & Sinus	Bayer Healthcare	sr
Aleve Sinus & Headache	Bayer Healthcare	sr
Allegra-D 12 Hour	Senofi-Aventis	sr
Allegra-D 24 Hour	Senofi-Aventis	sr
Allerx	Cornerstone	sr
Allerx-D	Cornerstone	sr
Allfen	MCR American	sr
Allfen-DM	MCR American	sr
Alophen	Numark	ec
Altex-PSE	Alphagen	sr
Altoprev	First Horizon	sr
Ambi 1000/55	Ambi	sr
Ambi 45/800	Ambi	sr
Ambi 45/800/30	Ambi	sr
Ambi 60/580	Ambi	sr
Ambi 60/580/30	Ambi	sr
Ambi 80/700	Ambi	sr
Ambi 80/700/40	Ambi	sr
Ambifed-G	Ambi	sr
Ambifed-G DM	Ambi	sr
Amdry-C	Prasco	sr
Amdry-D	Parsco	sr
Amibid DM	Amide	sr
Amibid LA	Amide	sr
Amidal	Amide	sr
Aminoxin	Tyson Neutraceuticals	ec

Drug	Manufacturer	Form
Ami-Tex PSE	Amide	sr
Anextuss	Cypress	sr
Aquabid-DM	Alphagen	sr
Aquatab C	Adams	sr
Aquatab D	Adams	sr
Aquatab DM	Adams	sr
Arithrotec	Pharmacia	ec
Asacol	Procter & Gamble	ec
Ascocid-1000	Key	sr
Ascocid-500-D	Key	sr
Ascriptin Enteric	Novartis Consumer	ec
ATP	Tyson Neutraceuticals	ec
Atrohist Pediatric	Celltech	sr
Augmentin XR	GlaxoSmithKline	sr
Avinza	Ligand	sr
Azulfidine Entabs	Pharmacia	ec
Bayer Aspirin Regimen	Bayer Healthcare	ec
Bellahist-D LA	Cypress	sr
Bellatal ER	Qualitest	sr
Biaxin XL	Abbott	sr
Bidex-DM	Stewart-Jackson	sr
Bidhist	Cypress	sr
Bidhist-D	Cypress	sr
Biohist LA	Ivax	sr
Bisac-Evac	G & W	ec
Biscolax	Global Source	ec
Blanex-A	Blansett	sr
Bontril Slow-Release	Valeant	sr
Bromfed	Victory	sr
Bromfed-PD	Victory	sr
Bromfenex	Ethex	sr
Bromfenex PD	Ethex	sr
Bromfenex PE	Ethex	sr
Bromfenex PE Pediatric	Ethex	sr
Budeprion SR	Teva	sr
Buproban	Teva	sr
Calan SR	Pharmacia	sr
Campral	Forest	ec
Carbatrol	Shire US	sr
Cardene SR	Roche	sr
Cardizem CD	Biovall	sr
Cardizem LA	KOS	sr
Carox Plus	Seneca	sr
Cartia XT	Andrx	sr
Catemine	Tyson Neutraceuticals	ec
Cemill 1000	Miller	sr
Cemill 500	Miller	sr
Certuss-D	Capellon	sr
Cevi-Bid	Lee	sr
Chlorex-A	Cypress	sr
Chlor-Phen	Truxton	sr
Chlor-Trimeton Allergy	Schering Plough	sr
Chlor-Trimeton Allergy Decongestant	Schering Plough	sr
Cipro XR	Schering Plough	sr
Clarinex-D 24 Hour	Schering Plough	sr
Coldamine	Breckenridge	sr
Coldec D	Breckenridge	sr
Coldec TR	Breckenridge	sr

(*Continued on next page*)

Drug	Manufacturer	Form
Coldex-A	United Research	sr
ColdMist DM	Breckenridge	sr
ColdMist Jr	Breckenridge	sr
ColdMist LA	Breckenridge	sr
Colfed-A	Breckenridge	sr
Concerta	McNeil Consumer	sr
Contac 12-Hour	GlaxoSmithKline	sr
Correctol	Schering Plough	ec
Cotazym-S	Organon	ec
Covera-HS	Pharmacia	sr
CPM 8/PE 20/MSC 1.25	Cypress	sr
Crantex ER	Breckenridge	sr
Crantex LA	Breckenridge	sr
Crantex Lac	Breckenridge	sr
Creon 10	Solvay	ec
Creon 20	Solvay	ec
Creon 5	Solvay	ec
Cymbalta	Eli Lilly	ec
Cypex-LA	Cypress	sr
Dacex-PE	Cypress	sr
Dairycare	Plainview	ec
Dallergy	Laser	sr
Dallergy-Jr	Laser	sr
D-Amine-SR	Alphagen	sr
Deconamine SR	Kenwood Therapeutics	sr
Deconex	Poly	sr
Decongest II	Qualitest	sr
De-Congestine	Qualitest	sr
Deconsal II	Cornerstone	sr
Depakote	Abbott	ec
Depakote ER	Abbott	sr
Depakote Sprinkles	Abbott	ec
Despec SR	Int'l Ethical	sr
Detrol LA	Pharmacia	sr
Dexaphen SA	Major	sr
Dexcon-PE	Cypress	sr
Dexedrine Spansules	GlaxoSmithKline	sr
D-Feda II	WE Pharm.	sr
Diabetes Trio	Mason Vitamins	sr
Diamox Sequels	Duramed	sr
Dilacor XR	Watson	sr
Dilantin Kapseals	Pfizer	sr
Dilatrate-SR	Schwarz Pharma	sr
Diltia XT	Andrx	sr
Dilt-XR	Apotex	sr
Dimetane Extentabs	Wyeth	sr
Disophrol Chronotab	Schering Plough	sr
Ditropan XL	Ortho-McNeil	sr
Donnatal Extentabs	PBM	sr
Doryx	Warner Chilcott	ec
Drexophed SR	Qualitest	sr
Drihist SR	Prasco	sr
Drixomed	Iopharm	sr
Drixoral	Schering Plough	sr
Drixoral Plus	Schering Plough	sr
Drixoral sinus	Schering Plough	sr
Drize-R	Monarch	sr
Drysec	A. G. Marin	sr
Dulcolax	Boehr. Ingelheim	ec
Duomax	Capellon	sr

Drug	Manufacturer	Form
Duradex	Proethic	sr
Duradryl Jr	Breckenridge	sr
Durahist	Proethic	sr
Durahist D	Proethic	sr
Durahist PE	Proethic	sr
Duraphen DM	Proethic	sr
Duraphen Forte	Proethic	sr
Duraphen II	Proethic	sr
Duraphen II DM	Proethic	sr
Duratuss	Victory	sr
Duratuss GP	Victory	sr
Dynabac	Muro	ec
Dynabac D5-Pak	Muro	ec
Dynacirc CR	Reliant	sr
Dynahist-ER Pediatric	Breckenridge	sr
Dynex	Athlon	sr
Dytan-CS	Hawthorn	sr
Easprin	Harvest	ec
EC Naprosyn	Roche	ec
Ecotrin	GlaxoSmithKline	ec
Ecotrin Adult Low Strength	GlaxoSmithKline	ec
Ecotrin Maximum Strength	GlaxoSmithKline	ec
Ecpirin	Prime Marketing	ec
Ed A-Hist	Edwards	sr
Ed-Chlor-Tan	Edwards	sr
Effexor-XR	Wyeth	sr
Efidac 24 Chlorpheniramine	Novartis Consumer	sr
Efidac 24 Pseudoephedrine	Novartis Consumer	sr
Enablex	Novartis	sr
Endal	Pediamed	sr
Entab-DM	Rising	sr
Entercote	Global Source	ec
Entex ER	Andrx	sr
Entex LA	Andrx	sr
Entex PSE	Andrx	sr
Entocort EC	Prometheus	ec
Equetro	Shire US	sr
ERYC	Warner Chilcott	ec
Ery-Tab	Abbott	ec
Eskalith-CR	GlaxoSmithKline	sr
Exefen-DM	Larken	sr
Exefen-PD	Larken	sr
Extendryl Jr	Fleming	sr
Extendryl SR	Fleming	sr
Extress-30	Key	sr
Extuss LA	Cypress	sr
Feen-A-Mint	Schering Plough	ec
Femilax	G & W	ec
Fero-Folic-500	Abbott	sr
Fero-Grad-500	Abbott	sr
Ferro-Sequels	Inverness Medical	sr
Ferro-Time	Time-Cap	sr
Ferrous Fumarate DS	Vita-Rx	sr
Fetrin	Lunsco	sr
Flagyl ER	Pharmacia	sr
Fleet Bisacodyl	Fleet, C. B.	ec
Focalin XR	Novartis	sr
Folitab 500	Rising	sr
Fortamet	First Horizon	sr

(*Continued on next page*)

Drug	Manufacturer	Form
Fumatinic	Laser	sr
G/P 1200/75	Cypress	sr
Genacote	Ivax	ec
GFN 1000/DM 50	Cypress	sr
GFN 1200/DM 20/PE 40	Cypress	sr
GFN 1200/DM 60/PSE 60	Cypress	sr
GFN 1200/Phenylephrine 40	Cypress	sr
GFN 1200/PSE 50	Cypress	sr
GFN 500/DM 30	Cypress	sr
GFN 550/PSE 60	Cypress	sr
GFN 550/PSE 60/DM 30	Cypress	sr
GFN 595/PSE 48	Cypress	sr
GFN 595/PSE 48/DM 32	Cypress	sr
GFN 795/PSE 85	Cypress	sr
GFN 800/DM 30	Cypress	sr
GFN 800/PE 25	Cypress	sr
GFN 800/PSE 60	Cypress	sr
Gilphex TR	Gil	sr
Giltuss TR	Gil	sr
Glucophage XR	Bristol-Myers Squibb	sr
Glucotrol XL	Pfizer	sr
GP-1200	Iopharm	sr
Guaifed	Victory	sr
Guaifed-PD	Victory	sr
Guaifenex DM	Ethex	sr
Guaifenex GP	Ethex	sr
Guaifenex PSE 120	Ethex	sr
Guaifenex PSE 60	Ethex	sr
Guaifenex PSE 80	Ethex	sr
Gualmax-D	Schwarz Pharma	sr
Gua-SR	Seatrace	sr
Guia-D	Breckenridge	sr
Guiadex D	Breckenridge	sr
Guiadex PD	Breckenridge	sr
Guiadrine DM	Breckenridge	sr
Guiadrine G-1200	Breckenridge	sr
Guiadrine GP	Breckenridge	sr
Guiadrine PSE	Breckenridge	sr
H 9600 SR	Hawthorn	sr
Halfprin	Kramer	ec
Hemax	Pronova	sr
Histacol LA	Breckenridge	sr
Histade	Breckenridge	sr
Histade MX	Breckenridge	sr
Hista-Vent DA	Ethex	sr
Hista-Vent PSE	Ethex	sr
Histex CT	Teamm	sr
Histex I/E	Teamm	sr
Histex SR	Teamm	sr
Humavent LA	WE Pharm.	sr
Humibid DM	Carolina	sr
Humibid L.A.	Carolina	sr
Hydro Pro DM SR	Breckenridge	sr
Hyoscyamine TR	Breckenridge	sr
Iberet-500	Abbott	sr
Iberet-Folic-500	Abbott	sr
Icar-C Plus SR	Hawthorn	sr
Imdur	Schering Plough	sr
Inderal LA	Wyeth	sr
Indocin SR	Forte Pharma	sr

Drug	Manufacturer	Form
Innopran XL	Reliant	sr
Iobid DM	Iopharm	sr
Ionamin	Celltech	sr
Iosal II	Iopharm	sr
Iotex PSE	Iopharm	sr
Isochron	Forest	sr
Isoptin SR	FSC	sr
Kadian	Alphagen	sr
Kaon-Cl 10	Savage	sr
K-Dur 10	Schering Plough	sr
K-Dur 20	Schering Plough	sr
Klor-Con 10	Upsher-Smith	sr
Klor-Con 8	Upsher-Smith	sr
Klor-Con M10	Upsher-Smith	sr
Klor-Con M15	Upsher-Smith	sr
Klor-Con M20	Upsher-Smith	sr
Klotrix	Bristol-Myers Squibb	sr
Kronofed-A	Ferndale	sr
Kronofed-A-Jr	Ferndale	sr
K-Tab	Abbott	sr
K-Tan	Prasco	sr
Lescol XL	Novartis	sr
Levall G	Athlon	sr
Levbid	Schwarz Pharma	sr
Levsinex	Schwarz Pharma	sr
Lexxel	Astra Zeneca	sr
Lipram 4500	Global	ec
Lipram-CR10	Global	ec
Lipram-CR20	Global	ec
Lipram-CR5	Global	ec
Lipram-PN10	Global	ec
Lipram-PN16	Global	ec
Lipram-PN20	Global	ec
Lipram-UL12	Global	ec
Lipram-UL18	Global	ec
Lipram-UL20	Global	ec
Liquibid-D	Capellon	sr
Liquibid-D 1200	Capellon	sr
Liquibid-PD	Capellon	sr
Lithobid	JDS Pharm.	sr
Lodine XL	Wyeth	sr
Lodrane 12 Hour	ECR	sr
Lodrane 12D	ECR	sr
Lodrane 24	ECR	sr
Lohist-12	Larken	sr
Lohist-12D	Larken	sr
Lusonex	Wraser	sr
Mag Delay	Major	ec
Mag64	Rising	ec
Mag-SR	Cypress	sr
Mag-SR Plus Calcium	Cypress	sr
Mag-Tab SR	Niche	sr
Maxifed	MCR American	sr
Maxifed DM	MCR American	sr
Maxifed DMX	MCR American	sr
Maxifed-G	MCR American	sr
Maxiphen DM	Ambi	sr
Maxovite	Tyson Neutraceuticals	sr
Medent DM	Stewart-Jackson	sr

(*Continued on next page*)

Drug	Manufacturer	Form
Medent LD	Stewart-Jackson	sr
Mega-C	Merit	sr
Melfiat	Numark	sr
Menopause Trio	Mason Vitamins	sr
Mestinon Timespan	Valeant	sr
Metadate CD	Celltech	sr
Metadate ER	Celltech	sr
Methylin ER	Mallinckrodt	sr
Micro-K	Ther-Rx	sr
Micro-K 10	Ther-Rx	sr
Mild-C	Carison, J. R.	sr
Mindal	Breckenridge	sr
Mindal DM	Breckenridge	sr
Mintab C	Breckenridge	sr
Mintab D	Breckenridge	sr
Mintab DM	Breckenridge	sr
Miraphen PSE	Caraco	sr
Modane	Savage	ec
MS Contin	Purdue	sr
MSP-BLU	Cypress	ec
Mucinex	Adams	sr
Muco-Fen DM	Ivax	sr
Multi-Ferrous Folic	United Research	sr
Multiret Folic-500	Amide	sr
Myfortic	Novartis	ec
Nacon	Cypress	sr
Nalex-A	Blansett	sr
Nasatab LA	ECR	sr
Nasex	Cypress	sr
Nd Clear	Seatrace	sr
Nescon-PD	Cypress	sr
New Ami-Tex LA	Amide	sr
Nexium	Astra Zeneca	ec
Niaspan	KOS	sr
Nicomide	Sirius	sr
Nifediac CC	Teva	sr
Nifedical XL	Teva	sr
Nitrocot	Truxton	sr
Nitro-Time	Time-Cap	sr
Nohist	Larken	sr
Norel SR	U.S. Pharm. Corp.	sr
Norpace CR	Pharmacia	sr
Obstetrix EC	Seyer Pharmatec	ec
Omnihist L.A.	WE Pharm.	sr
Oramorph SR	AAI Pharma	sr
Oruvail	Wyeth	sr
Oxycontin	Purdue	sr
Palcaps 10	Breckenridge	ec
Palcaps 20	Breckenridge	ec
Palgic-D	Pamlab	sr
Pancrease	McNeil Consumer	ec
Pancrease MT 10	McNeil Consumer	ec
Pancrease MT 16	McNeil Consumer	ec
Pancrease MT 20	McNeil Consumer	ec
Pancrecarb MS-16	Digestive Care	ec
Pancrecarb MS-4	Digestive Care	ec
Pancrecarb MS-8	Digestive Care	ec
Pangestyme CN-10	Ethex	ec
Pangestyme CN-20	Ethex	ec
Pangestyme EC	Ethex	ec

Drug	Manufacturer	Form
Pangestyme MT16	Ethex	ec
Pangestyme UL12	Ethex	ec
Pangestyme UL18	Ethex	ec
Pangestyme UL20	Ethex	ec
Panmist DM	Pamlab	sr
Panmist Jr	Pamlab	sr
Panmist LA	Pamlab	sr
Pannaz	Pamlab	sr
Panocaps	Breckenridge	ec
Panocaps MT 16	Breckenridge	ec
Panocaps MT 20	Breckenridge	ec
Papacon	Consolidated Midland	sr
Para-Time SR	Time-Cap	sr
Paser	Jacobus	sr
Pavacot	Truxton	sr
Paxil CR	GlaxoSmithKline	sr
PCE Dispertab	Abbott	sr
PCM LA	Cypress	sr
Pendex	Cypress	sr
Pentasa	Shire US	sr
Pentopak	Zoetica	sr
Pentoxil	Upsher-Smith	sr
Pharmadrine	Breckenridge	sr
Phenabid	Gil	sr
Phenabid DM	Gil	sr
Phenavent	Ethex	sr
Phenavent D	Ethex	sr
Phenavent LA	Ethex	sr
Phenavent PED	Ethex	sr
Phendiet-105	Truxton	sr
Phenytek	Mylan Bertek	sr
Plendil	Astra Zeneca	sr
Poly Hist Forte	Poly	sr
Poly-Vent	Poly	sr
Poly-Vent Jr	Poly	sr
Prehist D	Marnel	sr
Prelu-2	Roxane	sr
Prevacid	Tap	ec
Prilosec	Astra Zeneca	ec
Prilosec OTC	Procter & Gamble	sr
Procanbid	Monarch	sr
Procardia XL	Pfizer	sr
Profen Forte	Ivax	sr
Profen Forte DM	Ivax	sr
Profen II	Ivax	sr
Profen II DM	Ivax	sr
Prolex PD	Blansett	sr
Prolex-D	Blansett	sr
Pronestyl-SR	Bristol-Myers Squibb	sr
Prosed EC	Star	ec
Proset-D	Blansett	sr
Protid	Lunsco	sr
Protonix	Wyeth	ec
Prozac Weekly	Eli Lilly	ec
Pseubrom	Alphagen	sr
Pseubrom-PD	Alphagen	sr
Pseudatex	Breckenridge	sr
Pseudocot-C	Truxton	sr
Pseudocot-G	Truxton	sr

(*Continued on next page*)

Drug	Manufacturer	Form
Pseudovent	Ethex	sr
Pseudovent 400	Ethex	sr
Pseudovent DM	Ethex	sr
Pseudovent PED	Ethex	sr
P-Tuss DM	Prasco	sr
Qdall	Atley	sr
Quibron-T/SR	Monarch	sr
Quindal	Qualitest	sr
Ralix	Cypress	sr
Razadyne ER	Ortho-McNeil	sr
Reliable Gentle Laxative	Ivax	ec
Rescon-Jr	Capellon	sr
Rescon-MX	Capellon	sr
Respa-1ST	Respa	sr
Respa-AR	Respa	sr
Respa-DM	Respa	sr
Respahist	Respa	sr
Respaire-120 SR	Laser	sr
Respaire-60 SR	Laser	sr
Respa-PE	Respa	sr
Rhinabid	Breckenridge	sr
Rhinabid PD	Breckenridge	sr
Rhinacon A	Breckenridge	sr
Ribo-2	Tyson Neutraceuticals	ec
Risperdal Consta	Janssen	sr
Ritalin LA	Novartis	sr
Ritalin-SR	Novartis	sr
Rodex Forte	Legere	sr
Rondec-TR	Biovail	sr
Ru-Tuss 800	Sage	sr
Ru-Tuss 800 DM	Sage	sr
Ru-Tuss Jr	Sage	sr
Ryneze	Stewart-Jackson	sr
Rythmol SR	Reliant	sr
Sam-E	Pharmavite	ec
Sinemet CR	Bristol-Myers Squibb	sr
Sinutuss DM	WE Pharm.	sr
Sinuvent PE	WE Pharm.	sr
Sitrex	Vindex	sr
Slo-Niacin	Upsher-Smith	sr
Slow Fe	Novartis Consumer	sr
Slow Fe With Folic Acid	Novartis Consumer	sr
Slow-Mag	Purdue	ec
Spacol T/S	Dayton	sr
St. Joseph Pain Reliever	McNeil Consumer	ec
Sta-D	Magna	sr
Stahist	Magna	sr
Stamoist E	Magna	sr
Sudafed 12 Hour	Pfizer	sr
Sudafed 24 Hour	Pfizer	sr
Sudal DM	Atley	sr
Sudal SR	Atley	sr
Sular	First Horizon	sr
Sulfazine EC	Qualitest	ec
Symax Duotab	Capellon	sr
Symax-SR	Capellon	sr
Tarka	Abbott	sr
Taztia XT	Andrx	sr
Tegretol-XR	Novartis	sr
Tenuate Dospan	Sanofi-Aventis	sr

Drug	Manufacturer	Form
Theo-24	UCB	sr
Theocap	Forest	sr
Theochron	Forest	sr
Theo-Time	Major	sr
Thiamilate	Tyson Neutraceuticals	ec
Tiazac	Forest	sr
Time-Hist	MCR American	sr
Toprol XL	Astra Zeneca	sr
TotalDay	Nat'l Vitamin Co.	sr
Touro Allergy	Dartmouth	sr
Touro CC	Dartmouth	sr
Touro CC-LD	Dartmouth	sr
Touro DM	Dartmouth	sr
Touro HC	Dartmouth	sr
Touro LA	Dartmouth	sr
Touro LA-LD	Dartmouth	sr
Tranxene-SD	Ovation	sr
Trental	Sanofi-Aventis	sr
Trikof-D	Respa	sr
Trinalin Repetabs	Schering Plough	sr
Trituss-ER	Everett	sr
Tussafed-LA	Everett	sr
Tussall-ER	Everett	sr
Tussbid	Breckenridge	sr
Tussi-Bid	Capellon	sr
Tussitab	Iopharm	sr
Tylenol Arthritis	McNeil Consumer	sr
Ultrabrom	WE Pharm.	sr
Ultrabrom PD	WE Pharm.	sr
Ultracaps MT 20	Breckenridge	ec
Ultrase	Axcan Scandipharm	ec
Ultrase MT12	Axcan Scandipharm	ec
Ultrase MT18	Axcan Scandipharm	ec
Ultrase MT20	Axcan Scandipharm	ec
Uniphyl	Purdue	sr
Uni-Tex	United Research	sr
Urimax	Xanodyne	ec
Urocit-K 10	Mission	sr
Urocit-K 5	Mission	sr
Uroxatral	Sanofi-Aventis	sr
Ultra	Hawthron	sr
V-Dec-M	Seatrace	sr
Veracolate	Numark	ec
Verelan	Schwarz Pharma	sr
Verelan PM	Schwarz Pharma	sr
Versacaps	Seatrace	sr
Videx EC	Bristol-Myers Squibb	ec
Vivotif Berna	Berna Products	ec
Voltaren	Novartis	ec
Voltaren-XR	Novartis	sr
Vospire ER	Odyssey	sr
We Mist II LA	WE Pharm.	sr
We Mist LA	WE Pharm.	sr
Wellbid-D	Prasco	sr
Wellbid-D 1200	Prasco	sr
Wellbutrin SR	GlaxoSmithKline	sr
Wellbutrin XL	GlaxoSmithKline	sr
Wobenzym N	Marlyn	ec
Xanax XR	Pharmacia	sr

(*Continued on next page*)

Drug	Manufacturer	Form
Xiral	Hawthorn	sr
XpeCT-At	Hawthorn	sr
XpeCT-HC	Hawthorn	sr
Z-Cof LA	Zyber	sr
Z-Cof LAX	Zyber	sr
Zephrex LA	Sanofi-Aventis	sr
Zorprin	Par	sr
Zyban	GlaxoSmithKline	sr
Zymase	Organon	ec
Zyrtec-D	Pfizer	sr

Reprinted with permission from *The Drug Topics Red Book*. Montvale NJ: Thomson Medical Economics, 2006.

Sugar-Free Products

Listed below, by therapeutic category, is a selection of drug products that contain no sugar. When recommending these products to diabetic patients, keep in mind that many may contain sorbitol, alcohol, or other sources of carbohydrates. This list should not be considered all-inclusive. Generics and alternate brands of some products may be available. Check product labeling for a current listing of inactive ingredients.

Analgesics	Manufacturer
Actamin Maximum Strength Liquid	Cypress
Addaprin Tablet	Dover
Aminofen Tablet	Dover
Aminofen Max Tablet	Dover
Aspirtab Tablet	Dover
Back Pain-Off Tablet	Textilease Medique
Backprin Tablet	Hart Health and Safety
Buffasal Tablet	Dover
Dyspel Tablet	Dover
Febrol Liquid	Scot-Tussin
I-Prin Tablet	Textilease Medique
Medi-Seltzer Effervescent Tablet	Textilease Medique
Ms.-Aid Tablet	Textilease Medique
PMS Relief Tablet	Textilease Medique
Silapap Children's Elixir	Silarx

Antacids/Antiflatulents	
Almag Chewable Tablet	Textilease Medique
Alcalak Chewable Tablet	Textilease Medique
Aldroxicon I Suspension	Textilease Medique
Aldroxicon II Suspension	Textilease Medique
Baby Gasz Drops	Lee
Dimacid Chewable Tablet	Otis Clapp & Son
Diotame Chewable Tablet	Textilease Medique
Diotame Suspension	Textilease Medique
Gas-Ban Chewable	Textilease Medique
Mallamint Chewable	Textilease Medique
Mylanta Gelcaplet	Johnson & Johnson/Merck
Neutralin Tablet	Dover
Tums E-X Chewable Tablet	GlaxoSmithKline Consumer

Antiasthmatic/Respiratory Agents

Jay-Phyl Syrup	Pharmakon

Antidiarrheals

Diarrest Tablet	Dover
Di-Gon II Tablet	Textilease Medique
Imogen Liquid	Pharmaceutical Generic

Blood Modifiers/Iron Preparations

I.L.X. B-12 Elixir	Kenwood
Irofel Liquid	Dayton
Nephro-Fer Tablet	R & D

Corticosteroids

Pediapred Solution	Celltech

Cough/Cold/Allergy Preparations

Accuhist DM, Pediatric Drops	Pediamed
Accuhist Pediatric Drops	Pediamed
Alacol DM Syrup	Ballay
Amerifed DM Liquid	MCR American
Amerifed Liquid	Ambi
Amerituss AD Solution	Ambi
Anaplex DM Syrup	ECR
Anaplex DMX Syrup	ECR
Anaplex HD Syrup	ECR
Andehist DM Liquid	Cypress
Andehist DM NR Liquid	Cypress
Andehist DM NR Syrup	Cypress
Andehist DM Syrup	Cypress
Andehist Liquid	Cypress
Andehist NR Liquid	Cypress
Andehist NR Syrup	Cypress
Andehist Syrup	Cypress
Atuss EX Liquid	Atley
Atuss NX Solution	Atley
Baltussin Solution	Ballay
Bellahist-D LA Tablet	Cypress
Benadryl Allergy/Sinus Children's Solution	Warner-Lambert Consumer
Boidec DM Drops	Bio-Pharm
Bromaxefed DM RF Syrup	Morton Grove
Bromaxefed RF Syrup	Morton Grove
Bromdec Solution	Scientific Laboratories
Bromdec DM Solution	Scientific Laboratories
Bromhist-DM Solution	Cypress
Bromhist Pediatric Solution	Cypress
Bromophed DX Syrup	Qualitest
Bromphenex DM Solution	Breckendridge
Bromphenex HD Solution	Breckenridge
Bromplex DM Solution	Prasco
Bromplex HD Solution	Prasco
Broncotron Liquid	Seyer Pharmatec
Broncotron-D Suspension	Seyer Pharmatec
Brovex HC Solution	Athlon
B-Tuss Liquid	Blansett
Carbaphen 12 Ped Suspension	Gil
Carbaphen 12 Suspension	Gil
Carbatuss-CL Solution	GM
Carbetaplex Solution	Breckenridge
Carbihist Solution	Boca Pharmacal

(*Continued on next page*)

Carbinoxamine PSE Solution	Boca Pharmacal
Carbofed DM Liquid	Hi-Tech
Carbofed DM Syrup	Hi-Tech
Carbofed DM Drops	Hi-Tech
Carboxine Solution	Cypress
Carboxine-PSE Solution	Cypress
Cardec DM Syrup	Qualitest
Cetafen Cold Tablet	Hart Health and Safety
Cheratussin DAC Liquid	Qualitest
Chlordex GP Syrup	Cypress
Codal-DM Syrup	Cypress
Colace Solution	Purdue Pharma
ColdCough EXP Solution	Breckenridge
ColdCough HC Solution	Breckenridge
ColdCough PD Solution	Breckenridge
ColdCough Solution	Breckenridge
ColdCough XP Solution	Breckenridge
Coldec DS Solution	Breckenridge
ColdMist DM Syrup	Breckenridge
Coldonyl Tablet	Dover
Colidrops Pediatric Liquid	A.G. Marin
Cordron-D Solution	Cypress
Cordron-DM Solution	Cypress
Cordron-HC Solution	Cypress
Corfen DM Solution	Cypress
Co-Tussin Liquid	American Generics
Cotuss-V Syrup	Alphagen
Coughtuss Solution	Breckenridge
Crantex HC Syrup	Breckenridge
Crantex Syrup	Breckenridge
Cypex-LA Tablet	Cypress
Cytuss HC Syrup	Cypress
Dacex-A Solution	Cypress
Dacex-DM Solution	Cypress
Dacex-PE Solution	Cypress
Decahist-DM Solution	Cypress
De-Chlor DM Solution	Cypress
De-Chlor DR Solution	Cypress
De-Chlor G Solution	Cypress
De-Chlor HC Solution	Cypress
De-Chlor HD Solution	Cypress
De-Chlor MR Solution	Cypress
De-Chlor NX Solution	Cypress
Decorel Forte Tablet	Textilease Medique
Denaze Solution	Cypress
Despec Liquid	International Ethical
Despec-SF Liquid	International Ethical
Dexcon-DM Solution	Cypress
Diabetic Tussin Allergy Relief Liquid	Health Care Products
Diabetic Tussin Allergy Relief Gelcaplet	Health Care Products
Diabetic Tussin C Expectorant Liquid	Health Care Products
Diabetic Tussin Cold & Flu Gelcaplet	Health Care Products
Diabetic Tussin DM Liquid	Health Care Products
Diabetic Tussin EX Liquid	Health Care Products
Dimetapp Allergy Children's Elixir	Wyeth Consumer
Diphen Capsule	Textilease Medique
Double-Tussin DM Liquid	Reese
Drocon-CS Solution	Cypress
Duratuss DM Solution	Victory
Dynatuss Syrup	Breckenridge
Dynatuss HC Solution	Breckenridge
Dynatus HCG Solution	Breckenridge

Dytan-CS Tablet	Hawthorn
Emagrin Forte Tablet	Otis Clapp & Son
Endacof DM Solution	Larken Laboratories
Endacof HC Solution	Larken Laboratories
Endacof XP Solution	Larken Laboratories
Endacof-PD Solution	Larken Laboratories
Endal HD Liquid	Pediamed
Endal HD Plus Liquid	Pediamed
Endotuss-HD Syrup	American Generics
Enplus-HD Syrup	Alphagen
Entex Syrup	Andrx
Entex HC Syrup	Andrx
Exo-Tuss Syrup	American Generics
Ganidin NR Liquid	Cypress
Gani-Tuss NR Liquid	Cypress
Gani-Tuss-DM NR Liquid	Cypress
Genebronco-D Liquid	Pharm Generic Developers
Genecof-HC Liquid	Pharmaceutical Generic
Genecof-XP Liquid	Pharmaceutical Generic
Genedel Syrup	Pharmaceutical Generic
Genedotuss-DM Liquid	Pharmaceutical Generic
Genelan Liquid	Pharm Generic Developers
Genetuss-2 Liquid	Pharm Generic Developers
Genexpect DM Liquid	Pharmaceutical Generic
Genexpect-PE Liquid	Pharmaceutical Generic
Genexpect-SF Liquid	Pharmaceutical Generic
Gilphex TR Tablet	Gil
Giltuss Liquid	Gil
Giltuss HC Syrup	Gil
Giltuss Pediatric Liquid	Gil
Giltuss TR Tablet	Gil
Guai-Co Liquid	Alphagen
Gualcon DMS Liquid	Textilease Medique
Guai-DEX Liquid	Alphagen
Guaitussin AC Solution	Scientific Laboratories
Guaitussin DAC Solution	Scientific Laboratories
Guapetex HC Solution	Scientific Laboratories
Guapetex Syrup	Scientific Laboratories
Guiatuss AC Syrup	Alpharma
Guiatuss AC Syrup	Ivax
Halotussin AC Liquid	Watson
Hayfebrol Liquid	Scot-Tussin
Histacol DM Pediatric Solution	Breckenridge
Histex PD Liquid	TEAMM
Histex PD 12 Suspension	Teamm
Histinex HC Syrup	Ethex
Histinex PV Syrup	Ethex
Histuss HC Solution	Scientific Laboratories
Histuss PD Solution	Scientific Laboratories
Hydex-PD Solution	Cypress
Hydone Liquid	Hyrex
Hydro-DP Solution	Cypress
Hydro-GP Syrup	Cypress
Hydro PC Syrup	Cypress
Hydro PC II Plus Solution	Cypress
Hydro Pro Solution	Breckenridge
Hydrocof-HC Solution	Morton Grove
Hydron CP Syrup	Cypress
Hydron EX Syrup	Cypress
Hydron KGS Liquid	Cypress

(*Continued on next page*)

Hydron PSC Liquid	Cypress
Hydro-Tussin CBX Solution	Ethex
Hydro-Tussin DM Elixir	Ethex
Hydro-Tussin HC Syrup	Ethex
Hydro-Tussin HD Liquid	Ethex
Hydro-Tussin XP Syrup	Ethex
Hytuss Tablet	Hyrex
Hytuss 2X Capsule	Hyrex
Jaycof Expectorant Syrup	Pharmakon
Jaycof-HC Liquid	Pharmakon
Jaycof-XP Liquid	Pharmakon
Kita LA Tos Liquid	R.I.D.
Lodrane Liquid	ECR
Lodrane D Suspension	ECR
Lodrane XR Suspension	ECR
Lohist-LQ Solution	Larken
Lortuss DM Solution	Proethic Laboratories
Lortuss HC Solution	Proethic Laboratories
Marcof Expectorant Syrup	Marnel
Maxi-Tuss HCX Solution	MCR American
M-Clear Syrup	McNeil, R.A.
M-Clear Jr Solution	McNeil, R.A.
Metanx Tablet	Pamlab
Mintex PD Liquid	Breckenridge
Mintuss NX Solution Syrup	Breckenridge
Mytussin DAC Syrup	Morton Grove
Nalex DH Liquid	Blansett
Nalex-A Liquid	Blansett
Nasop Suspension	Hawthorn
Neotuss S/F Liquid	A.G. Marin
Nescon-PD Tablet	Cypress
Niferex Elixir	Ther-Rx
Norel DM Liquid	U.S. Corp
Nycoff Tablet	Dover
Onset Forte Tablet	Textilease Medique
Orgadin Liquid	American Generics
Orgadin-Tuss Liquid	American Generics
Orgadin-Tuss DM Liquid	American Generics
Organidin NR Liquid	Wallace
Organidin NR Tablet	Wallace
Palgic-DS Syrup	Pamlab
Pancof Syrup	Pamlab
Pancof EXP Syrup	Pamlab
Pancof HC Solution	Pamlab
Pancof XP Liquid	Pamlab
Pancof XP Solution	Pamlab
Panmist DM Syrup	Pamlab
Pediatex Solution	Zyber
Pediatex D	Zyber
Pediatex DM Liquid	Zyber
Pediatex DM Solution	Zyber
Pediatex HC Solution	Zyber
Phanasin Syrup	Pharmakon
Phanasin Diabetic Choice Syrup	Pharmakon
Phanatuss Syrup	Pharmakon
Phanatuss DM Diabetic Choice Syrup	Pharmakon
Phanatuss-HC Diabetic Choice Solution	Pharmakon
Phena-HC Solution	GM
Phenabid DM Tablet	Gil
Phenydryl Solution	Scientific Laboratories
Pneumotussin 2.5 Syrup	ECR

Poly Hist DM Solution	Poly
Poly Hist PD Solution	Poly
Poly-Tussin Syrup	Poly
Poly-Tussin DM Syrup	Poly
Poly-Tussin HD Syrup	Poly
Poly-Tussin XP Syrup	Poly
Pro-Clear Solution	Pro-Pharma
Pro-Cof D Liquid	Qualitest
Pro-Red Solution	Pro-Pharma
Prolex DH Liquid	Blansett
Prolex DM Liquid	Blansett
Protex Solution	Scientific Laboratories
Protex D Solution	Scientific Laboratories
Protuss Liquid	First Horizon
Quintex Syrup	Qualitest
Quintex HC Syrup	Qualitest
Relacon-DM Solution	Cypress
Relacon-HC Solution	Cypress
Rescon-DM Liquid	Capellon
Rhinacon A Solution	Breckenridge
Rhinacon DH Solution	Breckenridge
Rindal HD Liquid	Breckenridge
Rindal HD Plus Solution	Breckenridge
Rindal HPD Solution	Breckenridge
Romilar AC Liquid	Scot-Tussin
Romilar DM Liquid	Scot-Tussin
Rondamine DM Liquid	Major
Rondec Syrup	Biovail
Rondec DM Syrup	Biovail
Rondec DM Drops	Biovail
Ru-Tuss A Syrup	Sage
Ru-Tuss DM Syrup	Sage
Scot-Tussin Allergy Relief Formula Liquid	Scot Tussin
Scot-Tussin DM Cough Chasers Lozenge	Scot-Tussin
Scot-Tussin Original Liquid	Scot Tussin
Siladryl Allergy Liquid	Silarx
Siladryl DAS Liquid	Silarx
Sildec Syrup	Silarx
Sildec Drops	Silarx
Sildec-DM Syrup	Silarx
Silexin Syrup	Otis Clapp & Son
Silexin Tablet	Otis Clapp & Son
Sil-Tex Liquid Liquid	Silarx
Siltussin DM DAS Cough Formula Syrup	Silarx
S-T Forte 2 Liquid	Scot-Tussin
Statuss Green Liquid	Magna
Sudodrin Tablet	Textilease Medique
Sudafed Children's Cold & Cough Solution	Pfizer
Sudafed Children's Solution	Pfizer
Sudafed Children's Tablet	Pfizer
Sudanyl Tablet	Dover
Sudatuss-SF Liquid	Pharm Generic Developers
Sudodrin Tablet	Textilease Medique
Supress DX Pediatric Drops	Kramer-Novis
Suttar-SF Syrup	Gil
Triant-HC Solution	Hawthorn
Tricodene Syrup	Pfeiffer
Trispec-PE Liquid	Deliz
Trituss DM Solution	Breckenridge
Trituss Solution	Everett

(*Continued on next page*)

Tri-Vent DM Solution	Ethex
Tusdec-DM Solution	Cypress
Tusdec-HC Solution	Cypress
Tusnel Solution	Llorens
Tussafed Syrup	Everett
Tussafed-EX Pediatric Drops	Everett
Tussafed-HC Syrup	Everett
Tussafed-HCG Solution	Everett
Tussall Solution	Everett
Tuss-DM Liquid	Seatrace
Tuss-ES Syrup	Seatrace
Tussi-Organidin DM NR Liquid	Wallace
Tussi-Organidin NR Liquid	Wallace
Tussi-Organidin-S NR Liquid	Wallace
Tussi-Pres Liquid	Kramer-Novis
Tussirex Liquid	Scot-Tussin
Uni Cof EXP Solution	United Research Labs
Uni Cof Solution	United Research Labs
Uni-Lev 5.0 Solution	United Research Labs
Vazol Solution	Wraser
Vi-Q-Tuss Syrup	Qualitest
Vitussin Expectorant Syrup	Cypress
Welltuss EXP Solution	Prasco
Welltuss HC Solution	Prasco
Z-Cof HC Solution	Zyber
Z-Cof HC Syrup	Zyber
Ztuss Expectorant Solution	Magna
Zyrtec Syrup	Pfizer

Fluoride Preparations

Ethedent Chewable Tablet	Ethex
Fluor-A-Day Tablet	Pharmascience
Fluor-A-Day Lozenge	Pharmascience
Flura-Loz Tablet	Kirkman
Lozi-Flur Lozenge	Dreir
Sensodyne w/Fluoride Gel	GlaxoSmithKline Consumer
Sensodyne w/Fluoride Tartar Control Toothpaste	GlaxoSmithKline Consumer
Sensodyne w/Fluoride Toothpaste	GlaxoSmithKline Consumer

Laxatives

Citrucel Powder	GlaxoSmithKline Consumer
Colace Solution	Purdue Pharma
Fiber Ease Liquid	Plainview
Fibro-XL Capsule	Key
Genfiber Powder	Ivax
Konsyl Easy Mix Formula Powder	Konsyl
Konsyl-Orange Powder	Konsyl
Metamucil Smooth Texture Powder	Procter & Gamble
Reguloid Powder	Rugby
Senokot Wheat Bran	Purdue Products

Miscellaneous

Acidoll Capsule	Key
Alka-Gest Tablet	Key
Bicitra Solution	Ortho-McNeil
Colidrops Pediatric Drops	A.G. Manin
Cytra-2 Solution	Cypress
Cytra-K Solution	Cypress
Cytra-K Crystals	Cypress
Melatin Tablet	Mason Vitamins

Methadose Solution	Mallinckrodt
Neutra-Phos Powder	Ortho-McNeil
Neutra-Phos-K Powder	Ortho-McNeil
Polycitra-K Solution	Ortho-McNeil
Polycitra-LC Solution	Ortho-McNeil
Questran Light Powder	Par

Mouth/Throat Preparations

Aquafresh Triple Protection Gum	GlaxoSmithKline Consumer
Cepacol Maximum Strength Spray	J.B. Williams
Cepacol Sore Throat Lozenges	J.B. Williams
Cheracol Sore Throat Spray	Lee
Cylex Lozenges	Pharmakon
Fisherman's Friend Lozenges	Mentholatum
Fresh N Free Liquid	Geritrex
Isodettes Sore Throat Spray	GlaxoSmithKline Consumer
Larynex Lozenges	Dover
Listerine Pocketpaks Film	Pfizer Consumer
Medikoff Drops	Textilease Medique
Oragesic Solution	Parnell
Orasept Mouthwash/Gargle Liquid	Pharmakon
Robitussin Lozenges	Wyeth Consumer
Sepasoothe Lozenges	Textilease Medique
Thorets Maximum Strength Lozenges	Otis Clapp & Son
Throto-Ceptic Spray	S.S.S.
Vademecum Mouthwash & Gargle Concentrate	Dermatone

Potassium Supplements

Cena K Liquid	Century
Kaon Elixir	Savage
Kaon-Cl 20% Liquid	Savage
Rum-K Liquid	Fleming

Vitamins/Minerals/Supplements

Action-Tabs Made For Men	Action Labs
Adaptosode For Stress Liquid	HVS
Adaptosode R + R for Acute Stress Liquid	HVS
Alamag Tablet	Textilease Medique
Alcalak Tablet	Textilease Medique
Aldroxicon I Suspension	Textilease Medique
Aldroxicon II Suspension	Textilease Medique
Aminoplex Powder	Tyson
Aminostasis Powder	Tyson
Aminotate Powder	Tyson
Apetigen Elixir	Kramer-Novis
Apptrim Capsule	Physician Therapeutics
Apptrim-D Capsule	Physician Therapeutics
B-C-Bid Caplet	Lee
Bevitamel Tablet	Westlake
Biosode Liquid	HVS
Biotect Plus Caplet	Gil
C & M Caps-375 Capsule	Key
Calbon Tablet	Emrex/Economed
Cal-Cee Tablet	Key
Calcet Plus Tablet	Mission Pharmacal
Calcimin-300 Tablet	Key
Cal-Mint Chewable Tablet	Freeda Vitamins
Cena K Solution	Century
Cerefolin Tablet	Pamlab

(*Continued on next page*)

Cevi-Bid Tablet	Lee
Choice DM Liquid	Bristol-Myers Squibb
Cholestratin Tablet	Key
Chromacaps Tablet	Key
Chromium K6 Tablet	Rexall Consumer
Citrimax 500 Plus Tablet	Mason Vitamins
Combi-Cart Tablet	Atrium Bio-Tech
Delta D3 Tablet	Freeda Vitamins
Detoxosode Liquids	HVS
Dexfol Tablet	Rising
DHEA Capsule	ADH Health Products
Diabeze Tablet	Key
Diatx Tablet	Pamlab
Diatx ZN Tablet	Pamlab
Diet System 6 Gum	Applied Nutrition
Dimacid Tablet	Otis Clapp & Son
Diucaps Capsule	Legere
Di-Phen-500 Capsule	Key
Electrolab Tablet	Hart Health And Safety
Endorphenyl Capsule	Tyson
Ensure Nutra Shake Pudding	Ross Products
Enterex Diabetic Liquid	Victus
Essential Nutrients Plus Silica Tablet	Actions Labs
Evening Primrose Oil Capsule	National Vitamin
Evolve Softgel	Bionutrics Health Products
Ex-L Tablet	Key
Extress Tablet	Key
Eyetamins Tablet	Rexall Consumer
Fem-Cal Tablet	Freeda Vitamins
Fem-Cal Plus Tablet	Freeda Vitamins
Ferrocite F Tablet	Breckenridge
Folacin-800 Tablet	Key
Folbee Plus Tablet	Breckenridge
Folplex 2.2 Tablet	Breckenridge
Foltx Tablet	Pamlab
Gabadone Capsule	Physician Therapeutics
Gram-O-Leci Tablet	Freeda Vitamins
Hemovit Tablet	Dayton
Herbal Slim Complex Capsule	ADH Health Products
Irofol Liquid	Dayton
Lynae Calcium/Vitamin C Chewable Tablet	Boscogen
Lynae Chondroitin/Glucosamine Capsule	Boscogen
Lynae Ginse-Cool Chewable Tablet	Boscogen
Mag-Caps Capsule	Rising
Mag-Ox 400 Tablet	Blaine
Mag-SR Tablet	Cypress
Magimin Tablet	Key Company
Magnacaps Capsule	Key Company
Mangimin Capsule	Key Company
Mangimin Tablet	Key Company
Medi-Lyte Tablet	Textilease Medique
Metanx Tablet	Pamlab
Multi-Delyn w/Iron Liquid	Silarx
Nephro-Fer Tablet	Watson
Neutra-Phos Powder	Ortho-Mcneil
Neutra-Phos-K Powder	Ortho-Mcneil
New Life Hair Tablet	Rexall Consumer
Niferex Elixir	Ther-Rx
Nutrisure OTC Tablet	Westlake
O-Cal Fa Tablet	Pharmics
Plenamins Plus Tablet	Rexall Consumer

Powervites Tablet	Green Turtle Bay Vitamin
Prostaplex Herbal Complex Capsule	ADH Health Products
Prostatonin Capsule	Pharmaton Natural Health
Protect Plus Liquid	Gil
Protect Plus NR Softgel	Gil
Pulmona Capsule	Physician T
Quintabs-M Tablet	Freeda Vitamins
Re/Neph Liquid	Ross Products
Replace Capsule	Key
Replace w/o Iron Capsule	Key
Resource Arginaid Powder	Novartis Nutrition
Ribo-100 T.D. Capsule	Key
Samolinic Softgel	Key
Sea Omega 30 Softgel	Rugby
Sea Omega 50 Softgel	Rugby
Sentra Am Capsule	Physician Therapeutics
Sentra PM Capsule	Physician Therapeutics
Soy Care for Bone Health Tablet	Inverness Medical
Soy Care for Menopause Capsule	Inverness Medical
Span C Tablet	Freeda Vitamins
Strovite Forte Syrup	Everett
Sunnie Tablet	Green Turtle Bay Vitamin
Sunvite Tablet	Rexall Consumer
Super Dec B100 Tablet	Freeda Vitamins
Super Quints-50 Tablet	Freeda Vitamins
Supervite Liquid	Seyer Pharmatec
Suplevit Liquid	Gil
Theramine Capsule	Physician Therapeutics
Triamin Tablet	Key
Triamino Tablet	Freeda Vitamins
Ultramino Tablet	Freeda Vitamins
Uro-Mag Capsule	Blaine
Vinatal 600 Kit	Breckenridge
Vitalize Liquid	Scot-Tussin
Vitamin C/Rose Hips Tablet	ADH Health Products
Vitrum Jr Chewable Tablet	Mason Vitamins
Xtramins Tablet	Key
Yohimbe Power Max 1500 For Women Tablet	Action Labs
Yohimbized 1000 Capsule	Action Labs
Ze-Plus Softgel	Everett

Alcohol-Free Products

The following is a selection of alcohol-free products by therapeutic category. The list is not comprehensive. Generic and alternate brands may exist. Always check product labeling for definitive information on specific ingredients.

Analgesics	Manufacturer
Acetaminophen Infants Drops	Ivax
Actamin Maximum Strength Liquid	Cypress
Addaprin Tablet	Dover
Advil Children's Suspension	Wyeth Consumer
Aminofen Tablet	Dover
Aminofen Max Tablet	Dover
APAP Elixir	Bio-Pharm
Aspirtab Tablet	Dover

(*Continued on next page*)

Buffasal Tablet	Dover
Demerol Hydrochloride Syrup	Sanofi-Synthelabo
Dolono Elixir	R.I.D.
Dyspel Tablet	Dover
Genapap Children Elixir	Ivax
Genapap Infant's Drop	Ivax
Motrin Children's Suspension	McNeil Consumer
Motrin Infant's Suspension	McNeil Consumer
Silapap Children's Elixir	Silarx
Silapap Infant's Drops	Silarx
Tylenol Children's Suspension	McNeil Consumer
Tylenol Extra Strength Solution	McNeil Consumer
Tylenol Infant's Drops	McNeil Consumer
Tylenol Infant's Suspension	McNeil Consumer

Antiasthmatic Agents

Dilor-G Liquid	Savage
Dy-G Liquid	Cypress
Elixophyllin-GG Liquid	Forest

Anticonvulsants

Zarontin Syrup	Pfizer

Antiviral Agents

Epivir Oral Solution	GlaxoSmithKline

Cough/Cold/Allergy Preparations

Accuhist Pediatric Drops	Propst
Alacol DM Syrup	Ballay
Allergy Relief Medicine Children's Elixir	Hi-Tech Pharmacal
Altarussin Syrup	Altaire
Amerifed DM Liquid	MCR American
Amerifed Liquid	Ambi
Anaplex DM Syrup	ECR
Anaplex DMX Suspension	ECR
Anaplex HD Syrup	ECR
Andehist DM Drops	Cypress
Andehist DM Syrup	Cypress
Andehist DM NR Liquid	Cypress
Andehist DM NR Syrup	Cypress
Andehist NR Syrup	Cypress
Andehist Syrup	Cypress
Aquatab DM Syrup	Adams
Atuss DR Syrup	Atley
Atuss EX Liquid	Atley
Atuss G Liquid	Atley
Atuss HC Syrup	Atley
Atuss MS Syrup	Atley
Baltussin Solution	Ballay Pharm
Benadryl Allergy Solution	Pfizer Consumer
Benadryl Allergy/Sinus Children's Solution	Pfizer
Biodec DM Drops	Bio-Pharm
Bromaline Solution	Rugby
Bromaline DM Elixir	Rugby
Bromanate Elixir	Alpharma USPD
Bromatan-DM Suspension	Cypress
Bromaxefed DM RF Syrup	Morton Grove
Bromaxefed RF Syrup	Morton Grove
Broncotron Liquid	Seyer Pharmatec
Bromdec Solution	Scientific Laboratories

Bromdec DM Solution	Scientific Laboratories
Bromhist Pediatric Solution	Cypress
Bromhist-DM Pediatric Syrup	Cypress
Bromhist-DM Solution	Cypress
Bromphenex HD Solution	Breckenridge
Bromplex DM Solution	Prasco Laboratories
Broncotron-D Suspension	Seyer Pharmatec
Bron-Tuss Liquid	American Generics
Brovex HC Solution	Athlon
B-Tuss Liquid	Blansett
Carbaphen 12 Ped Suspension	Gil
Carbaphen 12 Suspension	Gil
Carbatuss Liquid	GM
Carbatuss-CL Solution	GM
Carbaxefed DM RF Liquid	Morton Grove
Carbetaplex Solution	Breckenridge
Carbihist Solution	Boca Pharmacal
Carbofed DM Drops	Hi-Tech Pharmacal
Carbofed DM Syrup	Hi-Tech Pharmacal
Carboxine Solution	Cypress
Carboxine-PSE Solution	Cypress
Cardec Syrup	Qualitest
Cardec DM Syrup	Qualitest
Cepacol Sore Throat Liquid	J. B. Williams
Chlordex GP Syrup	Cypress
Chlor-Mes D Solution	Cypress
Chlor-Trimeton Allergy Syrup	Schering Plough
Codal-DH Syrup	Cypress
Codal-DM Syrup	Cypress
Codotuss Liquid	Major
Coldec DS Solution	Breckenridge
Coldec-DM Syrup	United Research Labs
Coldmist DM Solution	Breckenridge
Coldmist DM Syrup	Breckenridge
Coldmist S Syrup	Breckenridge
Coldonyl Tablet	Dover
Coldtuss DR Syrup	United Research Labs
Colidrops Pediatric Liquid	A. G. Marin
Complete Allergy Elixir	Cardinal Health
Cordron-D Solution	Cypress
Cordron-DM Solution	Cypress
Cordron-HC Solution	Cypress
Corfen DM Solution	Cypress
Co-Tussin Liquid	American Generics
Cotuss-V Syrup	Alphagen
Crantex HC Syrup	Breckenridge
Crantex Syrup	Breckenridge
Creomulsion Complete Syrup	Summit Industries
Creomulsion Cough Syrup	Summit Industries
Creomulsion For Children Syrup	Summit Industries
Creomulsion Pediatric Syrup	Summit Industries
Cytuss HC Syrup	Cypress
Dacex-A Solution	Cypress
Dacex-DM Solution	Cypress
Decahist-DM Solution	Cypress
De-Chlor DM Solution	Cypress
De-Chlor DR Solution	Cypress
Dehistine Syrup	Cypress
Deka Liquid	Dayton
Deka Pediatric Drops Solution	Dayton

(*Continued on next page*)

Deltuss Liquid	Deliz
Denaze Solution	Cypress
Despec Liquid Labs	International Ethical
Dex PC Syrup	Boca Pharmacal
Dexcon-DM Solution	Cypress
Diabetic Tussin Allergy Relief Liquid	Healthcare Products
Diabetic Tussin C Expectorant Liquid	Healthcare Products
Diabetic Tussin Cold & Flu Tablet	Healthcare Products
Diabetic Tussin DM Liquid	Healthcare Products
Diabetic Tussin DM Maximum Strength Liquid	Healthcare Products
Diabetic Tussin DM Maximum Strength Capsule	Healthcare Products
Diabetic Tussin EX Liquid	Healthcare Products
Dimetapp Allergy Children's Elixir	Whitehall-Robins
Dimetapp Cold & Fever Children's Suspension	Wyeth Consumer
Dimetapp Decongestant Pediatric Drops	Wyeth Consumer
Double-Tussin DM Liquid	Reese
Drocon-CS Solution	Cypress
Duradal HD Plus Syrup	Prasco Laboratories
Duratan DM Suspension	Proethic Laboratories
Duratuss DM Solution	Victory
Dynatuss Syrup	Breckenridge
Dynatuss EX Syrup	Breckenridge
Dynatuss HC Solution	Breckenridge
Dynatuss HCG Solution	Breckenridge
Endacof DM Solution	Larken Laboratories
Endacof HC Solution	Larken Laboratories
Endacof XP Solution	Larken Laboratories
Endagen-HD Syrup	Monarch
Endal HD Solution	Pediamed
Endal HD Syrup	Propst
Endal HD Plus Syrup	Propst
Endotuss-HD Syrup	American Generics
Enplus-HD Syrup	Alphagen
Entex Syrup	Andrx
Entex HC Syrup	Andrx
Exo-Tuss	American Generics
Father John's Medicine Plus Drops	Oakhurst
Friallergia DM Liquid	R.I.D.
Friallergia Liquid	R.I.D.
Ganidin NR Liquid	Cypress
Gani-Tuss NR Liquid	Cypress
Gani-Tuss-DM NR Liquid	Cypress
Genahist Elixir	Ivax
Genebronco-D Liquid	Pharm Generic
Genecof-HC Liquid	Pharm Generic
Genecof-XP Liquid	Pharm Generic
Genecof-XP Syrup	Pharm Generic
Genedel Syrup	Pharm Generic
Genedotuss-DM Liquid	Pharm Generic
Genepatuss Liquid	Pharm Generic
Genetuss-2 Liquid	Pharm Generic
Genexpect-DM Liquid	Pharm Generic
Genexpect-PE Liquid	Pharm Generic
Genexpect-SF Liquid	Pharm Generic
Giltuss HC Syrup	Gil
Giltuss Liquid	Gil
Giltuss Pediatric Liquid	Gil
Guai-Co Liquid	Alphagen
Guaicon DMS Liquid	Textilease Medique
Guai-Dex Liquid	Alphagen
Guaifed Syrup	Muro

Guaitussin AC Solution	Scientific Laboratories
Guaitussin DAC Solution	Scientific Laboratories
Guapetex HC Solution	Scientific Laboratories
Guapetex Syrup	Scientific Laboratories
Halotussin AC Liquid	Watson Pharma
Hayfebrol Liquid	Scot-Tussin
H-C Tussive Syrup	Vintage
Histacol DM Pediatric Solution	Breckenridge
Histacol DM Pediatric Syrup	Breckenridge
Histex HC Syrup	TEAMM
Histex Liquid	TEAMM
Histex PD Drops	TEAMM
Histex PD Liquid	TEAMM
Histinex HC Syrup	Ethex
Histinex PV Syrup	Ethex
Histuss HC Solution	Scientific Laboratories
Hi-Tuss Syrup	Hi-Tech Pharmacal
Hycomal DH Liquid	Alphagen
Hydex-PD Solution	Cypress
Hydone Liquid	Hyrex
Hydramine Elixir	Ivax
Hydro PC Syrup	Cypress
Hydro PC II Plus Solution	Cypress
Hydro Pro Solution	Breckenridge
Hydrocol-HC Solution	Morton Grove
Hydro-DP Solution	Cypress
Hydron CF Syrup	Cypress
Hydron EX Syrup	Cypress
Hydron KGS Liquid	Cypress
Hydron PSC Liquid	Cypress
Hydro-Tussin DM Elixir	Ethex
Hydro-Tussin HC Syrup	Ethex
Hydro-Tussin HD Liquid	Ethex
Hydro-Tussin XP Syrup	Ethex
Hyphen-HD Syrup	Alphagen
Jaycof Expectorant Syrup	Pharmakon
Jaycof-HC Liquid	Pharmakon
Jaycof-XP Liquid	Pharmakon
Kita La Tos Liquid	R.I.D.
Levall Liquid	Andrx
Levall 5.0 Liquid	Andrx
Lodrane Liquid	ECR
Lodrane D Suspension	ECR
Lodrane XR Suspension	ECR
Lohist D Syrup	Larken Laboratories
Lohist-LQ Solution	Larken
Lortuss DM Solution	Proethic
Lortuss HC Solution	Proethic
Marcof Expectorant Syrup	Marnel
Maxi-Tuss HCX Solution	MCR American
M-Clear Jr Solution	McNeil, R.A.
M-Clear Syrup	McNeil, R.A.
Medi-Brom Elixir	Medicine Shoppe
Mintex Liquid	Breckenridge
Mintex PD Liquid	Breckenridge
Mintuss DM Syrup	Breckenridge
Mintuss EX Syrup	Breckenridge
Mintuss G Syrup	Breckenridge
Mintuss HD Syrup	Breckenridge
Mintuss MR Syrup	Breckenridge

(*Continued on next page*)

Mintuss MS Syrup	Breckenridge
Mintuss NX Solution	Breckenridge
Motrin Cold Children's Suspension	McNeil Consumer
Mytussin-PE Liquid	Morton Grove
Nalex DH Liquid	Blansett Pharmacal
Nalex-A Liquid	Blansett Pharmacal
Nalspan Senior DX Liquid	Morton Grove
Nasop Suspension	Hawthorn
Neotuss S/F Liquid	A.G. Marin
Neotuss-D Liquid	A.G. Marin
Norel DM Liquid	U.S. Pharmaceutical
Nucofed Syrup	Monarch
Nycoff Tablet	Dover
Orgadin Liquid	American Generics
Orgadin-Tuss Liquid	American Generics
Orgadin-Tuss DM Liquid	American Generics
Organidin NR Liquid	Wallace
Palgic-DS Syrup	Pamlab
Pancof Syrup	Pamlab
Pancof EXP Syrup	Pamlab
Pancof HC Liquid	Pamlab
Pancof HC Solution	Pamlab
Pancof XP Liquid	Pamlab
Pancof XP Solutuion	Pamlab
Panmist DM Syrup	Pamlab
Panmist-S Syrup	Pamlab
PediaCare Cold + Allergy Children's Liquid	Pharmacia
PediaCare Cough + Cold Children's Liquid	Pharmacia
PediaCare Decongestant Infants Drops	Pharmacia
PediaCare Decongestant Plus Cough Drops	Pharmacia
PediaCare Multi-Symptom Liquid	Pharmacia
PediaCare Nightrest Liquid	Pharmacia
Pediahist DM Syrup	Boca
Pedia-Relief Liquid	Major
Pediatex Liquid	Zyber
Pediatex Solution	Zyber
Pediatex-D Liquid	Zyber
Pediatex D Solution	Zyber
Pediatex DM Solution	Zyber
Pediox Liquid	Atley
Phanasin Syrup	Pharmakon
Phanatuss Syrup	Pharmakon
Phanatuss-HC Diabetic Choice Solution	Pharmakon Labs
Phena-HC Solution	GM
Phena-S Liquid	GM
Pneumotussin 2.5 Syrup	ECR
Poly Hist DM Solution	Poly
Poly Hist PD Solution	Poly
Poly-Tussin Syrup	Poly
Poly-Tussin DM Syrup	Poly
Poly-Tussin HD Syrup	Poly
Poly-Tussin XP Syrup	Poly
Primsol Solution	Medicis
Pro-Clear Solution	Pro-Pharma
Pro-Cof Liquid	Qualitest
Pro-Cof D Liquid	Qualitest
Prolex DH Liquid	Blansett Pharmacal
Prolex DM Liquid	Blansett Pharmacal
Pro-Red Solution	Pro-Pharma
Protex Solution	Scientific Laboratories

Protex D Solution	Scientific Laboratories
Protuss Liquid	First Horizon
Protuss-D Liquid	First Horizon
Pyrroxate Extra Strength Tablet	Lee
Q-Tussin PE Liquid	Qualitest
Qual-Tussin DC Syrup	Pharm. Associates
Quintex Syrup	Qualitest
Quintex HC Syrup	Qualitest
Relacon-DM Solution	Cypress
Relacon-HC Solution	Cypress
Rescon-DM Liquid	Capellon
Rescon-GG Liquid	Capellon
Rhinacon A Solution	Breckenridge
Rhinacon DH Solution	Breckenridge
Rindal HD Liquid	Breckenridge
Rindal HD Plus Solution	Breckenridge
Rindal HPD Solution	Breckenridge
Robitussin Cough & Congestion Liquid	Wyeth Consumer
Robitussin DM Syrup	Wyeth Consumer
Robitussin PE Syrup	Wyeth Consumer
Robitussin Pediatric Drops	Wyeth Consumer
Robitussin Pediatric Cough Syrup	Wyeth Consumer
Robitussin Pediatric Night Relief Liquid	Wyeth Consumer
Romilar AC Liquid	Scot-Tussin
Romilar DM Liquid	Scot-Tussin
Rondamine DM Liquid	Major
Rondec Syrup	Biovail
Rondec DM Drops	Biovail
Rondec DM Syrup	Biovail
Ru-Tuss A Syrup	Sage
Ru-Tuss DM Syrup	Sage
Scot-Tussin Allergy Relief Formula Liquid	Scot-Tussin
Scot-Tussin DM Liquid	Scot-Tussin
Scot-Tussin Expectorant Liquid	Scot-Tussin
Scot-Tussin Original Syrup	Scot-Tussin
Scot-Tussin Senior Liquid	Scot-Tussin
Siladryl Allergy Liquid	Silarx
Siladryl DAS Liquid	Silarx
Sildec Liquid	Silarx
Sildec Syrup	Silarx
Sildec-DM Drops	Silarx
Sildec-DM Syrup	Silarx
Sil-Tex Liquiduid Liquid	Silarx
Siltussin DAS Liquid	Silarx
Siltussin DM Syrup	Silarx
Siltussin DM DAS Cough Formula Syrup	Silarx
Siltussin SA Syrup	Silarx
Simply Cough Liquid	McNeil Consumer
Simply Stuffy Liquid	McNeil Consumer
S-T Forte 2 Liquid	Scot-Tussin
Statuss DM Syrup	Magna
Sudafed Children's Cold & Cough Solution	Pfizer
Sudafed Children's Solution	Pfizer
Sudafed Children's Tablet	Pfizer
Sudanyl Tablet	Dover
Sudatuss DM Syrup	Pharmaceutical Generic
Sudatuss-2 Liquid	Pharmaceutical Generic
Sudatuss-SF Liquid	Pharmaceutical Generic
Triaminic Infant Decongestant Drops	Novartis Consumer
Triant-HC Solution	Hawthorn

(*Continued on next page*)

Trispec-PE Liquid	Deliz
Trituss DM Solution	Breckenridge
Trituss Solution	Everett
Tri-Vent DM Solution	Ethex
Tri-Vent DPC Syrup	Ethex
Tusdec-DM Solution	Cypress
Tusdec-HC Solution	Cypress
Tusnel Pediatric Solution	Llorens Pharma
Tusnel Solution	Llorens Pharma
Tussafed Syrup	Everett
Tussafed-EX Syrup	Everett
Tussafed-EX Pediatric Liquid	Everett
Tussafed-HC Syrup	Everett
Tussafed-HCG Solution	Everett
Tussall Solution	Everett
Tussbid Capsule	Breckenridge
Tuss-DM Liquid	Seatrace
Tuss-ES Syrup	Seatrace
Tussex Syrup	H. L. Moore
Tussinate Syrup	Pediamed
Tussi-Organidin DM NR Liquid	Wallace
Tussi-Organidin NR Liquid	Wallace
Tussi-Pres Liquid	Kramer-Novis
Tussirex Liquid	Scot-Tussin
Tussirex Syrup	Scot-Tussin
Tylenol Allergy-D Children's Liquid	McNeil Consumer
Tylenol Cold Children's Liquid	McNeil Consumer
Tylenol Cold Children's Suspension	McNeil Consumer
Tylenol Cold Infants' Drops	McNeil Consumer
Tylenol Cold Plus Cough Children's Liquid	McNeil Consumer
Tylenol Cold Plus Cough Infants' Suspension	McNeil Consumer
Tylenol Flu Children's Suspension	McNeil Consumer
Tylenol Flu Night Time Max Strength Liquid	McNeil Consumer
Tylenol Sinus Children's Liquid	McNeil Consumer
Uni-Lev 5.0 Solution	United Research
Vanex-HD Syrup	Monarch
Vazol Solution	Wraser Pharm
Vicks 44E Pediatric Liquid	Procter & Gamble
Vicks 44M Pediatric Liquid	Procter & Gamble
Vicks Dayquil Multi-Symptom Liquicap	Procter & Gamble
Vicks Dayquil Multi-Symptom Liquid	Procter & Gamble
Vicks 44 Liquid Capsules Cold, Flu, Cough	Procter & Gamble
Vicks Nyquil Children's Liquid	Procter & Gamble
Vicks Sinex 12 Hour Spray	Procter & Gamble
Vicks Sinex Spray	Procter & Gamble
Vi-Q-Tuss Syrup	Vintage
V-Tann Suspension	Breckenridge
Vitussin Expectorant Syrup	Cypress
Vortex Syrup	Superior
Welltuss EXP Solution	Prasco Laboratories
Welltuss HC Solution	Prasco Laboratorues
Z-Cof DM Syrup	Zyber
Z-Cof DMX Solution	Zyber
Z-Cof HC Syrup	Zyber
Ztuss Expectorant Solution	Magna

Ear/Nose/Throat Products

4-Way Saline Moisturizing Mist Spray	Bristol-Myers
Ayr Baby Saline Spray	B.F. Ascher
Bucalcide Solution	Seyer Pharmatec

Bucalcide Spray	Seyer Pharmatec
Bucalsep Solution	Gil
Bucalsep Spray	Gil
Cepacol Sore Throat Liquid	Combe
Cheracol Sore Throat Spray	Lee
Fresh N Free Liquid	Geritrex
Gly-Oxide Liquid	GlaxoSmithKline
Isodettes Sore Throat Spray	GlaxoSmithKline
Lacrosse Mouthwash Liquid	Aplicare
Larynex Lozenges	Dover
Listermint Liquid	Pfizer Consumer
Nasal Moist Gel	Blairex
Orajel Baby Liquid	Del
Orajel Baby Nighttime Gel	Del
Oramagic Oral Wound Rinse Powder for Suspension	MPM Medical
Orasept Mouthwash/Gargle Liquid	Pharmakon Labs
Tanac Liquid	Del
Tech 2000 Dental Rinse Liquid	Care-Tech
Throto-Ceptic Spray	S.S.S.
Zilactin Baby Extra Strength Gel	Zila Consumer

Gastrointestinal Agents

Axid	Pediamed Pharm
Axid Solution	Reliant
Baby Gasz Drops	Lee
Colidrops Pediatric Drops	A.G. Marin
Colace Solution	Purdue Pharma
Diarrest Tablet	Dover
Imogen Liquid	Pharmaceutical
Kaodene NN Suspension	Pfeiffer
Liqui-Doss Liquid	Ferndale
Mylicon Infants' Suspension	J&J-Merck
Neoloid Liquid	Kenwood
Neutralin Tablet	Dover
Senokot Children's Syrup	Purdue Frederick

Hematinics

Irofol Liquid	Dayton

Miscellaneous

Cytra-2 Solution	Cypress
Cytra-K Solution	Cypress
Emetrol Solution	Pharmacia
Fluorinse Solution	Oral B
Primsol Solution	FSC
Rum-K Liquid	Fleming

Psychotropics

Thorazine Syrup	

Topical Products

Aloe Vesta 2-N-1 Antifungal Ointment	Convatec
Blistex Complete Moisture Stick	Blistex
Blistex Fruit Smoothies Stick	Blistex
Blistex Herbal Answer Gel	Blistex
Blistex Herbal Answer Stick	Blistex
Dermatone Lips N Face Protector Ointment	Dermatone
Dermatone Moisturizing Sunblock Cream	Dermatone
Dermatone Outdoor Skin Protection Cream	Dermatone

(*Continued on next page*)

Dermatone Skin Protector Cream	Dermatone
Eucapsulein Facial Lotion	Beiersdorf, Inc.
Evoclin Foam	Connetics
Fleet Pain Relief Pads	Fleet
Fresh & Pure Douche Solution	Unico
Handclens Solution	Woodward
Joint-Ritis Maximum Strength Ointment	Naturopathic Laboratories
Neutrogena Acne Wash Liquid	Neutrogena
Neutrogena Antiseptic Liquid	Neutrogena
Neutrogena Clear Pore Gel	Neutrogena
Neutrogena T/Derm Liquid	Neutrogena
Neutrogena Toner Liquid	Neutrogena
Podiciens Spray	Woodward
Propa pH Foaming Face Wash Liquid	Del
Sea Breeze Foaming Face Wash Gel	Clairol
Shade Uvaguard Lotion	Schering Plough
Sportz Bloc Cream	Med-Derm
Stri-Dex Maximum Strength Pad	Blistex
Stri-Dex Sensitive Skin Pad	Blistex
Stri-Dex Super Scrub Pad	Blistex
Therasoft Anti-Acne Cream	SFC/Solvent Free
Therasoft Skin Protectant Cream	SFC/Solvent Free
Tiger Balm Arthritis Rub Lotion	Prince of Peace Enterprises

Vitamins/Minerals/Supplements

Adaptosode For Stress Liquid	HVS
Adaptosode R + R For Acute Stress Liquid	HVS
Apetigen Elixir	Kramer-Novis
Biosode Liquid	HVS
Detoxosode Products Liquid	HVS
Folbic Tablet	Breckenridge
Folplex 2.2 Gel	Breckenridge
Genesupp-500 Liquid	Pharmaceutical
Genetect Plus Liquid	Pharmaceutical
Multi-Delyn w/Iron Liquid	Silarx
Poly-Vi Sol Drops	Mead Johnson
Poly-Vi Sol w/Iron Drops	Mead Johnson
Poly-Vi Solution Liquid	Mead Johnson
Poly-Vi Solution w/Iron Liquid	Mead Johnson
Protect Plus Liquid	Gil
Soluvite-F Drops	Pharmics
Strovite Forte Syrup	Everett
Supervite Liquid	Seyer Pharmatec
Suplevit Liquid	Gil
Tri-Vi-Sol Drops	Mead Johnson
Tri-Vi-Sol w/Iron Drops	Mead Johnson
Vitafol Syrup	Everett
Vitalize Liquid	Scot-Tussin
Vitamin C/Rose Hips Tablet, Extended Release	ADH Health Products

Drugs That May Cause Photosensitivity

The drugs in this table are known to cause photosensitivity in some individuals. Effects can range from itching, scaling, rash, and swelling to skin cancer, premature skin aging, skin and eye burns, cataracts, reduced immunity, blood vessel damage, and allergic reactions.

The list is not all-inclusive, and shows only representative brands of each generic. When in doubt, always check specific product labeling. Individuals should be advised to wear protective clothing and to apply sunscreens while taking the medications listed below.

Generic	Brand
Acamprosate	Campral
Acetazolamide	Diamox
Acitretin	Soriatane
Acyclovir	Zovirax
Alendronate	Fosamax
Alitretinoin	Panretin
Almotriptan	Axert
Amilloride/hydrochlorothiazide	Moduretic
Aminolevulinic acid	Levulan Kerastick
Amiodarone	Cordarone, Pacerone
Amitriptyline	Elavil
Amitriptyline/chlordiazepoxide	Limbitrol
Amitriptyline/perphenazine	Triavil
Amlodipine/atorvastatin	Caduet
Amoxapine	
Anagrelide	Agrylin
Apripiprazole	Abilify
Atazanavir	Reyataz
Atenolol/chlorthalidone	Tenoretic
Atorvastasin	Lipitor
Atovaquone/proguanil	Malarone
Azatadine/pseudoephedrine	Ryanatan, Trinalin
Azithromycin	Zithromax
Benazepril	Lotensin
Benazepril/hydrochlorothiazide	Lotensin HCT
Bendroflumethiazide/nadolol	Corzide
Bexarotene	Targretin
Bismuth/metronidazole/tetracycline	Helidac
Bisoprolol/hydrochlorothiazide	Ziac
Brompheniramine/dextromethorphan/phenylephrine	Alacol DM
Brompheniramine/dextromethorphan/pseudoephedrine	Bromfed-DM
Buffered aspirin/pravastatin	Pravigard PAC
Bupropion	Wellbutrin, Zyban
Candesartan/hydrochlorothiazide	Atacand HCT
Capecitabine	Xeloda
Captopril	Capoten
Captopril/hyrdrochlorothiazide	Capozide
Carbamazepine	Carbatrol, Tegretol, Tegretol-XR
Carbinoxamine/pseudoephedrine	Palgic-D, Palgic-DS, Pediatex-D
Carvedilol	Coreg
Celecoxib	Celebrex
Cetirizine	Zyrtec
Cetirizine/pseudoephedrine	Zyrtec-D
Cevimeline	Evoxac
Chlorhexidine gluconate	Hibistat
Chloroquine	Aralen
Chlorothiazide	Diuril
Chlorpheniramine/hydrocodone/pseudoephedrine	Tussend
Chlorpheniramine/phenylephrine/pyrilamine	Rynatan
Chlorpromazine	Thorazine
Chlorpropamide	Diabinese
Chlorthalidone	Thalitone
Chlorthalidone/clonidine	Clorpres
Cidofovir	Vistide
Ciprofloxacin	Cipro
Citalopram	Celexa

(*Continued on next page*)

Generic	Brand
Clemastine	Tavist
Clonidine/chlorthalidone	Clorpres
Clozapine	Clozaril, Fazaclo
Cromolyn sodium	Gastrocrom
Cyclobenzaprine	Flexeril
Cyproheptadine	Cyproheptadine
Dacarbazine	DTIC-Dome
Dantrolene	Dantrium
Demeclocycline	Declomycin
Desipramine	Norpramin
Diclofenac potassium	Cataflam
Diclofenac sodium	Voltaren
Diclofenac sodium/misoprostol	Arthrotec
Diflunisal	Dolobid
Dihydroergotamine	D.H.E. 45
Diltiazem	Cardizem, Tiazac
Diphenhydramine	Benadryl
Divalproex	Depakote
Doxepin	Sinequan
Doxycycline hyclate	Doryx, Periostat, Vibra-Tabs,Vibramycin
Doxycycline monohydrate	Monodox
Duloxetine	Cymbalta
Enalapril	Vasotec
Enalapril/felodipine	Lexxel
Enalapril/hydrochlorothiazide	Vaseretic
Enalaprilat	Vasotec I.V.
Epirubicin	Ellence
Eprosartan mesylate/hydrochlorothiazide	Teveten HCT
Erythromycin/sulfisoxazole	Pediazole
Estazolam	ProSom
Estradiol	Gynodiol, Estrogel
Eszopiclone	Lunesta
Ethionamide	Trecator-SC
Etodolac	Lodine
Felbamate	Felbatol
Fenofibrate	Tricor, Lofibra
Floxuridine	Sterile FUDR
Flucytosine	Ancobon
Fluorouracil	Efudex
Fluoxetine	Prozac, Sarafem
Fluphenazine	Prolixin
Flutamide	Eulexin
Fluvastatin	Lescol
Fluvoxamine	Luvox
Fosinopril	Monopril
Fosphenytoin	Cerebyx
Furosemide	Lasix
Gabapentin	Neurontin
Gatifloxacin	Tequin
Gemfibrozil	Lopid
Gemifloxacin mesylate	Factive
Gentamicin	Garamycin
Glatiramer	Copaxone
Glimepiride	Amaryl
Glipizide	Glucotrol
Glyburide	DiaBeta, Glynase, Micronase
Glyburide/metformin HCl	Glucovance
Griseofulvin	Fulvicin P/G, Grifulvin, Gris-PEG
Haloperidol	Haldol

Generic	Brand
Hexachlorophene	pHisoHex
Hydralazine/hydrochlothiazide	Hydra-zide
Hydrochlorothiazide	HydroDIURIl, Microzide, Oretic
Hydrochlorothiazide/fosinopril	Monopril HCT
Hydrochlorothiazide/irbesartan	Avalide
Hydrochlorothiazide/lisinopril	Prinzide, Zestoretic
Hydrochlorothiazide/losartan potassium	Hyzaar
Hydrochlorothiazide/methyldopa	Aldoril
Hydrochlorothiazide/moexipril	Uniretic
Hydrochlorothiazide/propanolol	Inderide
Hydrochlorothiazide/quinapril	Accuretic
Hydrochlorothiazide/spironolactone	Aldactazide
Hydrochlorothiazide/telmisartan	Micardis HCT
Hydrochlorothiazide/timolol	Timolide
Hydrochlorothiazide/triamterene	Dyazide, Maxzide
Hydrochlorothiazide/valsartan	Diovan HCT
Hydroflumethiazide	Hydroflumethiazide
Hydroxychloroquine	Plaquenil
Hypericum	Kira, St. John's Wort
Hypericum/vitamin B_1/vitamin C/kava-kava	One-A-Day Tension & Mood
Ibuprofen	Motrin
Imatinib Mesylate	Gleevec
Imipramine	Tofranil
Imiquimod	Aldara
Indapamide	Lozol
Interferon alfa-2b, recombinant	Intron A
Interferon alfa-n3 (human leukocyte derived)	Alferon-N
Interferon beta-1a	Avonex
Interferon beta-1b	Betaseron
Irbesartan/hydrochlorothiazide	Avalide
Isoniazid/pyrazinamide/rifampin	Rifater
Isotrentinoin	Accutane, Amnesteem
Itraconazole	Sporanox
Ketoprofen	Orudis, Oruvail
Lamotrigine	Lamictal
Leuprolide	Lupron
Levamisole	Levamisole
Lisinopril	Prinivil, Zestril
Lisinorpil/hydrochlorothiazide	Prinivil, Zestoretic
Lomefloxacin	Maxaquin
Loratadine	Claritin
Loratadine/pseudoephedrine	Claritin-D
Losartan	Cozaar
Losartan/hydrochlorothiazide	Hyzaar
Lovastatin	Altoprev, Mevacor
Lovastatin/niacin	Advicor
Maprotiline	Maprotiline
Mefenamic acid	Ponstel
Meloxicam	Mobic
Mesalamine	Pentasa
Methazolamide	
Methotrexate	Trexall
Methoxsalen	Uvadex, Oxsoralen 8-MOP
Methyclothiazide	Enduron
Methyldopa/hydrochlorothiazide	Aldoril
Metolazone	Mykrox, Zaroxolyn
Minocycline	Dynacin, Minocin
Mirtazapine	Remeron

(*Continued on next page*)

Generic	Brand
Moexipril	Univasc
Moexipril/hydrochlorothiazide	Uniretic
Moxilfloxacin	Avelox
Nabumetone	Relafen
Nadolol/bendroflumethiazide	Corzide
Nalidixic acid	Nalidixic acid
Naproxen	Naprosyn, EC-Naprosyn
Naproxen sodium	Anaprox, Naprelan
Naratriptan	Amerge
Nefazodone	Serzone
Nifedipine	Adalat CC, Procardia
Nisoldipine	Sular
Norfloxacin	Noroxin
Nortriptyline	Pamelor
Ofloxacin	Floxin
Olanzapine	Zyprexa
Olanzapine/fluoxetine	Symbyax
Olmesartan medoxomil/hydrochlorothiazide	Benicar HCT
Olsalazine	Dipentum
Oxaprozin	Daypro
Oxcarbazepine	Trileptal
Oxycodone	Roxicodone
Oxytetracycline	Terramycin
Pantoprazole	Protonix
Paroxetine	Paxil
Pastinaca sativa	Parsnip
Pentosan polysulfate	Elmiron
Pentostatin	Perphenazine
Pilocarpine	Salagen
Piroxicam	Feldene
Polythiazide	Renese
Polythiazide/prazosin	Minizide
Porfimer sodium	Photofrin
Pravastatin	Pravachol
Prochlorperazine	Compazine, Compro
Promethazine	Phenergan
Protriptyline	Vivactil
Pyrazinamide	Pyrazanamide
Quetiapine	Seroquel
Quinapril	Accupril
Quinapril/hydrochlorothiazide	Accuretic
Quinidine gluconate	Quinidine
Quinidine sulfate	Quinidex
Raberprazole sodium	Aciphex
Ramipril	Altace
Riluzole	Rilutek
Risperidone	Risperdal, Risperdal Consta
Ritonavir	Norvir
Rizatriptan	Maxalt
Ropinirole	Requip
Rosuvastatin	Crestor
Ruta graveolens	Rue
Saquinavir	Fortovase
Saquinavir mesylate	Invirase
Selegiline	Eldepryl
Sertraline	Zoloft
Sibutramine	Meridia
Sildenafil	Viagra
Simvastatin	Zocor
Simvastatin/ezetimibe	Vytorin

Generic	Brand
Somatropin	Serostim
Solatol	Betapace, Betapace AF
Sulfamethoxazole/trimethoprim	Bactrim, Septra
Sulfasalazine	Azulfidine
Sulindac	Clinoril
Sumatriptan	Imitrex
Tacrolimus	Prograf, Protopic
Tazarotene	Tazorac
Telmisartan/hydrochlorothiazide	Micardis HCT
Tetracycline	Sumycin
Thalidomide	Thalomid
Thioridazine hydrochloride	Mellaril
Thiothixene	Navane
Tiagabine	Gabitril
Tolazamide	Tolazamide
Tolbutamide	Tolbutamide
Topiramate	Topamax
Tretinoin	Retin-A
Triamcinolone	Azmacort
Triamterene	Dyrenium
Triamterene/hydrochlorothiazide	Dyazide, Maxzide
Trifluoperazine	Trifluoperazine
Trimipramine	Surmontil
Trovafloxacin	Trovan
Valacyclovir	Valtrex
Valdecoxib	Bextra
Valproate	Depacon
Valproic acid	Depakene
Valsartan/hydrochlorothiazide	Diovan HCT
Vardenafil	Levitra
Venlafaxine	Effexor
Verteporfin	Visudyne
Vinblastine	Vinblastine
Voriconazole	Vfend
Zalcitabine	Hivid
Zaleplon	Sonata
Ziprasidone	Geodon
Zolmitriptan	Zomig
Zolpidem	Ambien

Drug/Alcohol Interactions

Product	Interaction	Onset	Severity
ACETAMINOPHEN	ETHANOL Concurrent use of ACETAMINOPHEN and ETHANOL may result in an increased risk of hepatotoxicity.	2	2
ACETOPHENAZINE	ETHANOL Concurrent use of ACETOPHENAZINE and ETHANOL may result in increased CNS depression and an increased risk of extrapyramidal reactions.	1	2

(Continued on next page)

Product	Interaction	Onset	Severity
ACITRETIN	ETHANOL Concurrent use of ACITRETIN and ETHANOL may result in a prolonged risk of teratogenicity.	2	1
ALFENTANIL	ETHANOL Concurrent use of ALFENTANIL and ETHANOL may result in decreased therapeutic effects for alfentanil.	2	2
ALPRAZOLAM	ETHANOL Concurrent use of ALPRAZOLAM and ETHANOL may result in increased sedation.	1	2
AMITRIPITYLINE	ETHANOL Concurrent use of AMITRIPTYLINE and ETHANOL may result in enhanced CNS depression and impairment of motor skills.	1	2
AMOBARBITAL	ETHANOL Concurrent use of AMOBARBITAL and ETHANOL may result in excessive CNS depression.	1	2
AMOXAPINE	ETHANOL Concurrent use of AMOXAPINE and ETHANOL may result in enhanced drowsiness and impairment of motor skills.	1	2
AMPRENAVIR	ETHANOL Concurrent use of AMPRENAVIR and ETHANOL may result in an increased risk of propylene glycol toxicity (seizures, tachycardia, lactic acidosis, renal toxicity, and hemolysis).	2	1
APROBARBITAL	ETHANOL Concurrent use of APROBARBITAL and ETHANOL may result in excessive CNS depression.	1	2
ASPIRIN	ETHANOL Concurrent use of ASPIRIN and ETHANOL may result in increased gastrointestinal blood loss.	1	2
BUPROPION	ETHANOL Concurrent use of BUPROPION and ETHANOL may result in an increased risk of seizures.	2	1
BUTABARBITAL	ETHANOL Concurrent use of BUTABARBITAL and ETHANOL may result in excessive CNS depression.	1	2
BUTALBITAL	ETHANOL Concurrent use of BUTALBITAL and ETHANOL may result in excessive CNS depression.	1	2
CALAMUS	ETHANOL Concurrent use of CALAMUS and ETHANOL may result in increased sedation.	1	2
CANNABIS	ETHANOL Concurrent use of CANNABIS and ETHANOL may result in increased intoxication.	1	2

Product	Interaction	Onset	Severity
CEFAMANDOLE	ETHANOL Concurrent use of CEFAMANDOLE and ETHANOL may result in disulfiram-like reactions.	2	1
CEFMENOXIME	ETHANOL Concurrent use of CEFMENOXIME and ETHANOL may result in disulfiram-like reactions.	1	1
CEFOPERAZONE	ETHANOL Concurrent use of CEFOPERAZONE and ETHANOL may result in disulfiram-like reactions.	2	1
CEFOTETAN	ETHANOL Concurrent use of CEFOTETAN and ETHANOL may result in disulfiram-like reactions.	2	1
CHAPARRAL	ETHANOL Concurrent use of CHAPARRAL and ETHANOL may result in elevated liver transaminases with or without concomitant hepatic damage.	1	2
CHLORAL HYDRATE	ETHANOL Concurrent use of CHLORAL HYDRATE and ETHANOL may result in increased sedation.	1	3
CHLORDIAZEPOXIDE	ETHANOL Concurrent use of CHLORDIAZEPOXIDE and ETHANOL may result in increased sedation.	1	2
CHLORPROMAZINE	ETHANOL Concurrent use of CHLORPROMAZINE and ETHANOL may result in increased sedation.	1	2
CHLORPROPAMIDE	ETHANOL Concurrent use of CHLORPROPAMIDE and ETHANOL may result in disulfiram-like reactions.	1	1
CIMETIDINE	ETHANOL Concurrent use of CIMETIDINE and ETHANOL may result in increased ethanol concentrations.	1	3
CISAPRIDE	ETHANOL Concurrent use of CISAPRIDE and ETHANOL may result in increased blood levels of ethanol.	1	2
CITALOPRAM	ETHANOL Concurrent use of CITALOPRAM and ETHANOL may result in potentiation of the cognitive and motor effects of alcohol.	0	2
CLOMIPRAMINE	ETHANOL Concurrent use of CLOMIPRAMINE and ETHANOL may result in enhanced drowsiness and impairment of motor skills.	1	2
CLORAZEPATE	ETHANOL Concurrent use of CLORAZEPATE and ETHANOL may result in increased sedation.	1	2

(*Continued on next page*)

Product	Interaction	Onset	Severity
COCAINE	ETHANOL Concurrent use of COCAINE and ETHANOL may result in increased heart rate and blood pressure.	1	2
CODEINE	ETHANOL Concurrent use of CODEINE and ETHANOL may result in increased sedation.	1	2
COMFREY	ETHANOL Concurrent use of COMFREY and ETHANOL may result in elevated liver transaminases with or without concomitant hepatic damage.	1	1
CYCLOSERINE	ETHANOL Concurrent use of CYCLOSERINE and ETHANOL may result in an increased risk of seizures.	1	1
DESIPRAMINE	ETHANOL Concurrent use of DESIPRAMINE and ETHANOL may result in enhanced drowsiness and impairment of motor skills.	1	2
DIAZEPAM	ETHANOL Concurrent use of DIAZEPAM and ETHANOL may result in increased sedation.	1	2
DIMETHINDENE	ETHANOL Concurrent use of DIMETHINDENE and ETHANOL may result in inceased sedation.	1	2
DIPHENHYDRAMINE	ETHANOL Concurrent use of DIPHENHYDRAMINE and ETHANOL may result in increased sedation.	1	2
DISULFIRAM	ETHANOL Concurrent use of DISULFIRAM and ETHANOL may result in ethanol intolerance.	1	1
DOTHIEPIN	ETHANOL Concurrent use of ETHANOL and DOTHIERIN may result in enhanced drowsiness and impairment of motor skills.	1	2
DOXEPIN	ETHANOL Concurrent use of DOXEPIN and ETHANOL may result in enhanced drowsiness and impairment of motor skills.	1	2
ESCITALOPRAM	ETHANOL Concurrent use of ESCITALOPRAM and ETHANOL may result in potentiation of the cognitive and motor effects of alcohol.	0	2
ESZOPICLONE	ETHANOL Concurrent use of ESZOPICLONE and ETHANOL may result in impaired psychomotor functions and risk of increased sedation.	1	2

Product	Interaction	Onset	Severity
ETEROBARB	ETHANOL Concurrent use of ETEROBARB and ETHANOL may result in excessive CNS depression.	1	2
ETHOPROPAZINE	ETHANOL Concurrent use of ETHOPROPAZINE and ETHANOL may result in increased CNS depression and an increased risk of extrapyramidal reactions.	1	2
FLUNITRAZEPAM	ETHANOL Concurrent use of FLUNITRAZEPAM and ETHANOL may result in excessive sedation and psychomotor impairment.	1	2
FLUPHENAZINE	ETHANOL Concurrent use of FLUPHENAZINE and ETHANOL may result in increased CNS depression and an increased risk of extrapyramidal reactions.	1	2
FOMEPIZOLE	ETHANOL Concurrent use of FOMEPIZOLE and ETHANOL may result in the reduced elimination of both drugs.	2	2
FOSPHENYTOIN	ETHANOL Concurrent use of FOSPHENYTOIN and ETHANOL may result in decreased phenytoin serum concentrations, increased seizure potential, and additive CNS depressant effects.	1	2
FURAZOLIDONE	ETHANOL Concurrent use of FURAZOLIDONE and ETHANOL may result in disulfiram-like reactions.	1	1
GERMANDER	ETHANOL Concurrent use of GERMANDER and ETHANOL may result in elevated liver transaminases with or without concomitant hepatic damage.	2	1
GLIPIZIDE	ETHANOL Concurrent use of GLIPIZIDE and ETHANOL may result in prolonged hypoglycemia and disulfiram-like reactions.	1	1
GLICLAZIDE	ETHANOL Concurrent use of ETHANOL and GLICLAZIDE may result in prolonged hypoglycemia and disulfiram-like reactions.	1	1
GLUTETHIMIDE	ETHANOL Concurrent use of GLUTETHIMIDE and ETHANOL may result in increased sedation.	1	2
GLYBURIDE	ETHANOL Concurrent use of GLYBURIDE and ETHANOL may result in prolonged hypoglycemia and disulfirma-like reactions.	1	1

(*Continued on next page*)

Product	Interaction	Onset	Severity
GOSSYPOL	ETHANOL Concurrent use of GOSSYPOL and ETHANOL may result in delayed effects of gossypol and/or increased toxic effects of ethanol.	1	2
GRISEOFULVIN	ETHANOL Concurrent use of GRISEOFULVIN and ETHANOL may result in disulfiram-like reactions.	1	1
GUAR GUM	ETHANOL Concurrent use of GUAR GUM and ETHANOL may result in increased intoxication effects of ethanol.	2	2
GUARANA	ETHANOL Concurrent use of GUARANA and ETHANOL may result in increased risk of ethanol intoxication.	1	3
HYDROCODONE	ETHANOL Concurrent use of HYDROCODONE and ETHANOL may result in increased sedation.	1	2
HYDROMORPHONE	ETHANOL Concurrent use of HYDROMORPHONE and ETHANOL may result in increased sedation.	1	2
IMIPRAMINE	ETHANOL Concurrent use of IMIPRAMINE and ETHANOL may result in enhanced drowsiness and impairment of motor skills.	1	2
INSULIN	ETHANOL Concurrent use of INSULIN and ETHANOL may result in increased hypoglycemia.	1	2
INSULIN LISPRO, HUMAN	ETHANOL Concurrent use of INSULIN LISPRO, HUMAN and ETHANOL and may result in increased hypoglycemia	1	2
ISONIAZID	ETHANOL Concurrent use of ISONIAZID and ETHANOL may result in decreased isoniazid concentrations and disulfiram-like reactions.	2	1
ISOTRETINOIN	ETHANOL Concurrent use of ISOTRETINOIN and ETHANOL may result in disulfiram-like reactions.	1	1
KAVA	ETHANOL Concurrent use of KAVA and ETHANOL may result in increased CNS depression and/or increased risk of hepatotoxicity.	1	2
KETOCONAZOLE	ETHANOL Concurrent use of KETOCONAZOLE and ETHANOL may result in disulfiram-like reactions (flushing, vomiting, increased respiratory rate, tachycardia).	1	1

Product	Interaction	Onset	Severity
LOFEPRAMINE	ETHANOL Concurrent use of LOFEPRAMINE and ETHANOL may result in enhanced drowsiness and impairment of motor skills.	1	2
LORAZEPAM	ETHANOL Concurrent use of LORAZEPAM and ETHANOL may result in increased sedation.	1	2
MA HUANG	ETHANOL Concurrent use of MA HUANG and ETHANOL may result in effects on mental status.	1	1
MATE	ETHANOL Concurrent use of MATE and ETHANOL may result in increased risk of ethanol intoxication.	1	3
MEPERIDINE	ETHANOL Concurrent use of MEPERIDINE and ETHANOL may result in increased sedation.	1	2
MEPHOBARBITAL	ETHANOL Concurrent use of MEPHOBARBITAL and ETHANOL may result in excessive CNS depression.	1	2
MEPROBAMATE	ETHANOL Concurrent use of MEPROBAMATE and ETHANOL may result in increased sedation.	1	2
MESORIDAZINE	ETHANOL Concurrent use of MESORIDAZINE and ETHANOL may result in increased CNS depression and an increased risk of extrapyramidal reactions.	1	2
METFORMIN	ETHANOL Concurrent use of METFORMIN and ETHANOL may result in an increased risk of lactic acidosis.	2	2
METHADONE	ETHANOL Concurrent use of METHADONE and ETHANOL may result in increased sedation.	1	2
METHOHEXITAL	ETHANOL Concurrent use of METHOHEXITAL and ETHANOL may result in excessive CNS depression.	1	2
METHOTREXATE	ETHANOL Concurrent use of METHOTREXATE and ETHANOL may result in increased hepatotoxicity.	2	2
METHOTRIMEPRAZINE	ETHANOL Concurrent use of METHOTRIMEPRAZINE and ETHANOL may result in increased CNS depression and an increased risk of extrapyramidal reactions.	1	2

(*Continued on next page*)

Product	Interaction	Onset	Severity
METRONIDAZOLE	ETHANOL Concurrent use of METRONIDAZOLE and ETHANOL may result in disulfiram-like reactions (flushing, increased respiratory rate, tachycardia) or sudden death.	1	1
MIRTAZAPINE	ETHANOL Concurrent use of MIRTAZAPINE and ETHANOL may result in psychomotor impairment.	1	2
MORPHINE	ETHANOL Concurrent use of MORPHINE and ETHANOL may result in increased risk of respiratory depression, hypotension, profound sedation, or coma.	1	2
MORPHINE SULFATE LIPOSOME	ETHANOL Concurrent use of MORPHINE SULFATE LIPOSOME and ETHANOL may result in increased risk of respiratory depression, hypotension, profound sedation, or coma.	1	1
MOXALACTAM	ETHANOL Concurrent use of ETHANOL and MOXALACTAM may result in disulfiram-like reactions.	2	1
NEFAZODONE	ETHANOL Concurrent use of NEFAZODONE and ETHANOL may result in an increased risk of CNS side effects.	1	3
NIACIN	ETHANOL Concurrent use of NIACIN and ETHANOL may result in increased side effects of flushing and pruritus.	0	2
NILUTAMIDE	ETHANOL Concurrent use of NILUTAMIDE and ETHANOL may result in an increased risk of ethanol intolerance (facial flushing, malaise, and hypotension).	1	3
NITROGLYCERIN	ETHANOL Concurrent use of NITROGLYCERIN and ETHANOL may result in hypotension.	1	2
NORTRIPTYLINE	ETHANOL Concurrent use of NORTRIPTYLINE and ETHANOL may result in enhanced drowsiness and impalment of motor skills.	1	2
OLANZAPINE	ETHANOL Concurrent use of OLANZAPINE and ETHANOL may result in excessive CNS depression.	1	2
OXYCODONE	ETHANOL Concurrent use of OXYCODONE and ETHANOL may result in increased sedation.	1	2
PARALDEHYDE	ETHANOL Concurrent use of PARALDEHYDE and ETHANOL may result in metabolic acidosis.	2	2

Product	Interaction	Onset	Severity
PAROXETINE	ETHANOL Concurrent use of PAROXETINE and ETHANOL may increase the risk of mental and motor-skill impairment.	1	3
PENNYROYAL	ETHANOL Concurrent use of PENNYROYAL and ETHANOL may result in elevated liver transaminases with or without concomitant hepatic damage.	1	1
PENTAZOCINE	ETHANOL Concurrent use of PENTAZOCINE and ETHANOL may result in increased sedation.	1	2
PERPHENAZINE	ETHANOL Concurrent use of PERPHENAZINE and ETHANOL may result in increased CNS depression and an increased risk of extrapyramidal reactions.	1	2
PHENELZINE	ETHANOL Concurrent use of PHENELZINE and ETHANOL may result in hypertensive urgency or emergency.	1	2
PHENOBARBITAL	ETHANOL Concurrent use of PHENOBARBITAL and ETHANOL may result in excessive CNS depression.	1	2
PHENYTOIN	ETHANOL Concurrent use of PHENYTOIN and ETHANOL may result in decreased phenytoin serum concentrations, increased seizure potential, and additive CNS depressant effects.	1	2
PIPOTIAZINE	ETHANOL Concurrent use of PIPOTIAZINE and ETHANOL may result in increased CNS depression and an increased risk of extrapyramidal reactions.	1	2
PRIMIDONE	ETHANOL Concurrent use of PRIMIDONE and ETHANOL may result in excessive CNS depression.	1	2
PROCARBAZINE	ETHANOL Concurrent use of PROCARBAZINE and ETHANOL may result in disulfiram-like reactions and increased sedation.	1	1
PROCHLORPERAZINE	ETHANOL Concurrent use of PROCHLORPERAZINE and ETHANOL may result in increased CNS depression and an increased risk of extrapyramidal reactions.	1	2
PROMAZINE	ETHANOL Concurrent use of PROMAZINE and ETHANOL may result in increased CNS depression and an increased risk of extrapyramidal reactions.	1	2

(*Continued on next page*)

Product	Interaction	Onset	Severity
PROPIOMAZINE	ETHANOL Concurrent use of PROPIOMAZINE and ETHANOL may result in increased CNS depression and an increased risk of extrapyramidal reactions.	1	2
PROTRIPTYLINE	ETHANOL Concurrent use of PROTRIPTYLINE and ETHANOL may result in enhanced drowsiness and impairment of motor skills.	1	2
QUETIAPINE	ETHANOL Concurrent use of QUETIAPINE and ETHANOL may result in potentiation of the cognitive and motor effects of alcohol.	1	2
SECOBARBITAL	ETHANOL Concurrent use of SECOBARBITAL and ETHANOL may result in excessive CNS depression.	1	2
SERTRALINE	ETHANOL Concurrent use of SERTRALINE and ETHANOL may increase the risk of mental and motor-skill impairment.	1	2
SULFAMETHOXAZOLE	ETHANOL Concurrent use of SULFAMETHOXAZOLE and ETHANOL may result in disulfiram-like reactions (flushing, sweating, palpitations, drowsiness).	1	1
TADALAFIL	ETHANOL Concurrent use of TADALAFIL and ETHANOL may result in an increased risk of hypotension and orthosiatic signs and symptoms.	1	2
TEMAZEPAM	ETHANOL Concurrent use of TEMAZEPAM and ETHANOL may result in impaired psychomotor functions.	1	2
THIETHYLPERAZINE	ETHANOL Concurrent use of THIETHYLPERAZINE and ETHANOL may result in increased CNS depression and an increased risk of extrapyramidal reactions.	1	2
THIOPENTAL	ETHANOL Concurrent use of THIOPENTAL and ETHANOL may result in excessive CNS depression.	1	2
THIORIDAZINE	ETHANOL Concurrent use of THIORIDAZINE and ETHANOL may result in increased CNS depression and an increased risk of extrapyramidal reactions.	1	2
TIZANIDINE	ETHANOL Concurrent use of TIZANIDINE and ETHANOL may increase the risk of tizanidine adverse effects (excessive CNS depression).	1	2

Product	Interaction	Onset	Severity
TOLAZAMIDE	ETHANOL Concurrent use of TOLAZAMIDE and ETHANOL may result in prolonged hypoglycemia and disulfiram-like reactions.	1	1
TOLAZOLINE	ETHANOL Concurrent use of TOLAZOLINE and ETHANOL may result in disulfiram-like reactions.	2	1
TOLBUTAMIDE	ETHANOL Concurrent use of TOLBUTAMIDE and ETHANOL may result in prolonged hypoglycemia and disulfiram-like reactions.	1	1
TRAMADOL	ETHANOL Concurrent use of TRAMADOL and ETHANOL may increase the risk of excessive CNS depression.	1	2
TRANYLCYPROMINE	ETHANOL Concurrent use of TRANYLCYPROMINE and ETHANOL may result in hypertensive urgency or emergency.	1	2
TRIAZOLAM	ETHANOL Concurrent use of TRIAZOLAM and ETHANOL may result in increased sedation.	1	2
TRIFLUOPERAZINE	ETHANOL Concurrent use of TRIFLUOPERAZINE and ETHANOL may result in increased CNS depression and an increased risk of extrapyramidal reactions.	1	2
TRIFLUPROMAZINE	ETHANOL Concurrent use of TRIFLUPROMAZINE and ETHANOL may result in increased CNS depression and an increased risk of extrapyramidal reactions.	1	2
TRIMETHOPRIM	ETHANOL Concurrent use of ETHANOL and COTRIMOXAZOLE may result in disulfiram-like reactions.	1	1
TRIMIPRAMINE	ETHANOL Concurrent use of TRIMIPRAMINE and ETHANOL may result in enhanced drowsiness and impairment of motor skills.	1	2
VALERIAN	ETHANOL Concurrent use of VALERIAN and ETHANOL may result in increased sedation.	1	2
VENLAFAXINE	ETHANOL Concurrent use of VENLAFAXINE and ETHANOL may result in an increased risk of CNS effects.	1	3
VERAPAMIL	ETHANOL Concurrent use of VERAPAMIL and ETHANOL may result in enhanced ethanol intoxication (impaired psychomotor functioning).	1	2

(*Continued on next page*)

Product	Interaction	Onset	Severity
WARFARIN	ETHANOL Concurrent use of WARFARIN and ETHANOL may result in increased or decreased international normalized ratio (INR) or prothrombin time.	2	2
YOHIMBINE	ETHANOL Concurrent use of YOHIMBINE and ETHANOL may result in increased ethanol intoxication and increased anxiety and blood pressure.	1	2
ZALEPLON	ETHANOL Concurrent use of ZALEPLON and ETHANOL may result in impaired psychomotor functions.	1	2
ZOLPIDEM	ETHANOL Concurrent use of ZOLPIDEM and ETHANOL may result in increased sedation.	1	2

ONSET: 0 = Unspecified
         1 = Rapid (within 24 hours)
         2 = Delayed (after 24 hours)
SEVERITY: 1 = Major (possibly life threatening or potential permanent damage)
           2 = Moderate (may exacerbate patient's condition)
           3 = Minor (little if any clinical effect)
Note: Disulfiram-like reactions include nausea, vomiting, diarrhea, flushing, tachycardia, and hypotension.
Reprinted with permission from *The Drug Topics Red Book*. Montvale, NJ: Thomson Medical Economics, 2006.

Drug/Tobacco Interactions

Product	Interaction	Onset	Severity
ALPRAZOLAM	TOBACCO Concurrent use of ALPRAZOLAM and TOBACCO may result in decreased alprazolam plasma concentrations and efficacy.	0	2
CONTRACEPTIVES, COMBINATION	TOBACCO Concurrent use of CONTRACEPTIVES, COMBINATION and TOBACCO may result in an increased risk of cardiovascular disease.	2	3
ERLOTINIB	TOBACCO Concurrent use of ERLOTINIB and TOBACCO may result in increased erlotinib clearance and reduced serum concentrations.	0	2
FLUVOXAMINE	TOBACCO Concurrent use of FLUVOXAMINE and TOBACCO may result in increased fluvoxamine metabolism.	2	3

Product	Interaction	Onset	Severity
IMIPRAMINE	TOBACCO Concurrent use of IMIPRAMINE and TOBACCO may result in decreased imipramine concentrations.	2	2
PENTAZOCINE	TOBACCO Concurrent use of PENTAZOCINE and TOBACCO may result in decreased pentazocine concentrations.	2	2
PROPOXYPHENE	TOBACCO Concurrent use of PROPOXYPHENE and TOBACCO may result in decreased propoxyphene concentrations.	2	2
ROPINIROLE	TOBACCO Concurrent use of ROPINIROLE and TOBACCO may result in decreased ropinirole plasma concentrations and efficacy.	0	2
THEOPHYLLINE	TOBACCO Concurrent use of THEOPHYLLINE and TOBACCO may result in decreased theophylline concentrations.	2	2
TOLBUTAMIDE	TOBACCO Concurrent use of TOLBUTAMIDE and TOBACCO may result in decreased tolbutamide concentrations.	2	2
WARFARIN	TOBACCO Concurrent use of WARFARIN and TOBACCO may result in increased or decreased international normalized ratio (INR) or prothrombin time.	2	2

ONSET: 0 = Unspecified
             1 = Rapid (within 24 hours)
             2 = Delayed (after 24 hours)
SEVERITY: 1 = Major (possibly life threatening or potential permanent damage)
             2 = Moderate (may exacerbate patient's condition)
             3 = Minor (little if any clinical effect)
Note: Disulfiram-like reactions include nausea, vomiting, diarrhea, flushing, tachycardia, and hypotension.
Reprinted with permission from *The Drug Topics Red Book*. Montvale, NJ: Thomson Medical Economics, 2006.

Use-In-Pregnancy Ratings

The U.S. Food and Drug Administration's Use-in-Pregnancy rating system weighs the degree to which available information has ruled out risk to the fetus against the drug's potential benefit to the patient. Below is a listing of drugs (by generic name) for which ratings are available.

X

CONTRAINDICATED IN PREGNANCY

Studies in animals or humans, or investigational or post-marketing reports, have demonstrated fetal risk which

clearly outweighs any possible benefit to the patient.

Acitretin
Amlodipine Besylate/
   Atorvastatin Calcium
Amprenavir
Anisindione
Atorvastatin Calcium

Bexarotene
Bicalutamide
Bosentan
Cetrorelix Acetate
Choriogonadotropin Alfa
Chorionic Gonadotropin
Clomiphene Citrate
Desogestrel/Ethinyl Estradiol

(Continued on next page)

Diclofenac Sodium/
  Misoprostol
Dihydroergotamine Mesylate
Dutasteride
Estazolam
Estradiol
Estradiol Acetate
Estradiol Cypionate/
  Medroxyprogesterone
  Acetate
Estradiol Valerate
Estradiol/Levonorgestrel
Estradiol/Norethindrone
  Acetate
Estrogens, Conjugated
Estrogens, Conjugated,
  Synthetic A
Estrogens, Conjugated/
  Medroxyprogesterone
  Acetate
Estrogens, Esterified
Estrogens, Esterified/
  Methyltestoterone
Estropipate
Ethinyl Estradiol/Drospirenone
Ethinyl Estradiol/Ethynodiol
  Diacetate
Ethinyl Estradiol/Etonogestrel
Ethinyl Estradiol/Ferrous
  Fumarate/Norethindrone
  Acetate
Ethinyl Estradiol/
  Levonorgestrel
Ethinyl Estradiol/
  Norelgestromin
Ethinyl Estradiol/
  Norethindrone
Ethinyl Estradiol/
  Norethindrone Acetate
Ethinyl Estradiol/Norgestimate
Ethinyl Estradiol/Norgestrel
Ezetimibe/Simvastatin
Finasteride
Fluorouracil
Flurazepam Hydrochloride
Fluvastatin Sodium
Follitropin Alfa
Follitropin Beta
Ganirelix Acetate
Goserelin Acetate
Histrelin Acetate
Hyrdromorphone
  Hydrochloride
Interferon Alfa-2B,
  Recombinant/Ribavirin
Iodine I 131 Tositumomab/
  Tositumomab
Isotretinoin
Leflunomide
Leuprolide Acetate
Levonorgestrel

Lovastatin
Lovastatin/Niacin
Medroxyprogesterone Acetate
Megestrol Acetate
Menotropins
Mequinol/Tretinoin
Mestranol/Norethindrone
Methotrexate Soduim
Methyltestosterone
Miglustat
Misoprostol
Nafarelin Acetate
Norethindrone
Norethindrone Acetate
Norgestrel
Oxandrolone
Oxymetholone
Plicamycin
Pravastatin Sodium
Pravastatin Sodium/Aspirin
  Buffered
Raloxifene Hydrochloride
Ribavirin
Rosuvastatin Calcium
Simvastatin
Tazarotene
Testosterone
Testosterone Enanthate
Thalidomide
Triptorelin Pamoate
Urofollitropin
Warfarin Sodium

D

POSITIVE EVIDENCE OF RISK

Investigational or postmarketing data show risk to the fetus. Nevertheless, potential benefits may outweigh the potential risk.

Alitretinoin
Alprazolam
Altretamine
Amiodarone Hydrochloride
Amlodipine Besylate/
  Benazepril Hydrochloride
Anastrozole
Arsenic Trioxide
Aspirin Buffered/Prevastatin
  Sodium
Aspirin/Dipryridamole
Atenolol
Azathioprine
Azathioprine Sodium
Benazepril Hydrochloride*
Benazepril Hydrochloride/
  Hydrochlorothiazide*

Bortezomib
Busulfan
Candesartan Cilexetil*
Candesartan Cilexetil/
  Hydrochlorothiazide*
Capecitabine
Captopril*
Carbamazepine
Carboplatin
Carmustine (Benu)
Chlorambucil
Cladribine
Clofarabine
Clonazepam
Cytarabine Liposome
Dactinomycin
Daunorubicin Citrate
  Liposome
Daunorubicin Hydrochloride
Demeclocycline
  Hydrochloride
Diazepam
Divalproex Sodium
Docetaxel
Doxorubicin Hydrochloride
Doxorubicin Hydrochloride
  Liposome
Doxycycline Calcium
Doxycycline Hyclate
Doxycycline Monohydrate
Efavirenz
Enalapril Maleate*
Enalapril Maleate/
  Hydrochlorothiazide*
Epirubicin Hydrochloride
Eprosartan Mesylate
Eriotinib
Exemestane
Felodipine/Enalapril Maleate
Floxuridine
Fludarabine Phosphate
Flutamide
Fosinopril Sodium*
Fosinopril Sodium/
  Hydrochlorothiazide*
Fosphenytoin Sodium
Fulvestrant
Gefitinib
Gemcitabine Hydrochloride
Gemtuzumab Ozogamicin
Goserelin Acetate
Ibritumomab Tiuxetan
Idarubicin Hydrochloride
Ifosfamide
Imatinib Mesylate
Irbesartan*
Irbesartan/
  Hydrochlorothiazide*

Irinotecan Hydrochloride
Letrozole
Lisinopril*
Lisinopril/
    Hydrochlorothiazide*
Lithium Carbonate
Losartan Potassium*
Losartan Potassium/
    Hydrochlorothiazide*
Mechlorethamine
    Hydrochloride
Melphalan
Melphalan Hydrochloride
Mephobarbital
Mercaptopurine
Methimazole
Midazolam Hydrochloride
Minocycline Hydrochloride
Mitoxantrone Hydrochloride
Moexipril Hydrochloride*
Moexipril Hydrochloride/
    Hydrochlorothiazide*
Neomycin Sulfate/Polymyxin
    B Sulfate
Nicotine
Olmesartan Medoxomil
Oxaliplatin
Pamidronate Disodium
Pemetrexed
Penicillamine
Pentobarbital Sodium
Pentostatin
Perindropil Erbumine*
Phenytoin
Procarbazine Hydrochloride
Quinapril Hydrochloride*
Quinapril Hydrochloride/
    Hydrochlorothiazide*
Ramipril
Streptomycin Sulfate
Tamoxifen Citrate
Telmisartan
Telmisartan/
    Hydrochlorothiazide
Temozolomide
Thioguanine
Tigecycline
Tobramycin
Topotecan Hydrochloride
Toremifene Citrate
Trandolaprill*
Trandolaprill/Verapamil
    Hydrochloride*
Tretinoin
Valproate Sodium
Valproic Acid
Valsartan*
Valsartan/
    Hydrochlorothiazide*
Vinorelbine Tartrate

Voriconazole
Zoledronic Acid

C

RISK CANNOT BE RULED OUT

Human studies are lacking, and animal studies are either positive for risk or are lacking as well. However, potential benefits may outweigh the potential risk.

Abacavir Sulfate
Abacavir Sulfate/Lamivudine
Abacavir Sulfate/Lamivudine/
    Zidovudine
Abciximab
Acamprosate Calcium
Acetaminophen
Acetaminophen/Butalbital/
    Caffeine
Acetaminophen/Caffeine/
    Chlorpheniramine Maleate/
    Hydrocodone Bitartrate/
    Phenylephrine
    Hydrochloride
Acetazolamide
Acetazolamide Sodium
Acyclovir
Adapalene
Adefovir Dipivoxil
Adenosine
Alatroflaxacin Mesylate
Albendazole
Albumin (Human)
Albuterol
Albuterol Sulfate
Albuterol Sulfate/Ipratropium
    Bromide
Alclometasone Dipropionate
Aldesleukin
Alemtuzumab
Alendronate Sodium
Alendronate Sodium/
    Cholecalciferol
Altopurinol Sodium
Almotriptan Malate
Alpha1-Proteinase Inhibitor
    (Human)
Alprostadil
Alteplase
Amantadine Hydrochloride
Amifostine
Aminocaproic Acid
Aminohippurate Sodium
Aminolevulinic Acid
    Hydrochloride

Aminosalicylic Acid
Amlodipine Besylate
Amlodipine Besylate/
    Benazepril Hydrochloride
Amoxicillin/Clarithromycin/
    Lansoprazole
Amphetamine Aspartate/
    Amphetamine Sulfate/
    Dextroamphetamine
    Saccharate/
    Dextroamphetamine Sulfate
Amprenavir
Anagrelide Hydrochloride
Anthralin
Antihemophilic Factor
    (Human)
Antihemophilic Factor
    (Recombinant)
Anti-inhibitor Coagulant
    Complex
Anti-Thymocyte Globulin
Apomorphine Hydrochloride
Aripiprazole
Arnica Montana/Herbals,
    Multiple/Sulfur
Asparaginase
Atomoxetine Hydrochloride
Atovaquone
Atovaquone/Proguanil
    Hydrochloride
Atropine Sulfate/Benzoic Acid/
    Hyoscyamine Sulfate/
    Methenamine/Methylene
    Blue/Phenyl Salicylate
Atropine Sulfate/Hyoscyamine
    Sulfate/Scopolamine
    Hydrobromide
Azelastine Hydrochloride
Bacitracin Zinc/Neomycin
    Sulfate/Polymyxin B Sulfate
Baclofen
Bcg. Live (Intravesical)
Becaplermin
Beclomethasone Dipropionate
Beclomethasone Dipropionate
    Monohydrate
Benzepril Hydrochloride*
Benazepril Hydrochloride/
    Hydrochlorothiazide*
Bendroflumethiazide
Benzocaine
Benzonatate
Benzoyl Peroxide
Benzoyl Peroxide/Clindamycin
Benzoyl Peroxide/
    Erythromycin
Betamethasone Dipropionate
Betamethasone Dipropionate/
    Chlotrimazole
Betamethasone Valerate
        (*Continued on next page*)

Betaxolol Hydrochloride
Bethanechol Chloride
Bevacizumab
Bimatoprost
Bisacodyl/Polyethylene
 Glycol/Potassium Chloride/
 Sodium Bicarbonate/
 Sodium Chloride
Bisoprolol Fumarate
Bisoprolol Fumarate/
 Hydrochlorothiazide
Bitolterol Mesylate
Black Widow Spider
 Antivenin (Equine)
Botulinum Toxin Type A
Botulinum Toxin Type B
Brinzolamide
Brompheniramine Maleate/
 Dextromethorphan
 Hydrobromide/
 Phenylephrine
 Hydrochloride
Budesonide
Bupivacaine Hydrochloride
Bupivacaine Hydrochloride/
 Epinephrine Bitartrate
Buprenorphine Hydrochloride
Buprenorphine Hydrochloride/
 Naloxone Hydrochloride
Butabarbital/Hyoscyamine
 Hydrobromide/
 Phenazopyridine
 Hydrochloride
Butalbital/Acetaminophen
Butenafine Hydrochloride
Butoconazole Nitrate
Butorphanol Tartrate
Caffeine Citrate
Calcipotriene
Calcitonin-Salmon
Calcitriol
Calcium Acetate
Candesarta Cilexetil*
Candesartan Cilexetil/
 Hydrochlorothiazide*
Capreomycin Sulfate
Captropil*
Carbetapentane Tannate/
 Chlorpheniramine Tannate
Carbetapentane Tannate/
 Chlorpheniramine Tannate/
 Ephedrine Tannate/
 Phenylephrine Tannate
Carbidopa/Entacapone/
 Levodopa
Carbidopa/Levodopa
Carbinoxamine Maleate/
 Dextromethorphan
 Hydrobromide/
 Pseudoephedrine
 Hydrochloride

Carteolol Hydrochloride
Carvedilol
Caspofungin Acetate
Celecoxib
Cetirizine Hydrochloride
Cetuximab
Cevimeline Hydrochloride
Chloramphenicol
Chloroprocaine
 Hydrochloride
Chlorothiazide
Chlorothiazide Sodium
Chlorpheniramine Maleate/
 Methscopolamine Nitrate/
 Phenylephrine
 Hydrochloride
Chlorpheniramine Maleate/
 Pseudoephedine
 Hydrochloride
Chlorpheniramine Polistirex/
 Hydrocodone Polistirex
Chlorpheniramine Tannate/
 Phenylephrine Tannate
Chlorpropamide
Chlorthalidone/Clonidine
 Hydrochloride
Choline Magnesium
 Trisalicylate
Cidofovir
Cilostazol
Cinacalcet Hydrochloride
Ciprofloxacin Hydrochloride
Ciprofloxacin Hydrochloride/
 Hydrocortisone
Ciprofloxacin/
 Dexamethasone
Citalopram Hydrobromide
Clarithromycin
Clobetasol Propionate
Clonidine
Clonidine Hydrochloride
Codeine Phosphate/
 Acetaminophen
Colistimethate Sodium
Colistin Sulfate/
 Hydrocortisone/Acetate/
 Neomycin Sulfate/
 Thonzonium Bromide
Corticorelin Ovine Triflutate
Cycloserine
Cyclosporine
Cytomegalovirus Immune
 Globulin
Dacarbazine
Daclizumab
Dantrolene Sodium
Dapsone
Darbepoetin Alia
Darifenacin
Deferoxamine Mesylate
Delavirdine Mesylate

Denileukin Diftitox
Desloratadine
Desloratadine/
 Pseudoephedrine Sulfate
Desoximetasone
Dexamethasone
Dexamethasone Sodium
 Phosphate
Dexmethylphenidate
 Hydrochloride
Dexrazoxane
Dextroamphetamine Sufate
Diazoxide
Dichlorphenamide
Diclofenac Potassium
Diclofenac Sodium
Diflorasone Diacetate
Diflunisal
Digoxin
Digoxin Immune Fab (Ovine)
Diltiazem Hydrochloride
Dimethyl Sulfoxide
Dinoprostone
Diphtheria & Tetanus Toxoids
 and Acellular Pertussis
 Vaccine Adsorbed
Diphtheria & Tetanus Toxoids
 and Acellular Pertussis
 Vaccine Adsorbed/Hepatitis
 B Vaccine, Recombinant/
 Poliovirus Vaccine
 Inactivated
Dirithromycin
Dofetilide
Donepezil Hydrochloride
Dorzolamide Hydrochloride
Dorzolamide Hydrochloride/
 Timolol Maleate
Doxazosin Mesylate
Dronabinol
Drotrecogin Alfa (Activated)
Duloxetine Hydrochloride
Echothiophate Iodide
Econazole Nitrate
Efalizumab
Eflornithine Hydrochloride
Eletriptan Hydrobromide
Enalapril Maleate*
Enalapril Maleate/Felodipine*
Enalapril Maleate/
 Hydrochlorothiazide*
Entacapone
Entecavir
Epinastine Hydrochloride
Epinephrine
Epoetin Alfa
Eprosartan Mesylate
Erythromycin Ethylsuccinate/
 Sulfisoxazole Acetyl
Escitalopram Oxalate
Esmolol Hydrochloride

Eszopiclone
Ethionamide
Ethotoin
Etidronate Disodium
Exenatide
Ezetimibe
Factor Ix Complex
Felodipine
Fenofibrate
Fentanyl
Fentanyl Citrate
Ferrous Fumarate/Folic
   Acid/Intrinsic Factor
   Concentrate/Liver
   Preparations/Vitamin B12/
   Vitamin C/Vitamins with
   Iron
Fexofenadine Hydrochloride
Fexofenadine Hydrochloride/
   Pseudoephedrine
   Hydrochloride
Filgrastim
Flecainide Acetate
Fluconazole
Flucytosine
Fludrocortisone Acetate
Flumazenil
Flunisolide
Fluocinolone Acetonide
Fluocinolone Acetonide/
   Hydroquinone/Tretinoin
Fluocinonide
Fluorometholone
Fluorometholone/
   Sulfacetamide Sodium
Fluoxetine Hydrochloride
Fluoxetine Hydrochloride/
   Olanzapine
Flurandrenolide
Flurbiprofen Sodium
Fluticasone Propionate
Fluticasone Propionate Hfa
Fluticasone Propionate/
   Salmeterol Xinafoate
Fomivirsen Sodium
Formoterol Fumarate
Fosamprenavir Calcium
Foscarnet Sodium*
Fosinopril Sodium*
Fosinopril Sodium/
   Hydrochlorothiazide*
Frovatriptan Succinate
Furosemide
Gabapentin
Gallium Nitrate
Ganciclovir
Ganciclovir Sodium
Gatifloxacin
Gemfibrozil
Gemifloxacin Mesylate
Gentamicin Sulfate

Gentamicin Sulfate/
   Prednisolone Acetate
Glimepiride
Glipizide
Glipizide/Metformin
   Hydrochloride
Globulin, Immune (Human)
Globulin, Immune (Human)/
   Rho (D) Immune Globulin
   (Human)
Glyburide
Gramicidin/Neomycin Sulfate/
   Polymyxin B Sulfate
Guaifenesin/Hydrocodone
   Bitartrate
Haemophilus B Conjugate
   Vaccine
Haemophilus B Conjugate
   Vaccine/Hepatitis B Vaccine,
   Recombinant
Halobetasol Propionate
Haloperidol Decanoate
Hemin
Heparin Sodium
Hepatitis A Vaccine, Inactivated
Hepatitis A Vaccine,
   Inactivated/Hepatitis B
   Vaccine, Recombinant
Hepatitis B Immune Globulin
   (Human)
Hepatitis B Vaccine,
   Recombinant
Homatropine Methylbromide/
   Hydrocodone Bitartrate
Homeophatic Formulations
Hydralazine Hydrochloride/
   Isosorbide Dinitrate
Hydrochlorothiazide
Hydrocodone Bitartrate
Hydrocodone Bitartrate/
   Acetaminophen
Hydrocodone Bitartrate/
   Ibuprofen
Hydrocortisone
Hydrocortisone Acetate
Hydrocortisone Acetate/
   Neomycin Sulfate/Polymyxin
   B Sulfate
Hydrocortisone Acetate/
   Pramoxine Hydrochloride
Hydrocortisone Butyrate
Hydrocortisone Probutate
Hydrocortisone/Neomycin
   Sulfate/Polymyxin B Sulfate
Hydromorphone Hydrochloride
Hydroquinone
Hyoscyamine Sulfate
Ibandronate Sodium
Ibutilide Fumarate
Iloprost
Imiglucerase

Imipenem/Cilastatin
Imiquimod
Immune Globulin Intravenous
   (Human)
Indinavir Sulfate
Indocyanine Green
Influenza Virus Vaccine
Insulin Aspart
Insulin Aspart Protamine,
   Human/Insulin Aspart,
   Human
Insulin Glargine
Insulin Glulisine
Interferon Alfa-2A,
   Recombinant
Interferon Alfa-2B,
   Recombinant
Interferon Alfacon-1
Interferon Alfa-N3 (Human
   Leukocyte Derived)
Interferon Beta-1A
Interferon Beta-1B
Interferon Gamma-1B
Iodoquinol/Hydrocortisone
Irbesartan*
Irbesartan/
   Hydrochlorothiazide*
Iron Dextran
Isoniazid/Pyrazinamide/
   Rifampin
Isosorbide Mononitrate
Isradipine
Itraconazole
Ivermectin
Ketoconazole
Ketorolac Tromethamine
Ketotifen Fumarate
Labetalol Hydrochloride
Lamivudine
Lamivudine/Zidovudine
Lamotrigine
Lanthanum Carbonate
Latanoprost
Levalbuterol Hydrochloride
Levalbuterol Tartrate
Levamisole Hydrochloride
Levetiracetam
Levobunolol Hydrochloride
Levofloxacin
Linezolid
Lisinopril*
Lisinopril/
   Hydrochlorothiazide*
Lopinavir/Ritonavir
Losartan Potassium*
Losartan Potassium/
   Hydrochlorothiazide*
Loteprednol Etabonate
Mafenide Acetate
   (*Continued on next page*)

Mefloquine Hydrochloride
Meloxicam
Meningoccal Polysaccharide
 Diphtheria Toxoid
 Conjugate Vaccine
Meningococcal
 Polysaccharide Vaccine
Meperidine Hydrochloride
Mepivacaine Hydrochloride
Metaproterenol Sulfate
Metaraminol Bitartrate
Metformin Hydrochloride/
 Pioglitazone Hydrochloride
Metformin Hydrochloride/
 Rosiglitazone Maleate
Methamphetamine
 Hydrochloride
Methazolamide
Methenamine Mandelate/
 Sodium Acid Phosphate
Methocarbamol
Methoxsafen
Methscopolamine Nitrate/
 Pseudoephedrine
 Hydrochloride
Methyldopa Chlorothiazide
Methyldopa/
 Hydrochlorothiazide
Methylphenidate
 Hydrochloride
Metipranolol
Metoprolol Succinate
Metoprolol Tartrate
Metoprolol Tartrate/
 Hydrochlorothiazide
Metyrosine
Mexiletine Hydrochloride
Micafungin Sodium
Mododrine Hydrochloride
Mivacurium Chloride
Modafinil
Moexipril Hydrochloride*
Moexipril Hydrochloride/
 Hydrochlorothiazide*
Mometasone Furoate
Mometasone Furoate
 Monohydrate
Morphine Sulfate
Morphine Sulfate, Liposomal
Moxifloxacin Hydrochloride
Mumps Virus Vaccine, Live
Muromonab-Cd3
Mycophenolate Mofetil
Mycophenolate Mofetil
 Hydrochloride
Mycophenolic Acid
Nabumetone
Nadolol
Nadolol/Bendroflumethiazide
Naloxone Hydrochloride/
 Pentazocine Hydrochloride

Naltrexone Hydrochloride
Naphazoline Hydrochloride
Naproxen
Naproxen Sodium
Naratriptan Hydrochloride
Natamycin
Nateglinide
Nefazodone Hydrochloride
Neomycin Sulfate/
 Dexamethasone Sodium
 Phosphate
Neomycin Sulfate/Polymyxin
 B Sulfate/Prednisolone
 Acetate
Nesiritide
Nevirapine
Niacin
Nicardipine Hydrochloride
Nifedipine
Nilutamide
Nimodipine
Nisoldipine
Nitroglycerin
Norfloxacin
Ofloxacin
Olanzapine
Olmesartan Medoxomil/
 Hydrochlorothiazide
Olopatadine Hydrochloride
Olsalazine Sodium
Omega-3-Acid Ethyl Esters
Omeprazole
Oprelvekin
Orphenadrine Citrate
Oseltamivir Phosphate
Oxcarbazepine
Oxycodone Hydrochloride/
 Acetaminophen
Oxycodone Hydrochloride/
 Ibuprofen
Oxymorphone Hydrochloride
Palifermin
Palivizumab
Pancrelipase
Paricalcitol
Paroxetine Hydrochloride
Paroxetine Mesylate
Peg-3350/Potassium Chloride/
 Sodium Bicarbonate/Sodium
 Chloride
Pegademase Bovine
Pegaspargase
Pegfilgrastim
Peginterferon Alfa-2A
Peginterferon Alfa-2B
Pemirolast Potassium
Pentazocine Hydrochloride/
 Acetaminophen
Pentoxifylline
Perindopril Erbumine*

Phenoxybenzamine
 Hydrochloride
Phentermine Hydrochloride
Pilocarpine Hydrochloride
Pimercrolimus
Pimozide
Pioglitazone Hydrochloride
Pirbuterol Acetate
Piroxicam
Plasma Fractions, Human/
 Rabies Immune Globulin
 (Human)
Plasma Protein Fraction
 (Human)
Pneumococcal Vaccine,
 Diphtheria Conjugate
Pneumococcal Vaccine,
 Polyvalent
Podofilox
Polyethylene Glycol
Polyethylene Glycol/
 Potassium Chloride/
 Sodium Bicarbonate/
 Sodium Chloride
Polyethylene Glycol/
 Potassium Chloride/Sodium
 Bicarbonate/Sodium
 Chloride/Sodium Sulfate
Polymyxin B Sulfate/
 Trimethoprim Sulfate
Polythiazide/Prazosin
 Hydrochloride
Porfimer Sodium
Potassium Acid Phosphate
Potassium Chloride
Potassium Citrate
Potassium Phosphate/Sodium
 Phosphate
Pralidoxime Chloride
Pramipexole Dihydrochloride
Pramlintide Acetate
Pramoxine Hydrochloride/
 Hydrocortisone Acetate
Prazosin Hydrochloride
Prednisolone Acetate
Prednisolone Acetate/
 Sulfacetamide Sodium
Prednisolone Sodium
 Phosphate
Pregabalin
Proclainamide Hydrochloride
Promethazine Hydrochloride
Propafenone Hydrochloride
Proparacaine Hydrochloride
Propranolol Hydrochloride
Pseudoephedrine
 Hydrochloride
Pyrimethamine
Quetiapine Fumerate
Quinapril Hydrochloride*
Quinidine Sulfate

Rabies Vaccine
Ramelteon
Ramipril*
Rasburicase
Remifentanil Hydrochloride
Repaglinide
Reteplase
Rho (D) Immune Globulin
    (Human)
Rifampin
Rifapentine
Rifamixin
Riluzole
Rimantadine Hydrochloride
Risedronate Sodium
Risedronate Sodium/Calcium
    Carbonate
Risperidone
Ritumixab
Rizatriptan Benzoate
Rocuronium Bromide
Rofecoxib
Ropinirole Hydrochloride
Rosiglitazone Maleate
Rubella Virus Vaccine, Live
Salmeterol Xinafoate
Sargamostim
Scopolamine
Selegiline Hydrochloride
Sertaconazole Nitrate
Sertraline Hydrochloride
Sevelamer Hydrochloride/
    Monohydrate
Sirolimus
Sodium Benzoate/Sodium
    Phenylacelate
Sodium Phenylbutyrate
Sodium Sulfacetamide/Sulfur
Solifenacin Succinate
Somatropin
Somatropin (rDNA Origin)
Stavudine
Streptokinase
Succimer
Sulfacetamide Sodium
Sulfamethoxazole
    Trimethoprim
Sulfanilamide
Sumatriptan
Sumatriptan Succinate
Tacrine Hydrochloride
Tacrolimus
Telithromycin
Telmisartan
Telmisartan/
    Hydrochlorothiazide*
Tenecteplase
Terazosin Hydrochloride
Teriparatide
Tetanus & Diphtheria Toxoids
    Adsorbed

Tetanus Immunde Globulin
    (Human)
Theophylline
Theophylline Anhydrous
Thiabendazole
Thrombin
Thyrotropin Alfa
Tiagabine Hydrochloride
Tiludronate Disodium
Timolol Hemihydrate
Timolol Maleate
Timolol Maleate
    Hydrochlorothiazide
Tinidazole
Tiotropium Bromide
Tipranavir
Tizanidine Hydrochloride
Tobramycin/Dexamethasone
Tobramycin/Loteprednol
    Etabonate
Tolcapone
Tolterodine Tartrate
Topiramate
Tramadol Hydrochloride
Tramodol Hydrochloride/
    Acetaminophen
Trandolapril*
Trandolapril/Verapamil
    Hydrochloride*
Travoprost
Tretinoin
Triamcinolone Acetonide
Triamterene
Triamterene/
    Hydrochlorothiazide
Trientine Hydrochloride
Triethanolamine Polypeptide
    Oleate-Condensate
Trifluridine
Trimethoprim Hydrochloride
Trimipramine Maleate
Tropicamide/
    Hydroxyamphetamine
    Hydrobromide
Trospium Chloride
Trovafloxacin Mesylate
Tuberculin Purified Protein
    Derivative, Diluted
Typhoid Vaccine Live Oral
    Ty21A
Unprostone Isopropyl
Urea
Valdecoxib
Valganciclovir Hydrochloride
Valsartan*
Valsartan/Hydrochlorothiazide*
Varicella Virus Vaccine, Live
Venlafaxine Hydrochloride
Verapamil Hydrochloride
Verteporfin
Vitamin K1

Yellow Fever Vaccine
Zalcitabine
Zaleplon
Zavamivir
Zidovudine
Zileuton
Ziprasidone Mesylate
Zolmitriptan
Zonisamide

B

NO EVIDENCE OF RISK IN HUMANS

Either animal findings show risk while human findings do not, or, if no adequate human studies have been done, animal findings are negative.

Acarbose
Acrivastine
Acyclovir
Acyclovir Sodium
Adalimumab
Agalsidase Beta
Alefacept
Alfuzosin Hydrochloride
Alosetron Hydrochloride
Amiloride Hydrochloride
Amiloride Hydrochloride/
    Hydrochlorthiazide
Amoxicillin
Amoxicillin/Clavulanate
    Potassium
Amphotericin B
Amphotericin B Lipid
    Complex
Amphotericin B, Liposomal
Amphotericin B/Cholesteryl
    Sulfate Complex
Ampicillin Sodium/Sulbactam
    Sodium
Anakinra
Anithrombin III
Aprepitant
Aprotinin
Argatroban
Arginine Hydrochloride
Atazanavir Sulfate
Azalaic Acid
Azithromycin
Azithromycin Dihydrate
Aztreonam
Balsalazide Disodium
Basiliximab
Bivalirudin
Brimonidine Tartrate
    (*Continued on next page*)

Budesonide
Bupropion Hydrochloride
Cabergoline
Carbenicillin Indanyl Sodium
Cefaclor
Cefazolin Sodium
Cefdinir
Cefditoren Pivoxil
Cefepime Hydrochloride
Cefixime
Cefoperazone Sodium
Cefotaxime Sodium
Cefotetan Disodium
Cefoxitin Sodium
Cefpodoxime Proxetil
Cefprozil
Ceftazidime Sodium
Ceftibuten Dihydrate
Ceftizoxime Sodium
Ceftriaxone Sodium
Cefuroxime
Cefuroxime Axetil
Cephalexin
Cetirizine Hdyrochloride
Ciclopirox
Ciclopirox Olamine
Cimetidine
Cimetidine Hydrochloride
Cisatracurium Besylate
Clindamycin Hydrochloride/
   Clindamycin Phosphate
Clindamycin Palmitate/
   Hydrochloride
Climdamycin Phosphate
Clopidogrel Bisulfate
Clotrimazole
Clozapine
Colesevelam Hydrochloride
Cromolyn Sodium
Cyclobenzaprine
   Hydrochloride
Cyproheptadine
   Hydrochloride
Dalfopristin/Quinupristin
Dalteparin Sodium
Dapiprazole Hydrochloride
Daptomycin
Desflurane
Desmopressin Acetate
Dicyclomine Hydrochloride
Didanosine
Diphenhydramine
   Hydrochloride
Dipivefrin Hydrochloride
Dipyridamole
Dolasetron Mesylate
Dornase Alfa
Doxapram Hydrochloride
Doxepin Hydrochloride
Doxercalciferol
Edetate Calcium Disodium

Emtricitabine
Emtricitabine/Tenofovir
   Disoproxil Fumarate
Enfuvirtide
Enoxaparin Sodium
Eplerenone
Epoprostenol Sodium
Ertapenem
Erythromycin
Erythromycin Ethylsuccinate
Erythromycin Stearate
Esomeprazole Magnesium
Esomeprazole Sodium
Etanercept
Ethacrynate Sodium
Ethacrynic Acid
Famciclovir
Famotidine
Fenoldopam Mesylate
Fondaparinux Sodium
Galantamine Hydrobromide
Glatiramer Acetate
Glucagon
Glyburide/Metformin
   Hydrochloride
Granisetron Hydrochloride
Hydrochlorothiazide
Ibuprofen
Indapamide
Infliximab
Insulin Lispro Protamine,
   Human/Insulin Lispro,
   Human
Insulin Lispro, Human
Ipratropium Bromide
Iron Sucrose
Isosorbide Mononitrate
Lactulose
Lansoprazole
Lansoprazole/Naproxen
Laronidase
Lepirudin
Levocarnitine
Lidocaine
Lidocaine Hydrochloride
Lidocaine/Prilocaine
Lindane
Loperamide Hydrochloride
Loracarbef
Loratadine
Malathion
Meclizine Hydrochloride
Memantine Hydrochloride
Meropenem
Mesalamine
Metformin Hydrochloride
Methohexital Sodium
Methyldopa
Metolazone
Metronidazole

Miglitol
Montelukast Sodium
Mupirocin
Mupirocin Calcium
Naftifine Hydrochloride
Nalbuphine Hydrochloride
Nalmefene Hydrochloride
Naloxone Hydrochloride
Naproxen Sodium
Nedocromil Sodium
Nevlfinavir Mesylate
Nitazoxanide
Nitrofurantoin Macrocrystals
Nitrofurantoin Macrocrystals/
   Nitrofurantoin
   Monohydrate
Nizatidine
Ocreotide Acetate
Omalizumab
Ondansetron
Ondansetron Hydrochloride
Orlistat
Oxiconazole Nitrate
Oxybutynin
Oxybutynin Chloride
Oxycodone Hydrochloride
Palonosetron Hydrochloride
Pancrelipase
Pantoprazole Sodium
Pegvisomant
Pemoline
Penciclovir
Penicillin G Benzathine
Penicillin G Benzathine/
   Peniciillin G Procaine
Penicillin G Potassium
Pentosan Polysulfate Sodium
Pergolide Mesylate
Permethrin
Piperacillin Sodium
Piperacillin Sodium/
   Tazabactam Sodium
Praziquantel
Progesterone
Propofol
Pseudoephedrine
   Hydrochloride
Pseudoephedrine Sulfate
Psyllium Preparations
Rabeprazole Sodium
Ranitidine Hydrochloride
Rifabutin
Ritonavir
Rivastigmine Tartrate
Ropivacaine Hydrochloride
Saquinvair
Saquinvair Mesylate
Sevoflurane
Sildenafil Citrate
Silver Sulfadiazine

Sodium Ferric Gluconate
Somatropin
Sotalol Hydrochloride
Sucralfate
Sulfasalazine
Tadalafil
Tamsulosin Hydrochloride
Tegaserod Maleate
Tenofovir Disoproxil Fumarate
Terbinafine Hydrochloride
Ticarcillin Disodium/
   Clavulanate Potassium

Ticlopidine Hydrochloride
Tirofiban Hydrochloride
Torsemide
Trastuzumab
Treprostinil Sodium
Urokinase
Ursodiol
Valacyclovir Hydrochloride
Vancomycin Hydrochloride
Vardefanil Hydrochloride
Zafirlukast
Zolpidem Tartrate

A

**CONTROLLED STUDIES
SHOW NO RISK**
*Adequate, well-controlled
studies in pregnant women
have failed to demonstrate
risk to the fetus.*
Levothyroxine Sodium
Liothyronine Sodium
Liotrix
Nystatin

Reprinted with permission from *The Drug Topics Red Book.* Montvale NJ: Thomson Medical Economics, 2006.

Drugs Excreted in Breast Milk

The following list is not comprehensive; generic forms and alternate brands of some products may be available. When recommending drugs to pregnant or nursing patients, always check product labeling for specific precautions.

Accolate
Accuretic
Aciphex
Actiq
Activella
Actonel with Calcium
ActoPlus Met
Actos
Adalat
Adderall
Advicor
Aggrenox
Aldactazide
Aldactone
Aldomet
Aldoril
Alesse
Allegra-D
Alfenta
Aloprim
Altace
Ambien
Anaprox
Ancef
Androderm
Antara
Apresoline
Aralen
Arthrotec
Asacol
Ativan
Augmentin
Avalide
Avandia
Avetox
Axid
Axocet
Azactam
Azasari

Azathloprine
Azulfidine
Bactrim
Baraclude
Benadryl
Bentyl
Betapace
Bextra
Bexxar
Bicllin
Biocadren
Boniva
Brethine
Brevicone
Brontex
Byetta
Caduet
Cafergot
Calan
Campral
Capoten
Capozide
Captopril
Carbatrol
Cardizem
Cataflam
Catapres
Ceclor
Cefizox
Cefobid
Cefotan
Ceftin
Celebrex
Celexa
Ceptaz
Cerebyx
Ceredase
Cipro
Ciprodex

Claforan
Clarinex
Claritin
Claritin-D
Cleocin
Climara
Clozaril
Codeine
CombiPatch
Combipres
Combivir
Combunox
Compazine
Cordarone
Corgard
Cortisporin
Corzide
Cosopt
Coumadin
Covera-HS
Cozaar
Crestor
Crinone
Cyclessa
Cymbalta
Cystospaz
Cytomel
Cytotec
Cytoxan
Dapsone
Daraprim
Darvon
Darvon-N
Decadron
Deconsal II
Demerol
Demulen
Depacon
Depakene

(*Continued on next page*)

Depakote
DepoDur
Depo-Provera
Desogen
Desoxyn
Desyrel
Dexedrine
DextroStat
D.H.E.45
Diabinese
Diastat
Diflucan
Digitek
Dilacor
Dilantin
Dilaudid
Diovan
Diprivan
Diuril
Dolobid
Dolophine
Doral
Doryx
Droxia
Duracion
Duragesic
Duramorph
Duratuss
Duricef
Dyazide
Dyrenium
E.E.S.
EC-Naprosyn
Ecotrin
Effexor
Elestat
EMLA
Enduron
Epzicom
Equetro
ERYC
EryPed
Ery-Tab
Erythrocin
Erythromycin
Esgic-plus
Eskalith
Estrogel
Estrostep
Ethmozine
Evista
FazaClo
Felbatol
Feldene
Femhrt
Florinal
Flagyl
Florinef
Floxin
Foradil
Fortamet

Fortaz
Fosamax Plus D
Furosemide
Gabitril
Galzin
Garamycin
Glucophage
Glyset
Guaifed
Halcion
Haldol
Helidac
Hydrocet
Hydrocortone
HydroDIURIL
Iberet-Folic
Ifex
Imitrex
Imuran
Inderal
Ideride
Indocin
INFed
Inspra
Invanz
Inversine
Isoptin
Kadlan
Keflex
Keppra
Kerlone
Ketek
Klonopin
Kronofed-A
Kutrase
Lamictal
Lamisil
Lamprene
Lanoxicaps
Lanoxin
Lariam
Lescol
Levbid
Levitra
Levlen
Levlite
Levora
Levothroid
Levoxyl
Levsin
Levsinex
Lexapro
Lexiva
Lexxel
Lindane
Lioresal
Lipitor
Lithium
Lithobid
Lo/Ovral
Loestrin

Lomotil
Loniten
Lopressor
Lortab
Lostensin
Lotrel
Luminal
Luvox
Lyrica
Macrobid
Macrodantin
Marinol
Maxipime
Maxzide
Mefoxin
Menostar
Methergine
Methotrexate
MetroCream/
    Gel/Lotion
Mexitil
Micronor
Microzide
Midamor
Migranal
Miltown
Minizide
Minocin
Mirapex
Mircette
M-M-R II
Mobic
Modicon
Moduretic
Monodox
Monopril
Morphine
MS Contin
MSIR
Myambutol
Mycamine
Mysoline
Namenda
Naprelan
Naprosyn
Nascobal
Necon
NegGram
Nembutal
Neoral
Niaspan
Nicotrol
Niravam
Nizoral
Norco
Nor-QD
Nordette
Norinyl
Noritate
Normodyne
Norpace

Norplant
Novantrone
Nubain
Nucofed
Nydrazid
Oramorph
Oretic
Ortho-Cept
Ortho-Cyclen
Ortho-Novum
Ortho Tri-Cyclen
Orudis
Ovcon
Oxistat
OxyContin
OxyFast
OxyIR
Pacerone
Pamelor
Pancrease
Paxil
PCE
Pediapred
Pediazole
Pediotic
Pentasa
Pepcid
Periostat
Persantine
Pfizerpen
Phenergan
Phenobarbital
Phrenilin
Pipracil
Plan B
Ponstel
Pravachol
Premphase
Prempro
Prevacid
Prevacid NapraPAC
PREVPAC
Prinzide
Procanbid
Prograf
Proloprim
Prometrium
Pronestyl
Propofol
Prosed/DS
Protonix
Provera
Prozac
Pseudoephedrine
Pulmicort
Pyrazinamide
Quinidex
Quinine
Raptiva
Reglan
Relpax

Renese
Requip
Reserpine
Restoril
Retrovir
Rifadin
Rifamate
Rifater
Rimactane
Risperdal
Rocaltrol
Rocephin
Roferon A
Roxanol
Rozerem
Sanctura
Sandimmune
Sarafem
Seconal
Sectral
Semprex-D
Septra
Seroquel
Sinequan
Slo-bid
Soma
Sonata
Spiriva
Sporanox
Stadol
Streptomycin
Stromectol
Symbyax
Symmetrel
Synthroid
Tagamet
Tambocor
Tapazole
Tarka
Tavist
Tazicef
Tazidime
Tegretol
Tenoretic
Tenormin
Tenuate
Tequin
Testoderm
Thalitone
Theo-24
The-Dur
Thorazine
Tiazac
Timolide
Timoptic
Tindamax
Tobi
Tofranil
Tolectin
Toprol-XL
Toradol

Trandate
Tranxene
Trental
Tricor
Triglide
Trilafon
Trileptal
Tri-Levlen
Trilisate
Tri-Norinyl
Triostat
Triphasil
Trivora
Trizivir
Trovan
Truvada
Tygacil
Tylenol
Tylenol with Codeine
Ultane
Ultram
Unasyn
Uniphyl
Uniretic
Unithroid
Urimax
Valium
Valtrex
Vanceril
Vancocin
Vantin
Vascor
Vaseretic
Vasotec
Ventavis
Verelan
Vermox
Versed
Vibramycin
Vibra-Tabs
Vicodin
Vigamox
Viramune
Voltaren
Vytorin
Wellbutrin
Xanax
Xolair
Zantac
Zarontin
Zaroxolyn
Zegerid
Zemplar
Zestoretic
Zetia
Ziac
Zinacef
Zithromax
Zocor
Zomig
Zonalon

(*Continued on next page*)

Zonegran	Zovirax	Zyloprim
Zosyn	Zyban	Zyprexa
Zovia	Zydone	Zyrtec

Reprinted with permission from *The Drug Products Red Book.* Montvale NJ: Thomson Medical Economics, 2006.

Low Potassium Diet

Potassium is a mineral found in most foods except sugar and lard. It plays a role in maintaining normal muscle activity and helps keep body fluids in balance. Too much potassium in the blood can lead to changes in the heartbeat and can lead to muscle weakness. The kidneys normally help keep blood potassium controlled, but in kidney disease or when certain drugs are taken, dietary potassium must be limited to maintain a normal level of potassium in the blood.

The following guidelines include 2–3 g of potassium per day.

- **Milk group.** Limit to 1 cup serving of milk or milk product (yogurt, cottage cheese, ice cream, pudding).
- **Fruit group.** Limit to two servings daily from the low potassium choices. Watch serving sizes. Avoid the high potassium choices.
- **Low potassium**

Apple, 1 small
Apple juice, applesauce $^1/_2$ cup
Apricot, 1 medium or $^1/_2$ cup canned in syrup
Blueberries, $^1/_2$ cup
Cherries, canned in syrup $^1/_3$ cup
Cranberries, cranberry juice $^1/_2$ cup
Fruit cocktail, canned in syrup $^1/_2$ cup
Grapes, 10 fresh
Lemon, lime 1 fresh
Mandarin orange, canned in syrup $^1/_2$ cup
Nectar: apricot, pear, peach $^1/_2$ cup
Peach, 1 small or $^1/_2$ cup canned with syrup
Pear, 1 small or $^1/_2$ cup canned with syrup
Pineapple, $^1/_2$ cup raw or canned with syrup
Plums, 1 small or $^1/_2$ cup canned with syrup
Tangerine, 1 small
Watermelon, $^1/_2$ cup

- **High potassium**

Avocado
Banana
Cantaloupe
Cherries, fresh
Dried fruits
Grapefruit, fresh and juice
Honeydew melon
Kiwi
Mango
Nectarine
Orange, fresh and juice
Papaya
Prunes, prune juice
Raisins

- **Avoid.** Avoid using the following salt substitutes owing to their high potassium content: Adolph's, Lawry's Season Salt Substitute, No Salt, Morton Season Salt Free, Nu Salt, Papa Dash, and Morton Lite Salt.

Copyright © 1978–2006 Lexi-Comp Inc. All Rights Reserved. Updated 11/16/05.

Tyramine Content of Foods

Food	Allowed	Minimize Intake	Not Allowed
Beverages	Milk, decaffeinated coffee, tea, soda	Chocolate beverage, caffeine-containing drinks, clear spirits	Acidophilus milk, beer, ale, wine, malted beverages
Breads/cereals	All except those containing cheese	None	Cheese bread and crackers
Dairy products	Cottage cheese, farmers or pot cheese, cream cheese, ricotta cheese, all milk, eggs, ice cream, pudding (except chocolate)	Yogurt (limit to 4 oz. per day)	All other cheeses (aged cheese, American, Camembert, Cheddar, Gouda, Gruyère, mozzarella, parmesan, provolone, Romano, Roquefort, stilton)
Meat, fish, and poultry	All fresh or frozen	Aged meats, hot dogs, canned fish and meat	Chicken and beef liver, dried and pickled fish, summer or dry sausage, pepperoni, dried meats, meat extracts, bologna, liverwurst
Starches— potatoes/rice	All	None	Soybean (including paste)
Vegetables	All fresh, frozen, canned, or dried vegetable juices except those not allowed	Chili peppers, Chinese pea pods	Fava beans, sauerkraut, pickles, olives, Italian broad beans
Fruit	Fresh, frozen, or canned fruits and fruit juices	Avocado, banana, raspberries, figs	Banana peel extract
Soups	All soups not listed to limit or avoid	Commercially canned soups	Soups which contain broad beans, fava beans, cheese, beer, wine, any made with flavor cubes or meat extract, miso soup
Fats	All except fermented	Sour cream	Packaged gravy
Sweets	Sugar, hard candy, honey, molasses, syrups	Chocolate candies	None
Desserts	Cakes, cookies, gelatin, pastries, sherbets, sorbets	Chocolate desserts	Cheese-filled desserts
Miscellaneous	Salt, nuts, spices, herbs, flavorings, Worcestershire sauce	Soy sauce, peanuts	Brewer's yeast, yeast concentrates, all aged and fermented products, monosodium glutamate, vitamins with brewer's yeast

Copyright © 1978-2006 Lexi-Comp Inc. All Rights Reserved. Updated 11/2/05.

NATIONAL AND STATE BOARDS OF PHARMACY CONTACT INFORMATION

This appendix contains the most recent contact information for the national and state boards of pharmacy. A current listing of contact information for state boards of pharmacy is maintained at the National Association of Boards of Pharmacy website, www.napb.com. In addition, contact information for all the pharmacy schools in the United States can be found at the American Association of Colleges of Pharmacy Web site, www.aacp.org.

National Association of Boards of Pharmacy
Carmen A. Catizone
Executive Director
1600 Feehanville Drive
Mount Prospect, IL 60056
Phone: 847/391-4406
Fax: 847/391-4502
Web site: www.nabp.net

State Boards of Pharmacy
Alabama State Board of Pharmacy
Louise Foster Jones
Executive Secretary
10 Inverness Center, Suite 110
Birmingham, AL 35242
Phone: 205/981-2280
Fax: 205/981-2330
Web site: www.albop.com
E-mail: ljones@albop.com

Alaska Board of Pharmacy
Sher Zinn
Licensing Examiner
PO Box 110806
Juneau, AK 99811-0806
Phone: 907/465-2589
Fax: 907/465-2974
Web site: www.commerce.state.ak.us/occ/ppha.htm
E-mail: sher_zinn@commerce.state.ak.us
(through the Division of Occupational Licensing)

Arizona State Board of Pharmacy
Harlan Wand
Executive Director
4425 West Olive Avenue, Suite 140
Glendale, AZ 85302-3844
Phone: 623/463-2727
Fax: 623/934-0583
Web site: www.pharmacy.state.az.us
E-mail: hwand@azsbp.com

Arkansas State Board of Pharmacy
Charles S. Campbell
Executive Director
101 East Capitol, Suite 218
Little Rock, AR 72201
Phone: 501/682-0190
Fax: 501/682-0195
Web site: www.arkansas.gov/asbp
E-mail: charlie.campbell@arkansas.gov

California State Board of Pharmacy
Patricia F. Harris
Executive Officer
1625 North Market Boulevard, N219
Sacramento, CA 95834
Phone: 916/574-7900
Fax: 916/574-8618
Web site: www.pharmacy.ca.gov/
E-mail: patricia_harris@dca.ca.gov

Colorado State Board of Pharmacy
Susan L. Warren
Program Director
1560 Broadway, Suite 1310
Denver, CO 80202-5143
Phone: 303/894-7800
Fax: 303/894-7764
Web site: www.dora.state.co.us/pharmacy
E-mail: susan.warren@dora.state.co.us

Connecticut Commission of Pharmacy
Michelle Sylvestre
Drug Control Agent and Board Administrator
State Office Building, 165 Capitol Avenue Room 147
Hartford, CT 06106
Phone: 860/713-6070
Fax: 860/713-7242
Web site: www.ct.gov/dcp/site/default.asp
E-mail: michelle.sylvestre@ct.gov

Delaware State Board of Pharmacy
David W. Dryden
Executive Secretary
Division of Professional Regulation
Cannon Bulding
861 Silver Lake Boulevard, Suite 203
Dover, DE 19904
Phone: 302/744-4526
Fax: 302/739-2711
Web site: www.dpr.delaware.gov
E-mail: debop@state.de.us

District of Columbia Board of Pharmacy
Bonnie Rampersaud
Executive Director
717 Fourteenth Street NW, Suite 600
Washington, DC 20005
Phone: 202/724-4900
Fax: 202/727-8471
Web site: www.dchealth.dc.gov
E-mail: graphelia.ramseur@dc.gov

Florida Board of Pharmacy
Rebecca Poston
Executive Director
4052 Bald Cypress Way, Bin #C04
Tallahassee, FL 32399-3254
Phone: 850/245-4292
Fax: 850/413-6982
Web site: www.doh.state.fl.us/mga
E-mail: rebecca_poston@doh.state.fl.us

Georgia State Board of Pharmacy
Sylvia L. "Sandy" Bond
Executive Director
Professional Licensing Boards
237 Coliseum Drive
Macon, GA 31217-3858
Phone: 478/207-1640
Fax: 478/207-1660
Web site: www.sos.state.ga.us/plb/pharmacy
E-mail: sibond@sos.state.ga.us

Guam Board of Examiners for Pharmacy
Jane M. Diego
Secretary for the Board
PO Box 2816
Hagatna, GU 96932
Phone: 671/735-7406 ext 11
Fax: 671/735-7413
E-mail: jmdiego@dphss.govguam.net

Hawaii State Board of Pharmacy
Lee Ann Teshima
Executive Officer
PO Box 3469
Honolulu, HI 96801
Phone: 808/586-2694
Fax: 808/586-2874
Web site: www.hawaii.gov/dcca/areas/pvl/
   boards/pharmacy
E-mail: pharmacy@dcca.hawaii.gov

Idaho Board of Pharmacy
Richard Markuson
Executive Director
3380 Americana Terrace, Suite 320
Boise, ID 83706
Phone: 208/334-2356
Fax: 208/334-3536
Web site: www.accessidaho.org/bop/
E-mail: rmarkuson@bop.state.id.us

Illinois Department of Financial and Professional
   Regulation, Division of Professional
   Regulation-State Board of Pharmacy
Kim Scott
Pharmacy Board Liaison
320 West Washington, 3rd Floor
Springfield, IL 62786
Phone: 217/782-8556
Fax: 217/782-7645
Web site: www.idfpr.com
E-mail: PRFGROUP10@idfpr.com
(through Department of Professional
   Regulation)

Indiana Board of Pharmacy
Marty Allain, Director
Director
402 West Washington Street, Room W072
Indianapolis, IN 46204-2739
Phone: 317/234-2067
Fax: 317/233-4236
Web site: http://www.in.gov/pla/bandc/isbp/
E-mail: pla4@pla.IN.gov

Iowa Board of Pharmacy Examiners
Lloyd K. Jessen
Executive Director/Secretary
400 Southwest Eighth Street, Suite E
Des Moines, IA 50309-4688
Phone: 515/281-5944
Fax: 515/281-4609
Web site: www.state.ia.us/ibpe
E-mail: Lloyd.jessen@ibpe.state.ia.us

Kansas State Board of Pharmacy
Debra L. Billingsley
Executive Secretary/Director
Landon State Office Building, 900 Jackson,
   Room 560
Topeka, KS 66612-1231
Phone: 785/296-4056 Fax: 785/296-8420
Web site: http://www.kansas.gov/pharmacy
E-mail: pharmacy@pharmacy.state.ks.us

Kentucky Board of Pharmacy
Michael A. Burleson
Executive Director
Spindletop Administration Building, Suite 302,
2624 Research Park Drive,
Lexington, KY 40511
Phone: 859/246-2820
Fax: 859/246-2823
Web site: http://pharmacy.ky.gov/
E-mail: mike.burleson@ky.gov

Louisiana Board of Pharmacy
Malcolm J. Broussard
Executive Director
5615 Corporate Boulevard, Suite 8E
Baton Rouge, LA 70808-2537
Phone: 225/925-6496
Fax: 225/925-6499
Web site: www.labp.com
E-mail: mbroussard@labp.com

Maine Board of Pharmacy
Geraldine Betts
Board Administrator
Department of Professional/Financial Regulation
35 State House Station
Augusta, ME 04333
Phone: 207/624-8689
Fax: 207/624-8637
Hearing Impaired: 207/624-8563
PFR/OLR Web site:
    www.maineprofessionalreg.org
E-mail: for all Licensing and Board Meeting
    Information/Inquires and for Application
    packets: kelly.l.mclaughlin@maine.gov
Enforcement inquiries:
    gregory.w.cameron@maine.gov
Administration and all other Inquiries:
    geraldine.l.betts@maine.gov

Maryland Board of Pharmacy
La Verne George Naesea
Executive Director
4201 Patterson Avenue
Baltimore, MD 21215-2299
Phone: 410/764-4755
Fax: 410/358-6207
Web site: http://www.dhmh.state.md.us/
    pharmacyboard/
E-mail: lnaesea@dhmh.state.md.us

Massachusetts Board of Registration in
    Pharmacy
Charles R. Young
Executive Director
239 Causeway Street, 2nd Floor
Boston, MA 02114
Phone: 617/973-0800
Fax: 617/973-0983
Web site: www.mass.gov/dpl/boards/ph/
    index.htm
E-mail: charles.young@state.ma.us

Michigan Board of Pharmacy
Rae Ramsdell
Director, Licensing Division
611 West Ottawa, 1st Floor
PO Box 30670
Lansing, MI 48909-8170
Phone: 517/335-0918
Fax: 517/373-2179
Web site: http://www.michigan.gov/healthlicense
Email: rhramsd@michigan.gov

Minnesota Board of Pharmacy
Cody C. Wiberg
Executive Director
2829 University Avenue SE, Suite 530
Minneapolis, MN 55414-3251
Phone: 612/617-2201
Fax: 612/617-2212
Web site: http://www.phcybrd.state.mn.us
E-mail: Cody.Wiberg@state.mn.us

Mississippi State Board of Pharmacy
Leland McDivitt
Executive Director
204 Key Drive, Suite C
Madison, MS 39110
Phone: 601/605-5388 Fax: 601/605-9546
Web site: www.mbp.state.ms.us
E-mail: lmcdivitt@mbp.state.ms.us

Missouri Board of Pharmacy
Kevin E. Kinkade
Executive Director
PO Box 625
Jefferson City, MO 65102
Phone: 573/751-0091
Fax: 573/526-3464
Web site: http://www.pr.mo.gov/pharmacists.asp
E-mail: kevin.kinkade@pr.mo.gov

Montana Board of Pharmacy
Executive Director
PO Box 200513
301 South Park Avenue, 4th Floor
Helena, MT 59620-0513
Phone: 406/841-2355
Fax: 406/841-2305
Web site: http://mt.gov/dli/bsd/license/
    bsd_boards/pha_board/board_page.asp
E-mail: dlibsdpha@state.mt.us

Nebraska Board of Pharmacy
Becky Wisell
Executive Secretary
PO Box 94986
Lincoln, NE 68509-4986
Phone: 402/471-2118
Fax: 402/471-3577
Web site: www.hhs.state.ne.us
E-mail: becky.wisell@hhss.ne.gov

Nevada State Board of Pharmacy
Larry L. Pinson
Executive Secretary
555 Double Eagle Circuit, Suite 1100
Reno, NV 89521
Phone: 775/850-1440
Fax: 775/850-1444
Web site: http://state.nv.us/pharmacy
E-mail: pharmacy@govmail.state.nv.us

New Hampshire Board of Pharmacy
Paul G. Boisseau
Executive Secretary
57 Regional Drive
Concord, NH 03301-8518
Phone: 603/271-2350
Fax: 603/271-2856
Web site: www.nh.gov/pharmacy
E-mail: pharmacy.board@nh.gov

New Jersey Board of Pharmacy
Joanne Boyer
Executive Director
124 Halsey Street
Newark, NJ 07101
Phone: 973/504-6450
Fax: 973/648-3355
Web site: http://www.state.nj.us/lps/ca/
    boards.htm
E-mail: boyerj@dca.lps.state.nj.us

New Mexico Board of Pharmacy
William Harvey
Executive Director/Chief Durg Inspector
5200 Oakland NE, Suite A
Albuquerque, NM 87113
Phone: 505/222-9830
Fax: 505/222-9845
Web site: www.state.nm.us/pharmacy
E-mail: William.Harvey@state.nm.us

New York Board of Pharmacy
Lawrence H. Mokhiber
Executive Secretary
89 Washington Avenue, 2nd Floor W
Albany, NY 12234-1000
Phone: 518/474-3817 ext. 130
Fax: 518/473-6995
Web site: www.op.nysed.gov
E-mail: pharmbd@mail.nysed.gov

North Carolina Board of Pharmacy
Jack W. Campbell IV
Executive Director
PO Box 4560
Chapel Hill, NC 27515-4560
Phone: 919/942-4454
Fax: 919/967-5757
Web site: www.ncbop.org
E-mail: jcampbell@ncbop.org

North Dakota State Board of Pharmacy
Howard C. Anderson Jr
Executive Director
PO Box 1354
Bismarck, ND 58502-1354
Phone: 701/328-9535
Fax: 701/328-9536
Web site: www.nodakpharmacy.com
E-mail: ndboph@btinet.net

Ohio State Board of Pharmacy
William T. Winsley
Executive Director
77 South High Street Room 1702
Columbus, OH 43215-6126
Phone: 614/466-4143
Fax: 614/752-4836
Web site: www.pharmacy.ohio.gov
E-mail: exec@bop.state.oh.us

Oklahoma State Board of Pharmacy
Bryan H. Potter
Executive Director
4545 Lincoln Boulevard, Suite 112
Oklahoma City, OK 73105-3488
Phone: 405/521-3815
Fax: 405/521-3758
Web site: www.pharmacy.ok.gov
E-mail: pharmacy@pharmacy.ok.gov

Oregon State Board of Pharmacy
Gary A. Schnabel
Executive Director
800 Northeast Oregon Street, Suite 150
Portland, OR 97232
Phone: 971/673-0001
Fax: 971/673-0002
Web site: www.pharmacy.state.or.us
E-mail: pharmacy.board@state.or.us

Pennsylvania State Board of Pharmacy
Melanie Zimmerman
Executive Secretary
PO Box 2649
Harrisburg, PA 17105-2649
Phone: 717/783-7156
Fax: 717/787-7769
Web site: www.dos.state.pa.us/pharm
E-mail: st-pharmacy@state.pa.us

Puerto Rico Board of Pharmacy
Madga Bouet
Executive Director, Department of Health, Board
    of Pharmacy
Call Box 10200, Santurce, PR 00908
Phone: 787/724-7282
Fax: 787/725-7903
E-mail: mbouet@salud.gov.pr

Rhode Island Board of Pharmacy
Catherine A. Cordy
Executive Director
3 Capitol Hill, Room 205
Providence, RI 02908-5097
Phone: 401/222-2837
Fax: 401/222-2158
Web site: http://www.health.ri.gov/hsr/
    professions/pharmacy.php
E-mail: cathyc@doh.state.ri.us

South Carolina Department of Labor, Licensing, and Regulation-Board of Pharmacy
LeeAnn Bundrick
Administrator
Kingstree Building
110 Centerview Drive, Suite 306
Columbia, SC 29210
Phone: 803/896-4700
Fax: 803/896-4596
Web site: www.llronline.com/POL/pharmacy
E-mail: bundrici@llr.sc.gov

South Dakota State Board of Pharmacy
Dennis M. Jones
Executive Secretary
4305 South Louise Avenue, Suite 104
Sioux Falls, SD 57106
Phone: 605/362-2737
Fax: 605/362-2738
Web site: www.state.sd.us/doh/pharmacy
E-mail: dennis.jones@state.sd.us

Tennessee Board of Pharmacy
Terry Webb Grinder
Interim Executive Director
Tennessee Department of Commerce and
    Insurance,
Board of Pharmacy
Davy Crockett Tower, 2nd Floor
500 James Robertson Pkwy
Nashville, TN 37243-1149
Phone: 615/741-2718
Fax: 615/741-2722
Web site: www.state.tn.us/commerce/boards/
    pharmacy
E-mail: terry.grinder@state.tn.us

Texas State Board of Pharmacy
Gay Dodson
Executive Director
333 Guadalupe, Tower 3, Suite 600
Austin, TX 78701-3942
Phone: 512/305-8000
Fax: 512/305-8082
Web site: www.tsbp.state.tx.us
E-mail: gay.dodson@tsbp.state.tx.us

Utah Board of Pharmacy
Diana L. Baker
Bureau Manager
PO Box 146741
Salt Lake City, UT 84114-6741
Phone: 801/530-6179
Fax: 801/530-6511
Web site: http://www.dopl.utah.gov/
E-mail: dbaker@utah.gov
(through Division of Occupational and
    Professional Licensing)

Vermont Board of Pharmacy
Peggy Atkins
Board Administrator
Office of Professional Regulation
26 Terrace Street
Montpelier, VT 05609-1106
Phone: 802/828-2373
Fax: 802/828-2465
Web site: www.vtprofessionals.org
E-mail: patkins@sec.state.vt.us

Virgin Islands Board of Pharmacy
Lydia T. Scott
Executive Assistant
Department of Health
Schneider Regional Center
48 Sugar Estate
St. Thomas, VI 00802
Phone. 340/774-0117
Fax: 340/777-4001
E-mail:lydia.scott@usvi-doh.org

Virginia Board of Pharmacy
Elizabeth Scott Russell
Executive Director
6603 West Broad Street, 5th Floor
Richmond, VA 23230-1712
Phone: 804/662-9911
Fax: 804/662-9313
Web site: www.dhp.state.va.us/pharmacy/
    deafault.htm
(or through Department of Health Professions at
    www.dhp.state.va.us)
E-mail: scotti.russell@dhp.virginia.gov

Washington State Board of Pharmacy
Steven M. Saxe
Executive Director
PO Box 47863
Olympia, WA 98504-7863
Phone: 360/236-4825
Fax: 360/586-4359
Web site: https://fortress.wa.gov/doh/hpqa1/hps4/
    pharmacy/default.htm
E-mail: Steven.Saxe@doh.wa.gov

West Virginia Board of Pharmacy
William T. Douglass Jr
Executive Director and General Counsel
232 Capitol Street
Charleston, WV 25301
Phone: 304/558-0558
Fax: 304/558-0572
Web site: http://www.wvbop.com/
E-mail: wdouglass@wvbop.com

Wisconsin Pharmacy Examining Board
Tom Ryan
Bureau Director
1400 East Washington
PO Box 8935
Madison, WI 53708-8935
Phone: 608/266-2112
Fax: 608/267-0644
Web site: http://www.drl.state.wi.us/
E-mail: thomas.ryan@drl.state.wi.us

Wyoming State Board of Pharmacy
James T. Carder
Executive Director
632 South David Street
Casper, WY 82601
Phone: 307/234-0294
Fax: 307/234-7226
Web site: http://pharmacyboard.state.wy.us/
E-mail: wybop@state.wy.us

Reprinted with permission from National Association of Boards of Pharmacy, Mount Prospect, IL.

BUDGETING FOR DRUG INFORMATION RESOURCES

Basic Library

References	Cost[a]
American Hospital Formulary Service (AHFS) Drug Information	$ 209.00
Drug Facts and Comparisons	$ 205.00
Handbook on Injectable Drugs	$ 219.00
Handbook of Non-Prescription Drugs: An Interactive Approach to Self-Care	$ 145.00
Martindale: The Complete Drug Reference	$ 470.00
Nonprescription Product Therapeutics	$ 90.00
Physicians' Desk Reference	$ 95.00
Remington's Pharmaceutical Sciences	$ 125.00
USP DI (three-volume set)	$ 412.00

Additional Resources

References	Cost[a]
Drug–drug interaction	
Drug Interactions Analysis and Management	$ 195.00
Drug Interaction Facts	$ 217.00
Evaluations of Drug Interactions	$ 230.00
Herbal	
PDR for Herbal Medicines	$ 60.00
The Review of Natural Products	$ 173.00
Internal medicine	
Cecil Textbook of Medicine	$ 149.00
Harrison's Principles of Internal Medicine	$ 135.00
Pediatrics	
Pediatric Dosage Handbook	$ 47.00
The Harriet Lane Handbook	$ 40.00
Pharmacokinetics	
Applied Biopharmaceutics and Pharmacokinetics	$ 60.00
Clinical Pharmacokinetics	$ 69.00
Concepts in Clinical Pharmacokinetics	$ 100.00
Applied Pharmacokinetics and Pharmacodynamics: Principles of Therapeutic Drug Monitoring	$ 73.00
Pharmacology	
Goodman and Gilman's The Pharmacological Basis of Therapeutics	$ 139.00
Pregnancy/breast-feeding	
Drugs in Pregnancy and Lactation	$ 99.00
Therapeutics	
Applied Therapeutics: The Clinical Use of Drugs	$ 206.00
Pharmacotherapy: A Pathophysiologic Approach	$ 200.00
Textbook of Therapeutics: Drug and Disease Management	$ 157.00

Continued.

References	Cost[a]
CD ROM computer systems/programs	
AHFS first WEB	$ 3,500.00
Clinical Pharmacology (online)	$ 495.00
Lexi–Comp online	$ 2,550.00
CliniTrend software	$ 722.00
DataKinetics software	$ 719.00
Facts and Comparisons 4.0 online (individual subscription)	$ 496.00
Iowa Drug Information System (online)	$ 9,600.00
IPA	$ 900.00
MD Consult (core collection, individual)	$ 220.00
Medline (primary component of PubMed)	0
MedTeach software	$ 565.00
Micromedex > 200 licensed bed facility	
Diseasedex	$16,000.00
Drugdex System	$16,500.00
Poisindex System	$16,900.00
Other Micromedex databases	
CareNotes System	$12,123.00
Drug–Reax	$ 2,081.00
Kinetidex	$ 4,126.00
Martindale: The Complete Drug Reference	$ 2,081.00
PDR	$ 6,954.00
P&T Quik	$ 1,669.00
Reprorisk	$ 3,164.00
UpToDate (stand-alone)	$1,495.00
Major online vendors	
Dialog	
EBSCOInformation Services	
Gale Group	
National Library of Medicine	
Ovid	
OCLC First Search	
Thomson Scientific	

[a]Costs are approximate and are based on 2005 figures. Costs depend on selection of format, site versus individual license fees, and concurrent users. Institutional subscriptions cost more than individual subscriptions.